The National Health Service and the Labour Market

Edited by
R.A. WILSON
J.A. STILWELL

With contributions by
S. CHARLES
K.G. KNIGHT
M. BOND
A.WESTAWAY

Avebury

Aldershot · Brookfield USA · Hong Kong · Singapore · Sydney

Published by
Avebury
Ashgate Publishing Limited
Gower House
Croft Road
Aldershot
Hants GU11 3HR
England

Ashgate Publishing Company
Old Post Road
Brookfield, Vermont 05036
USA

A CIP catalogue record for this book is available from the British Library and the US Library of Congress

ISBN 1 85628 390 9

Printed and Bound in Great Britain by
Athenaeum Press Ltd., Newcastle upon Tyne.

Contents

List of tables and figures

List of figures

Preface and acknowledgements

The research described in this book was conducted as part of a programme of work funded by the Department of Health. The purpose of this work has been to examine all aspects of the supply of *non-medical practitioner* labour to the NHS. Doctors are generally studied quite separately (see for example the work of the Advisory Committees on medical manpower referenced in Chapter 13). Possibly, in the future the demand for, and supply of, doctors will not be perceived as so separable. However, at the present time, the frontier between doctors' work and the work of other health care professionals remains a rather tabu issue. It therefore seems appropriate to retain this division and the present book focuses almost entirely on non-medical professions. Since the workforce with which this book deals is mainly female, the terms 'manpower' and 'manpower planning' are not as suitable as 'workforce' and 'workforce planning'. In general we have used the latter terminology, except where reference is made to work or committees referring to themselves by means of the former terms.

The research has been very much a team exercise. John Stilwell and Rob Wilson had overall responsibility for the project including editing this volume. Rob Wilson was the main author of Chapters 2-5 and contributed to Chapters 1, and 7-13. Sue Charles was the main author for Chapters 9-11 as well as contributing to Chapters 1 and 12. Tony Westaway played a similar role in Chapters 7 and 8, while Ben Knight was the prime author of Chapter 6. John Stilwell was the main author of Chapter 1 and contributed to Chapters 9-13. Meg Bond was the prime author of Chapter 13 in addition to providing valuable comments on many other parts of the book. Thanks are also due to Julia Conneely for research assistance in the early stages of the project, to Andrew Holden for clerical assistance, and to Carol Dobson and Barbara Wilson for their expert typing skills. The responsibility for the views expressed and for any remaining errors lies with the authors.

1 Introduction, aims and objectives

The National Health Service is the largest civilian employer in Europe. Employment in health services accounted for almost 1½ million jobs in 1990 most of which were in the public sector. This represents over 5 per cent of total employment in the UK. The bulk of these jobs are taken by females, the largest group of whom are nurses. The NHS is a key player in the labour market especially for female workers.

The past three years have seen a dramatic increase in the use within the NHS of concepts drawn from the free market tradition of private business. Whether these new grafts will be successful or unsuccessful, remains to be seen. However, the NHS has never been entirely insulated from market forces; it may not have charged for its services, but it has always had to buy its factors of production, whether nurses, doctors, medicines or bricks.

1.1 The plan of the book

The purpose of this book is to describe the results of research commissioned by the Department of Health aimed at examining the market for the labour of nurses, professions allied to medicine, and support workers. The research had four main aspects: a detailed assessment of supply and demand trends in the labour market generally in order to provide a useful picture for participants and policy makers of the labour market environment they are likely to face in the 1990s; a survey of theoretical and empirical work relevant to this labour market (both from the health labour market literature and the more general labour economics

1

area); an examination of the light to be thrown on the labour market both nationally and regionally, by hitherto under-exploited sources such as the Labour Force Survey; and finally, case studies of particular issues that were suggested by the other analysis, (the one highlighted here being an in depth study of the training of mature entrants, that is, women with children to be nurses). The labour market for doctors is not covered, since as noted in the Preface this issue is traditionally examined separately.

The general labour market environment

The book begins by exploring the external labour market conditions which the NHS is likely to face over the next decade. The next four chapters provide an overview of the labour market environment that the NHS is likely to face over the remainder of this decade. From a situation of substantial excess supply in the early 1980s, UK labour markets experienced a steady tightening up to 1989. In many parts of the country, and for certain types of labour, shortages had become severe. NHS employers, suddenly realizing that they would be among the most seriously affected both by competition from other employers and by the inexorable and (in the nature of past birth rates) irreversible diminution of their traditional labour pool, exploded into metaphor.

Subsequently, the Government's tight monetary and high interest rate policy, coupled with international economic developments, has resulted in a sharp recession. At the time of writing, the economy is only just showing signs of recovery. These events have meant that the predicted labour shortages have not really bitten.

The Institute for Employment Research (IER, 1991) nevertheless expects the longer-term picture to return to one of labour shortages for many skilled workers, particularly for those employers trying to recruit young, highly qualified, new entrants to the workforce. Chapters 2-6 attempt to identify some of the main issues and problems that will need to be addressed in order for the NHS to achieve its objectives regarding recruitment and retention of highly skilled and highly qualified personnel.

Likely developments in labour supply up to the turn of the century are discussed in Chapter 2. The demographic downturn in the number of young people and the offsetting growth in other categories are highlighted. Detailed projections, by age and gender are presented, based on official and other sources. Trends in the ethnic make-up of the labour force are also considered. Attention is focused on the supply of highly qualified persons and well qualified school leavers. The chapter draws on major studies by the Institute on the labour market for the highly qualified, as well as on official projections by the Department of Education and Science.

The main trends in labour demand from other employers for highly skilled and highly qualified persons are outlined in Chapter 3. This review concentrates on graduates and well qualified school leavers. It draws on the Institute's general labour market assessment work, as well as other

2

forecasts. The likely balance between supply and demand is discussed in Chapter 4. This draws upon research conducted by the Institute on behalf of the Department of Employment and the Department of Education and Science. The implications for NHS recruitment and retention are drawn out. Amongst the issues considered are: the impact of closer economic and political relationships in Europe ('1992' for short); the effects of technological change on the demand for skills; and the impact of demographic factors. The chapter also considers the reactions of other employers to the expected developments in labour markets over the medium term and summarises the main lessons to be learnt.

Chapter 5 represents a major change of focus. This reviews currently available evidence on career aspirations of the labour force and how these are changing, setting the context against which developments in the NHS need to be considered. Conditions of employment including pay, hours of work, length of contract, promotion prospects, pensions and other fringe benefits are discussed.

Theoretical and empirical evidence on labour market developments

In Chapter 6 issues connected with labour market participation are addressed. The chapter contains an in depth review of the general labour economics literature on labour supply and attempts to draw out the main implications as far as the NHS is concerned. One important aspect here is the links between labour supply decisions of members of the same household (notably man and wife) and how these may constrain labour supply. This discussion includes a summary of the main results from the empirical literature on the factors influencing labour supply.

The book also examines the internal labour market operating within the NHS, from both demand and supply perspectives. Chapters 7-9 focus more directly on developments within the NHS itself. They contain a critical review of the evidence from both theoretical and empirical studies of the market for labour within the NHS. Chapter 7 concentrates primarily on labour demand, including such topics as willingness to pay, substitution, skill mix and performance indicators. Chapter 8 moves on to consider supply side aspects including response to pay and other conditions of employment, nurse training and Project 2000. In Chapter 9 the discussion turns to wastage and labour turnover. A more general review of the role of so called manpower planning within the NHS is given in Chapter 10. As well as setting the NHS experience into a more general historical context, the chapter extends the discussion to cover doctors as well as nurses.

New evidence on supply from the labour force survey and a case study of mature entrants

The supply of potential skills to the NHS, especially in the nursing area, is a second key focus. The main aim of the research was to provide a broad-

3

brush review of readily available published evidence rather than developing new data. However, a substantial amount of new evidence is presented, based on information that has been extracted from the Labour Force Surveys (Chapters 11 and 12) and a pilot study of mature entrants (Chapter 13). Chapters 11 and 12 present new data on the supply of nursing skills using information from the Labour Force Survey. This valuable data resource has, to date, not been properly exploited. Chapter 11 presents information for the UK as a whole while Chapter 12 illustrates the potential for obtaining estimates for individual Regional Health Authorities. The results emphasise the large potential stocks of people with nursing skills who are economically inactive or who have moved into other jobs.

The evidence reviewed in Chapters 6-12 suggests that most employers will face an increasingly difficult labour market in the mid to late 1990s, as the demand for well qualified and well trained personnel continues to grow while the supply side is constrained by demographic factors. The main area of growth from the labour supply side is likely to be mature women, many only poorly qualified academically. It suggests that there may be considerable scope for meeting future demand for nursing and related skills by retraining mature entrants on the job to National Vocational Qualification Standards, rather than relying on the traditional flow of young, formally qualified new entrants. Chapter 13 presents the results of a pilot study aimed at examining the potential of such schemes. Finally, Chapter 14 brings the book to a close by providing a summary of the main points from each of the earlier chapters.

The remainder of this introductory chapter explores some of the key issues and attempts to draw some tentative conclusions. One of the key issues identified in the late 1980s was the so called 'demographic timebomb'. In the early 1990s there are some who believe that the problem has disappeared. However, it is argued that this view is premature, the timebomb remains undefused. Other important issues are the demand for professional status by many groups in the NHS workforce, the debate about new nursing and the role of the support worker, Project 2000, the pressures for tighter financial control and the effects of related reforms such as the introduction of independent trusts.

All these changes suggest that the NHS may need to radically reassess its recruitment and training strategies in the 1990s if it is to meet the needs for well qualified and motivated personnel that are crucial to the success of the service. The final section of this introductory chapter makes some suggestions as to how this might be achieved. It also identifies a number of areas where further research seems highly desirable.

1.2   Identifying the issues

The demographic timebomb - ticking or defused?

Demand for the services of the NHS is highly dependent on the size and age structure of the population. OPCS forecasts for the next 25 years are that there will be a small but significant growth in the size of the total population but, within that total, a dramatic change in the age distribution. There will be fewer young (usually healthy) adults and more very elderly (and usually frail) ones. The demand for the services of the NHS is therefore likely to rise, and since NHS production is highly labour intensive it follows that the NHS demand for labour -unless its budget is cut -will rise too.

At the point of initial recruitment the NHS draws an extraordinarily large percentage of its labour from a particular segment of the total labour force: those who are young, female and 'fairly well educated' (i.e. those who possess a minimum of 5 GCSEs). These are the characteristics which apply to the majority of those who are recruited into what are termed the associate professional groups of the NHS. Largest of these groups are the nurses, who alone make up approximately 50 per cent of its workforce. The 'professions allied to medicine' (PAMs) - i.e. radiographers, physiotherapists, and occupational therapists- and other related groups such as chiropodists, medical laboratory scientific officers, and dietitians, go to make up what is known as 'professional and technical manpower' (P&T for short).

Further, the NHS absorbs an extremely large percentage of this segment of the labour force. The Committee of Public Accounts (CPA, 1987, p.11) quotes DHSS figures for 1986 which imply that recruitment into nurse training alone took just under 25 per cent of 'fairly well educated' female school leavers. The projected contraction in the number of young adults implies a sizable reduction in the traditional pool for nurses and P&T staff. The NHS is already a dominant angler in this pool. It is unlikely to be able to cope simply by increasing its percentage of the catch. For example, the same source predicts that, simply to maintain the intake into nursing at 1986 levels in the face of the predicted decline in the number of suitable qualified female school leavers, the NHS would need to increase its share of the market from 25 per cent to something nearer 33 per cent. Allowing for a fairly limited amount of growth in the demand for nurses and some expansion in the demand for PAMs, the figure rises to something of the order of 45 per cent. Reid (1986) reaches much the same conclusion.

The statistical analysis in Chapters 2-5 confirms that, without radical changes in recruitment policies the National Health Service will find it increasingly difficult to meet its labour requirement. The Health Service is both highly labour intensive and a very large employer, and it might be reasonable to expect that it would have a strong and long-held interest in the labour market. But this has not been the case.

5

The shortages both experienced and expected in the late 1980s succeeded, temporarily at least, in concentrating minds upon this issue. All interested parties expressed concern: Parliament (Committee of Public Accounts, 1986 and 1987); management (National Association of Health Authorities, 1987; and Conroy and Stidston, 1988); workers (the Royal College of Nursing has stimulated a number of studies, such as Waite and Hutt, 1987; and Working Group of the RCN, 1987); consulted experts (Price Waterhouse, 1987); and the media (Brindle, 1989).The professional journals and magazines were full of articles on the topic, (see for example Pearce, 1988; and Delamothe, 1988a). However, the deep recession of 1990/91 has caused labour markets to slacken considerably and many commentators now appear to believe the problem has been solved. However, the long-term view expounded in Chapters 2-4 suggests that this could well be just a temporary reprieve.

Anticipated improvements in levels of educational attainment might or might not ease the situation in the medium-term as far as NHS recruitment is concerned. The review in Chapter 2 suggests that the social class structure among school leavers is also likely to change (the reduction in the size of this group being almost entirely due to the contraction in the birth rate amongst those in the lower socio-economic groups some 16 or so years earlier). This, coupled with DES forecasts of improvements in the quality of secondary education consequent upon its current reforms, could well mean that a greater percentage of school leavers achieve at least the minimum standard of 5 GCSEs required for entry into training for the relevant professions. However, that percentage increase is predicted to be nowhere near large enough to counteract the decline in the total size of the age cohort. Furthermore, the DES is also forecasting a substantial expansion in higher education, thereby syphoning off even more of the pool.

What is more, competition for this contracting segment of the labour force is likely to increase: the expanding service sector, and in particular the financial sector, trawls the same group. Across all industries and services it is the better qualified who will be in greatest demand. The NHS is therefore doubly likely to face a contraction in its labour supply. Thus the immediate crisis is seen as being demographically based. Underlying this essentially temporary (if not in political time scales) drama, however, a more permanent problem can be discerned. Even without an impending medium-term labour shortage, the NHS would still have had to become rather more concerned about its workforce than it has been in the past. The two conditions which once allowed it to take a fairly casual attitude towards questions of staffing - rising budgets and a plentiful supply of cheap and undemanding female labour - no longer obtain.

The rising budgets and easy labour market conditions of the seventies and early eighties allowed inefficiencies to flourish. First, the NHS was content to have a student fed, high wastage nursing and P&T workforce. With a plentiful supply of school leavers and the ready excuse that they

6

were female and inevitably going to leave for 'family reasons', the NHS made little attempt to retain and recruit trained staff. Thus it found itself overly dependent on one particular age band of the labour market. Second, it failed to develop systems for efficient workforce planning and demand determination. As discussed in Chapter 7, staffing determinations were regarded as low level responsibilities. In consequence, they tended to be historically determined and influenced by professional, but not economic, considerations. The result was a rapid growth in total employment with wide variations in employment patterns across Health Authorities (HAs) within the NHS.

The expansion in employment inevitably attracted attention. Parliament, in the shape of the Committee of Public Accounts, produced a series of reports in which this was a central issue (CPA, 1981, 1982, 1984, 1986 and 1987); see also National Audit Office (NAO, 1985a, 1985b and 1987) and three independent assessments by Gray and Smail (1982), Bosanquet and Gerard (1985) and Key (1986). These examined the following explanations:

- Increases in workload due, in general, to increases in demand arising from the ageing of the population and, in particular, to the effects of technological developments and changes in medical practice on the workloads of particular categories of workers, have made more labour hours necessary. (For example, new imaging techniques have increased the need for radiographers and reductions in the length of in-patient stay and the consequent increase in both patient throughput and average dependency mean a higher nurse/patient ratio is required on the wards.)

- Improvements in the 'Cinderella' services recognised as being understaffed (geriatrics, mental illness and mental handicap) obviously and straight-forwardly lead to expansions in employment.

- Reductions in hours per employee (due to reductions in the length of the working week, increases in holiday allowances and increasing use of part-time staff) imply that a greater number of staff was necessary to provide a given number of hours of labour service.

The general conclusion was that these factors offered some justification for part of the expansion in employment. However, in a situation of budget growth coupled with an absence of managerial incentives to spend it wisely, the NHS found it rather too easy to respond simply by hiring more staff without much consideration being given as to whether it could use those it was already employing rather more productively.

Furthermore, these factors were not thought to explain all of the expansion and the view was expressed that some of it was 'budget-led'. The problem is of course that the potential for the NHS to supply care is

7

boundless. The outputs of the NHS are difficult to quantify and the demand for its services is not restricted by a market price. In such a situation it can always do more - and so its budget becomes the major determinant of how much it does. 'The bigger the budget, the better the service and the bigger the workforce'. Again, these reports question whether the extra funds were always efficiently spent. They point to wide variations across the NHS in practices for determining staffing levels, grade mixes, duty rosters, etc.

These critical reports form part of the background which led to a change in the political environment in which the NHS operates. Now budgets are tighter, and getting ever more so, and a managerial revolution has been imposed upon it. Both changes mean that the NHS is now taking a far greater interest in the efficient use of its workforce. Indeed if budgets are restricted strongly enough, it is not just that there will be no more budget-led expansion in the workforce, but that the NHS will have to find ways of coping with changes which will undoubtedly increase its workload, such as a further ageing of the population, with a workforce which might even have to contract.

Tighter budgets, however, form only one blade of the pincers now beginning to squeeze the NHS. On the other side lie the rising professional aspirations of the nursing and P&T staff groups, this situation being an example of the changing position of women in the labour force. The early post-war period was characterised by an abundance of cheap female labour. This reflected a particular stage in the development of female participation in the labour market. It became more acceptable for women to work, and they did so in ever greater numbers. However, they continued to be satisfied with, or at least to acquiesce in, restrictions on their labour market opportunities to jobs which fitted a more traditional view of the female role - as unambitious carers. Thus traditional employers of the caring professions, like the NHS, were able to impose low wages and offer poor career structures for their mainly female work forces. (With respect to nursing, see Delamothe, 1988c, 1988d and in particular 1988e; and NUPE and LPU, 1989). For example, in 1986 the health departments felt able to argue in their submission to the pay review body for nurses and PAMs that there were no general difficulties in recruiting and retaining staff and therefore no reason to award large pay increases (Review Body for Nursing Staff, Midwives, Health Visitors and Professions Allied to Medicine, 1986a and 1986b).

But there were signs that the party was drawing to a close. The most obvious were the strikes in the late 1980s, over pay, by the nursing profession and ambulance drivers. Attracting less media attention, but probably of greater significance, were a whole series of moves by the relevant professional and training bodies to upgrade the standing of these skill groups. To quote a few instances:

8

-      During the late 1970s the College of Radiographers raised their
entry requirements to 5 'O' and 2 'A' levels. They also extended
the period of training from 2 to 3 years. They have proved willing
to control the level of intake into training (National Audit Office,
1987, p.16).

-      In 1986 the minimum requirement for entry into training for mental
illness and mental handicap nursing was raised from 2 to 5 'O'
levels (now GCSEs or equivalents) and 'Project 2000', advocating a
major reform of nurse training including the abandonment of the
less prestigious State Enrolled Nurse (SEN) grade, was published
(United Kingdom Central Council on Nursing, Midwifery and
Health Visiting, 1986; see also RCN, 1985a and 1985b; Price
Waterhouse, 1987; and Delamothe, 1988c).

-      Speech therapists, occupational therapists, chiropodists and
physiotherapists are all seeking degree status for their qualifications
(Council for Professions Supplementary to Medicine, 1981, pp.5-8;
and Harrison and Brooks, 1985) and most appear to be near to
achieving this aim.

-      Medical Laboratory Scientific Officers are attempting an all-
graduate intake to their profession (Audit Commission, 1990).

In short, these groups are aspiring to become the partners rather than
the servants of the medical profession. They are serving notice that they
want better pay, better career structures and, above all, higher status
(Long and Mercer, 1987, chs.5 and 6; and Mackay, 1988).

This drive towards professional status is a general trend. Yet managers
reveal a tendency to react with apparent -perhaps expedient-
incomprehension (Conroy and Stidston, 1988, pp.8-9; NAHA, 1987;
passim; and NAO, 1987, pp.16-17). They complain that these initiatives
are being promoted without reference to their effect on the supply of
trained labour into the NHS and with no apparent recognition of the
possibility that the relevant professional and training bodies might be
pursuing goals other than that of meeting the staffing needs of the NHS.

The latest annual reports of the pay review body for nurses and PAMs
suggest that there has been little change in the labour market situation over
the last year or two (Review Body for Nursing Staff, Midwifery, Health
Visitors and Professions Allied to Medicine, 1990a and 1990b and 1991a
and 1991b). With regard to nurses, the Review Body commissioned the
NHS Office of Manpower Economics to conduct a survey of vacancies
(the second such survey). The three months vacancy rate (i.e. the number
of whole time equivalent (WTE) funded posts vacant for more than three
months as a percentage of the total number of such posts) for Great Britain
at 31 March, 1989 was estimated as:

-    overall rate for nursing staff: 3.2 per cent
-    rate for qualified staff: 3.8 per cent
-    rate for unqualified staff: 1.6 per cent.

These estimates are very similar to those derived from the previous survey of a year earlier. The 1991 reports suggested little change. Comparable figures for PAMs were derived from an NHS Manpower Planning Advisory Group (MPAG) survey:

-    overall rate for PAMs: 5.5 per cent
-    rate for occupational therapists: 13.8 per cent
-    rate for physiotherapists: 5.5 per cent
-    overall rate, excluding occupational therapists: 3.4 per cent.

These figures are also similar to those derived in an Office of Manpower Economics survey. By the 1991 report, vacancy rates for PAMs had increased, but only very marginally. Thus far, therefore, there is little evidence of any *deterioration* in the ability of the NHS to fill such posts. The general recession and consequent slackening of the labour market was undoubtedly a major factor here. With regard to nurses, the management argument continues to be that the absence of evidence of any widespread shortage means that large across-the-board pay increases are not justified. The Review Body itself is a little less sanguine, saying that although there has been no dramatic change as yet, there is no room for complacency. Both are more worried about the situation with regard to PAMs, because the NHS demand for their labour is expected to rise.

Trent and West Midlands RHAs and Wales were approached for details on their activities in the human resource planning area. Each provided a number of reports. With respect to their analysis of the current situation, they confirm the impression gained from the Review Body reports: there was little sign of serious difficulty in filling posts. Indeed with the recession continuing much longer than many commentators had orginally anticipated the common cry was 'demographic timebomb - what demographic timebomb?'

Trent has set up what it terms a nurse manpower early warning system, with biennial report. These report and comment upon data collected from nurse training schools in the region. The first of these (Walker and Wren, 1990) revealed that, in the late 1980s/early 1990s, most schools were experiencing little difficulty in filling their intakes into training, though over the region as a whole they are recruiting a lower percentage of the 17-19 age cohort than was the case four years ago. As the reports point out, there are difficulties in interpreting the latter piece of information because the data are at the regional level and there are cross boundary flows of recruits. Incidentally, these reports also find an increase over the last four years in the number of older recruits into training, though admittedly from a low base. Trent's report on the national demand and supply of physiotherapists for the MPAG 'National Lead Regional Initiative' reveals a similar picture of a high number of applicants per place (2.5) for entry into physiotherapy training (Beaumont, Thornton and Sleney, 1989).

The aggregation of HA strategic plans for the future, however, reveal a growing demand for a number of the P&T staff groups and concern is expressed over whether this growth can be achieved, given the likely availability of labour and ability of HAs to pay for them. (Welsh Health Common Services Authority, Manpower Planning Division 1990; and DoH 1989). On the other hand, concern over a future shortage of nurses is now more muted. Both Trent (Jones, 1989) and the West Midlands (West Midlands RHA, Manpower Planning Section, 1989 and 1990) recognise that, though the number of young females in the workforce is set to decline, the number of older women will rise. Nursing training schools were not experiencing a decline in applications from any age groups, although there was a tendency for the mean age of training school entrants to rise.

The NHS may well have embarked upon a policy of attracting older women. But this cannot explain the unexpectedly high level of applications from girls from the traditional age group. The analysis in this book suggest that the timebomb is still ticking, and that the effects of demography are at present simply masked by the deep economic recession.

New nursing and the support worker

The pressure which led to Project 2000 was the rising aspirations of nurses for full professional status. The same pressure generated the 1988 regrading exercise, a move intended to provide nursing with a clinical, as opposed to an administrative, career structure. The recent nursing literature makes it clear that these two reforms should be seen as part of a much broader vision about the future role of the nursing profession (Beardshaw and Robinson, 1990; Binnie, 1987; Pembrey and Punton, 1990; Salvage, 1990; Robinson *et al.*, 1989; Audit Commission, 1991). A literature review is undertaken by Carr-Hill *et al.* (1991). The vision came originally from the United States and is called 'New Nursing'. It embodies a desire to move nursing away from a hierarchical, task-centred approach to a patient-centred, holistic one. That is, away from a situation in which one member of the shift is told to do all the bed baths, another to perform the round of temperature and blood pressure taking, and so on, to a situation in which a small team of nurses takes responsibility for each patient for the duration of their stay, drawing up a personalised care plan, providing for all their care needs, etc. This concept of nursing is, of course, in tune with modern ideas on the need for a holistic, caring approach towards patients rather than the traditional approach which tended to see the patient as an impersonal medical condition to be cured. Clearly, however it is also about the professionalisation of nursing; about carving out a sphere of influence separate from that of the medical profession, about becoming their equals rather than their handmaidens.

For current purposes, the interesting point about this concept of nursing is that it implies a nurse practitioner who does everything for her patient; everything from the most skilled of current nursing procedures to providing the basic care services of washing and feeding. It therefore flies somewhat in the face of moves to change the grade mix to make greater use of technically less well qualified personnel. It implies a desired grade mix of a high proportion of trained to untrained staff, with the role of those who are untrained being firmly restricted to non-patient-related duties. Thus, ward clerks and housekeepers are regarded as acceptable, but health care assistants with little or no training are not. This, of course, is at odds with the view that health care assistants can, by doing much of the 'basic nursing care' free the trained nurse to concentrate on the more technical elements.

This latter view suggests a desired grade mix of a much lower ratio of trained to untrained staff. This seems to be the official view, for one of the provisos for acceptance of Project 2000 appears to have been agreement that work should begin on the development of an NCVT (National Council for Vocational Training) training course for a new health support worker grade which will act, at least to some extent, as a substitute for the (in future) more highly skilled trained nurse and act as a replacement for students' contributions on wards when they become much more super-numeray.

It is important to note that by no means every nurse is an advocate of 'New Nursing'. As Francis, Peelo and Soothill (1988) make clear, only a proportion of nurses see themselves as pursuing a career. These tend to be the more academic, who are often those most vociferously in favour of professionalisation strategies. Nonetheless, results of the questionnaire in the study by Ball et al. (1989) suggest widespread agreement among nurses that the job of the trained nurse should not be restricted to just 'the technical bits'.

Accepting the qualification that not every nurse has radical views over the direction of development of her profession, it is nonetheless true to say that there are in this situation the seeds of a serious industrial relations problem. Seen from the perspective of the advocates of 'New Nursing' a management which seeks the substitution of unskilled for skilled nursing labour looks to be practising something close to Tayloristic scientific management ideas. As is now well established in the relevant economics literature, the effect can be a counterproductive loss of good will and cooperation. It is suggested therefore, that this literature might be of some interest to the NHS. Taylor's ideas on scientific management were originally set out 80 years ago (Taylor, 1947). A more recent general review of Taylorism is given in Littler (1985). Critiques of these ideas are to be found in Braverman (1974) and Edwards (1979).

12

The concept of the primary nurse is a compromise between the ultimate 'professional' model of the practitioner, and the task orientated, Taylorist, managerial model. The primary nurse co-ordinates the care for a small group of patients, who know that she is 'their' nurse, and gives them much but not all of their care. She will use the skills of other nurses or support workers, but not to such an extent as to break this psychological link. Primary nursing is being studied scientifically for the first time under a Welsh Office grant (to the Mid and West Wales College of Nursing) and by the Centre for Health Economics at York with a DoH grant. All these studies were due to report in Spring 1992. It is interesting to note that the Audit Commission (1991) has jumped the gun and commended the practice.

The NHS 'reforms'

The NHS reforms implemented in April 1991, including development of independent trusts, could eventually produce a rather more competitive labour market for the NHS. It is argued in Chapter 7 that the NHS is often a near monopsonistic employer of specialist skills, such as those possessed by nurses and many of the P&T staff groups. This has probably allowed it to pay wage rates which are below those which would emerge in a more competitive market. However, the creation of self governing hospitals, able to set their own rates of pay, could mean that eventually hospitals will compete against each other for labour and, in consequence, drive its price up to more like competitive levels. This intriguing idea is investigated by Mayston (1990). This view has to be seen as highly speculative because it is at least possible to argue that independent hospitals will continue to hold a lot of monopsonistic power within their *local* labour market. This is particularly likely to happen with respect to the female dominated professions, because their mobility is so often curtailed to fit in to their husband's choice of employer. Indeed studies from the United States suggest that hospitals do have considerable monopsonistic power in the market for nurses, even in this much more competitive health care system. For some recent examples of such studies, see: Sullivan (1989); and Robinson (1988). Nonetheless, there seems to have been very little attention paid to this aspect of the forthcoming reforms, and it is suggested that it is a topic worthy of further investigation.

It is also interesting to speculate on the possible labour market consequences for the NHS of the reforms to community care. These reforms will give local authorities prime responsibility for providing community care, and will thus make them alternative employers of a number of nursing and P&T skills, most notably health visitors and district nurses of course, but also presumably physiotherapists, chiropodists, etc. The facility of GPs to operate more independently is another potentially important factor. Perhaps in the long run there really will be at least some degree of competition in the labour markets from which the NHS draws so much of its trained staff.

1.3 The need to reassess recruitment and retention policies

If the NHS is to overcome the problems that in common with many other UK employers it is likely to face, it will need to reassess continually its recruitment and retention policies. A key issue that must be addressed is whether conventional recruitment practices actually deliver people with the required skills and competences. In particular, are the entry requirements that are currently employed strictly necessary in terms of the formal qualifications required to carry out the various duties that employees will be asked to perform? A second issue is whether these duties all have to be filled by recruiting young full-time females or whether some of the work can be done by other categories of personnel with suitable reorganization of workloads and recruitment strategies.

The package of pay benefits and employment conditions needs to be designed in such a way as to attract the various target groups identified as of potential value. While pay is a key element, other factors are also crucial. The image of the organization, perceptions of career prospects, flexibility as well as the details of the employment contract may also be very important. In the case of women the provision and costs of child care facilities are a key issue. Mechanisms for assessing the effect of changes in such elements on recruitment need to be established (if they do not already exist), in order that barriers to recruitment and causes of wastage can be identified.

The issue of flexibility is, as noted below, an important one. Greater flexibility is being demanded of employers, in the sense that to stick with old established rules of thumb will almost certainly fail to deal with the problems that the 1990s are likely to present. This may range from reassessing the target groups that are acceptable for recruitment, to reassessing entry requirements etc. It may also imply a need to adopt radical new solutions involving a significant break with the 'traditional' way in which things are done. The other aspect of flexibility is that employees are demanding a more flexible employment contract. Trends towards self-employment and part-time working are highlighted below.

Given the investment implicit in the recruitment of, particularly the more highly qualified new entrants, it is crucial that selection procedures are assessed to ensure the people with the desired characteristics are obtained and that having been recruited they are retained for sufficient time to recoup the investment in training and other costs. Many employers are now starting to take selection techniques much more seriously in order to ensure that objective decisions are made. The NHS may need therefore to reconsider its own policy in this area and to reassess whether it is keeping pace with developments in the private sector.

Having got the personnel and invested heavily in training it is important to ensure that wastage is carefully monitored in order to identify possible causes and to take policy initiatives to reduce it if it is becoming a serious problem. Many of the factors influencing wastage are within the control of the employing organization. However, it is important to systematically measure and analyse the nature and perceived causes of people leaving the organization. Only then can steps be taken to influence retention rates. This may involve changes in the way in which tasks are organized, working practices, payment systems, career progression, supervisory style and general organizational image/ambiance. Again however the NHS, to the extent that it remains part of the public sector, may have to operate within more fixed constraints than many other employers. This means that it will need to act even more effectively than its competitors in the labour market on those aspects which it is able to change.

Finally, retention may not be entirely divorced from the recruitment issue, since it is obviously most important to ensure that new entrants do not have unrealistic expectations of what the organization can offer.

1.4 Areas for further research

The current research reveals six main areas where further, more detailed, analysis would appear to be desirable.

(i) It has been noted that the pay review bodies currently examine pay in some detail. Nevertheless, there appears to be some room for further research, involving detailed examination of other aspects of terms and conditions of employment, such as fringe benefits, hours of work, etc., which may not have been fully covered by these reviews. The impact of changing labour market conditions generally, and within certain regional labour markets in particular, also deserves greater consideration.

(ii) It is probably felt within the NHS that the main reasons why people leave are well understood. However, despite the fact that much survey work has been conducted, there does not appear to be much quantitative analysis of the causes of wastage in the UK, comparable to that conducted in the US. As noted in Chapter 9, the problem of wastage is a complex one and a case can therefore be made for further research to exploit more fully the existing data and to confirm (or deny) the truth of various hypotheses. If the key determining factors can be identified, this will again facilitate policy changes to alleviate the problems. The review in Chapter 9, has identified various relevant studies in this area (mainly for the US), which point the way from a methodological viewpoint. Given suitable data there is scope for some quite sophisticated econometric analysis.

(iii) A similar set of remarks applies to the analysis of recruitment. There is considerable scope for research to identify the factors influencing the decision to enter the NHS, covering both those who do and those who do not choose to do so. This should focus on mature women, ethnic minorities and other possible target groups as well as the obvious young, female category. Responses are likely (from US evidence) to vary between such groups. This could be crucial in determining appropriate levels of incentives.

(iv) Related to (iii) is the apparent need for some form of regular survey of attitudes of those outside the NHS to employment therein. This could provide invaluable data, (in conjunction with the presently conducted surveys of attitudes of those within the NHS), with which to analyse recruitment problems.

(v) There would also appear to be some value in research to identify the effectiveness of advertising campaigns on recruitment. Given the need to target recruitment geographically, some consideration of the effectiveness of campaigns in different parts of the country seems appropriate. Further research on how advertising affects the perceptions of potential entrants could also be useful.

(vi) The results from Chapter 13 suggest the need for further research to examine the extent to which changes in the system for educating nurses (and PAMs) promote (or otherwise) the recruitment, career progression and retention of those with domestic responsibilities, especially those from black and other minority ethnic groups.

(vii) Finally, on the demand side, there appears to be a major gap in our knowledge of the degree of substitutability between labour inputs. Wide variations in skill mixes between different hospitals and localities suggest that contrary to the views of some practitioners there may be much more scope to vary the mix of nurses, paramedics, doctors and other staff. If efficient use is to be made of limited resources further exploration of this issue seems crucial.

2 The general labour supply picture

2.1 Demographic change

One of the few areas where forecasts can be made with reasonable certainty is in the area of demographic change. Although birth rates are notoriously difficult to predict, once born, the probability of any individual progressing to a ripe old age is known with relative accuracy. Indeed, the fortunes of many insurance companies rest on this fact. Given that losses to the home population due to net migration are relatively tiny, and do not greatly influence the total stock of people around at any one time, this means that the total stock of people of working age can be predicted up to 16 years ahead with considerable confidence.

All of those who are going to form part of the workforce of the 1990s have already been born. Indeed if we consider those with higher qualifications, such as a degree, the vast majority of those who will possess such qualifications in the year 2010 are already alive. Between 1964 and 1977 there was a 35 per cent fall in the number of births in the United Kingdom. Live births peaked at just over 1 million in 1964 and reached a trough of 660 thousand in 1977 (see Table 2.1). The implications of the pattern of births in the 1960s and 1970s are that there will be a very substantial fall in the number of young people entering the labour market in the 1990s. Between 1980 and 1993 the numbers of young people of 16 years of age will fall by 35 per cent and the numbers of young labour market entrants will remain relatively depressed to the turn of the decade and beyond. (See Figure 2.1.)

17

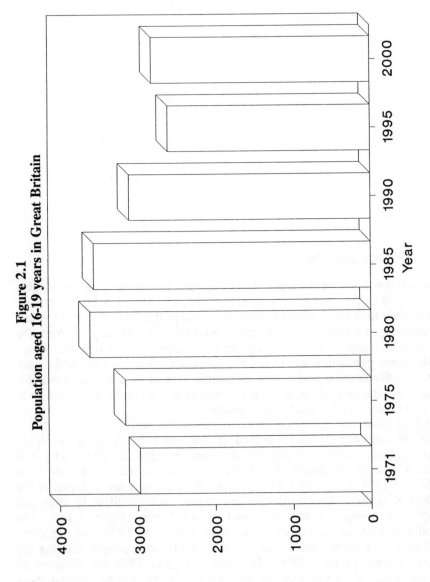

Figure 2.1
Population aged 16-19 years in Great Britain

Source: DE, Employment Gazette, May 1991

Table 2.1
Live births in the United Kingdom

	thousands
1951	797
1956	825
1961	944
1964	1,015
1966	980
1971	902
1976	676
1977	657
1981	731
1986	755
1988	788
1989	777
Projections:[a]	
1991	826
2001	768
2011	732
2025	772

Source: Office of Population Censuses and Surveys: Government Actuary's Department; General Register Office (Scotland), General Office (Northern Ireland). In *Social Trends* (1991) - Table 1-10.

Note: (a) 1989 based projections.

Table 2.2
Projections of 18 year olds by social class of parent

thousands

Year	Social Class						
	Professional I	Intermediate II	Skilled non-manual III N	Skilled manual III M	Semi-skilled IV	& Unskilled & V	Total
1980	39	93	93	325	225		775
1985	45	102	85	319	194		744
1990	46	109	70	265	140		630
1995	47	111	58	214	118		548
2000	56	127	64	230	126		602

Source: Department of Education and Science, unpublished estimates.

Note: Estimates based on data from Government Actuary's Department for England.

Table 2.3
Projected numbers of school leavers

thousands

| | 1980/81 | 1986/87 | 1988/89 | 1989/90 | Projections | |
					1993/94	2000/01
Young men						
All leavers	450	433	380	364	318	363
- for full-time education[a]	103	116	118	115	88	115
- for the labour market	346	317	262	249	236	248
Young women						
All leavers	426	410	358	344	300	344
- for full-time education[a]	137	143	141	138	110	136
- for the labour market	289	267	216	206	196	208
Young people						
All leavers	876	843	738	708	618	707
- for full-time education[a]	241	259	259	252	197	251
- for the labour market	635	584	419	456	432	456

Source: Department of Employment, *Employment Gazette*,
          (October 1991), pp.552-53.

Note: (a)   Those entering either full-time further education or temporary
            employment pending entry to full-time further education. In
            England and Wales, estimates are derived from schools'
            estimates of leavers intentions. In Scotland, estimates are
            derived from returns from colleges and the university record.

The decline in birth rates has particularly affected the manual social classes as indicated in Table 2.2. The decline for the professional and intermediate groups is relatively modest and indeed numbers will be higher in 2000 compared with 1980. For manual groups, however, the decline is, in some cases, almost 50 per cent from 1985 levels. These data suggest that the decline in the numbers of young people may not result in a significant fall in the number of those staying on into higher education, since the bulk of such people come from the higher social classes. The biggest changes will be for those least likely to enter post-compulsory education.

2.2 Numbers of school leavers

However, while the total number of young people of school leaving age can be projected with some accuracy, it is much more difficult to assess what proportion of this number will be available for work and what proportion will stay on to do post-compulsory education. This will depend upon a whole host of institutional and social and economic factors. The former include changes such as the introduction of YTS and GCSE, while the latter include changes in the social class structure and the perceived benefits of staying on as opposed to leaving school.

The Department of Education and Science has attempted to project the destinations of those leaving school (DES, 1990). These are summarised in Table 2.3 The **proportion** of those staying on at school beyond the minimum school leaving age is projected to rise from 35 per cent in 1986/87 to around 42 per cent by 2000/1. This is based on some assumptions about changing social class structure. However, the effects of factors such as unemployment, the relative returns to higher education and institutional changes such as GCSE and the National Curriculum are not taken into account. This latest evidence suggests an increase in educational participation, which many commentators have attributed to the contemporaneous changes in the examination system (notably the introduction of GCSE). However, research by Whitfield and Wilson (1991a and 1991b) suggests that the failure of earlier DES projections to properly account for the influence of various other socio-economic variables have lead to downward bias in their forecasts, especially in the short-run. The recent increase in staying on could therefore simply reflect the unwinding of a process of lagged adjustment to changes in various other socioeconomic factors (notably unemployment rates, the financial returns to staying on at school and the introduction of special employment and training measures such as the Youth Training Scheme (YTS)). If this interpretation is correct, the numbers staying on in full-time education could be significantly higher than DES project, thus exacerbating the recruitment problems of those trying to attract 16 and 17 year old school leavers. This would mean that the numbers entering the labour market will decline even more rapidly than indicated in Table 2.3, while the numbers entering further education would decline rather less.

Table 2.4
Estimates and projections of the resident population of Great Britain aged 16 and over

thousands

| | 1981 | 1985 | 1989 | Projections | | |
				1990	1995	2000
Males						
16-19	1,882	1,824	1,661	1,595	1347	1,455
20-24	2,107	2,341	2,295	2,249	1955	1,727
25-44	7,255	7,571	8,060	8,173	8322	8,367
45-64	5,947	5,963	5,908	5,944	6384	6,669
65+	3,253	3,294	3,456	3,517	3634	3,725
Working age[a]	17,192	17,698	17,925	17,961	18008	18,218
Females						
16-19	1,797	1,736	1,583	1,517	1268	1,374
20-24	2,052	2,271	2,219	2,173	1872	1,641
25-44	7,154	7,471	7,979	8,088	8,212	8,222
45-60	4,711	4,564	4,585	4,619	5,109	5,369
60+	6,588	6,691	6,738	6,738	6,705	6,708
Working age[b]	15,714	16,042	16,365	16,397	16461	16,606
All						
16-19	3,679	3,559	3,244	3,112	2615	2,829
20-24	4,159	4,612	4,514	4,423	3827	3,368
25-44	14,409	15,043	16,039	16,261	16534	16,587
45-64	12,180	12,141	11,968	12,028	12881	13,465
65+	8,288	8,371	8,760	8,790	8951	9,066
Working age[c]	31,686	33,741	34,290	34,614	34469	34,824

Source: Department of Employment; *Employment Gazette*, (May 1991), Table 2, pp.272-73.

Notes: (a) Men aged 16-64 years.
(b) Women aged 16-59 years.
(c) Men aged 16 to 64 and women aged 16 to 59 years.

23

Table 2.5
Estimates and projections of the economically active population

thousands

	1980	1990	Projections[d] 1995	2000
Males				
16-19	1,355	1,184	986	1,084
20-24	1,767	1,941	1,647	1,424
25-44	6,906	7,721	7,834	7,859
45-64	5,277	4,784	5,148	5,355
65+	332	301	249	210
Working age[a]	15,305	15,631	15,616	15,721
Females				
16-19	1,329	1,072	885	967
20-24	1,351	1,626	1,413	1,260
25-44	4,372	5,913	6,208	6,472
45-60	3,002	3,104	3,476	3,649
60+	507	507	453	445
Working age[b]	10,054	11,715	11,982	12,348
All				
16-19	2,684	2,256	1,871	2,051
20-24	3,118	3,567	3,061	2,684
25-44	11,277	13,635	14,042	14,331
45-64	8,608	7,147	8,929	9,315
65+	510	476	401	345
Working age[a,b]	25,359	27,345	27,598	28,069

Source: DE, *Employment Gazette*, (May 1991), p.269.

Notes: (a)   Men aged 16-64 years.
  (b)   Women aged 16-60 years.
  (c)   GB labour force definitions. Includes all persons aged 16 and over who are in employment or unemployed.
  (d)   ILO definitions. This excludes those unemployed who are not actively seeking work. More precise definitions are given in DE (1990).

24

The magnitude of this effect depends on the extent to which relative pay for 'stayers' as opposed to 'leavers' changes. The proportion of those staying on in school (or further education) will, of course, influence the numbers of those eventually emerging with higher qualifications such as degrees.

2.3 General prospect for labour supply

The emphasis so far has been on the number of young people entering the labour market. Although these flows are important, the vast majority of people who will be in the labour force in the year 2000 are already in the workforce. Demographic developments for the population generally are summarised in Table 2.4. This shows estimates and projections of the resident population of Great Britain aged 16 and above. The figures for the 16-19 and to a lesser extent the 20-24 year old age groups reflect the demographic changes we have already discussed. However, while the numbers of young people are projected to fall beween 1990 and 2000, the population of working age is actually expected to rise by 250 thousand for males and 200 thousand for females.

Such contrasts are accentuated when these population projections are translated into forecasts of the economically active population. This involves the projection of activity rates which are much more sensitive to economic, social and other factors than are demographic trends. The basic forecasts of activity rates by DE (1991) are based on a time series analysis of labour supply. This topic is examined in detail in Chapter 6 below. For the present, it is sufficient to focus on the official DE projections which relate economic activity to: the level of claimant unemployment (representing the pressure of demand in the labour market); the number of children aged under 10 (per woman in the relevant age group); and time trends representing a combination of factors which could not be adequately measured. The forecasts are based on an assumption of unchanged unemployment levels from January 1990 values. As noted in Chapter 6, these methods can be criticised on the grounds of not treating the labour supply decision within a household context and not incorporating various economic variables such as wages, although this can probably be justified on pragmatic grounds, given the problems of obtaining directly relevant data. However, a more robust specification has been developed by Briscoe and Wilson (1992). This model, based more firmly on a theoretical economic model of labour supply decisions within a household context, suggests more rapid declines in economic activity rates for older males while the converse is true for older females. The assumption of fixed unemployment levels in the DE forecasts is also contentious. Independent projections by IER (1991) allow for the fact that falling unemployment levels in the mid to late 1990s will probably increase economic activity rates. Both these considerations suggest that the numbers of mature females available for work in the late 1990s could be well above the levels suggested by the DE.

Figure 2.2

Changes in labour force, employment and unemployment, 1990-2000

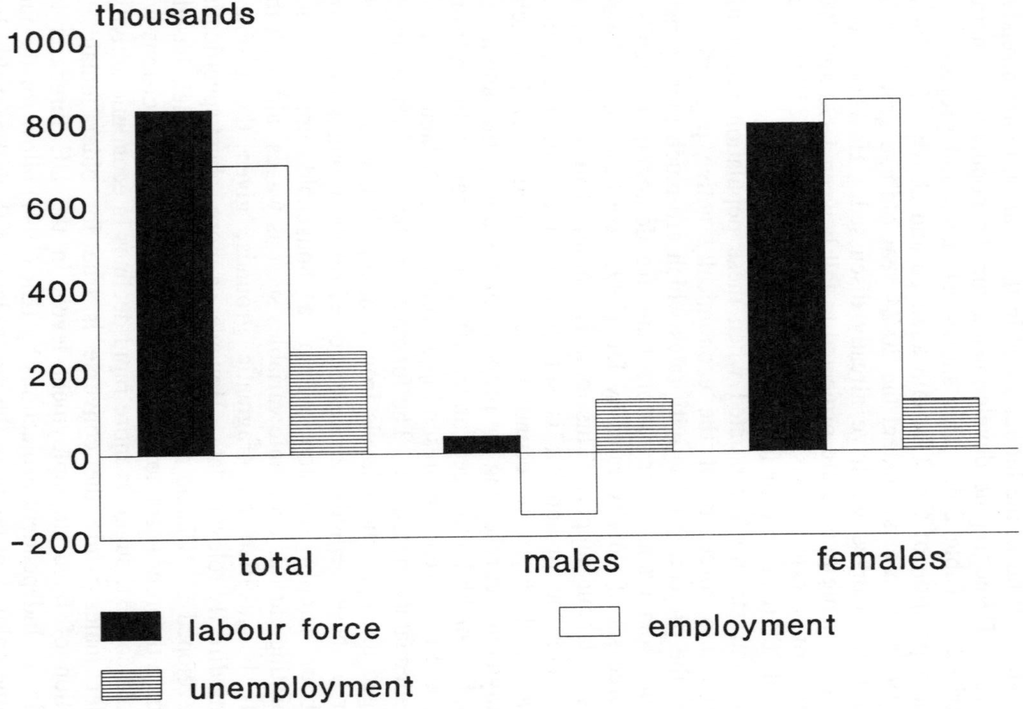

Legend: ■ labour force □ employment ▥ unemployment

Categories: total, males, females

y-axis (thousands): -200, 0, 200, 400, 600, 800, 1000

Source: IER Review of the Economy and Employment, 1991: Occupational Assessment

Table 2.6
Spatial variations in the projected labour force

Region	Projected changes 1988-2000				16-24 year olds: projected change as a percentage of unemployment[b]
	16-24 year olds		All those of working age[a]		
	thousands	%	thousands	%	
South East	-345	-17.3	591	6.8	219.7
East Anglia	-46	-19.7	140	14.1	255.6
South West	-74	-15.0	331	15.1	172.1
West Midlands	-152	-26.7	23	0.9	187.6
East Midlands	-94	-21.1	144	7.4	195.9
Yorkshire & Humberside	-122	-23.2	34	1.5	143.5
North West	-185	-26.3	-62	-2.0	158.5
North	-91	-26.7	-42	-2.9	149.2
Wales	-54	-19.2	33	2.6	114.9
Scotland	-163	-28.7	-36	-1.5	152.3
Great Britain	-1,327	-21.6	1,156	4.3	173.7

Source: Department of Employment (1990).

Notes: (a) Men aged 16-64, women aged 16-59.
(b) April 1988 figure.

Figure 2.3

Ethnic population by age and whether UK-born or overseas-born, 1986-1988 average

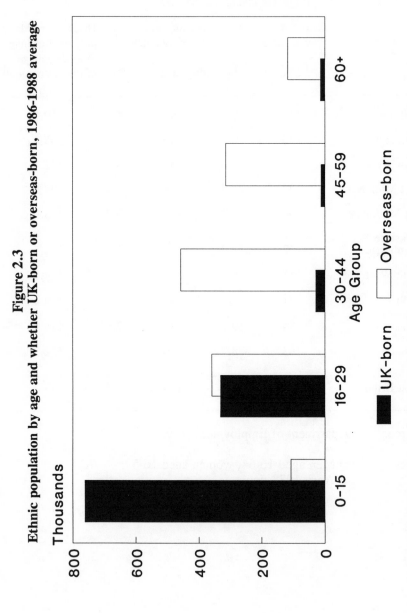

Source: Labour Force Survey, Office of Population Censuses and Surveys
[In Social Trends 1991]

Table 2.7
Population in Great Britain by ethnic origin and age, 1986-88

	Percentage in each age group					Total[a] all ages 60 or (= 100%)	
	Percentage						
	0-15	16-29	30-44	45-59	over	(thousands)	UK-born[b]
Ethnic group							
White	20	22	21	17	21	51,470	96
All ethnic minority groups of which West Indian or	32	23	25	13	7	3,049	43
Guyanese	25	32	16	20	7	495	53
Indian	31	27	24	14	5	787	36
Pakistani	44	25	18	11	2	428	42
Bangladeshi	49	22	14	13	2	108	31
Chinese	29	26	31	9	5	125	24
All ethnic groups	20	22	21	16	21	54,519	93

Source: *Labour Force Survey*, combined data for 1986 to 1988 inclusive, Office of Population Censuses and Surveys as reported in *Social Trends*.

Notes: (a) Population in private households.
(b) Refers to 1988 estimates.

The DE's projections of the numbers of economically active individuals are shown in Table 2.5. The results indicate an increase in the economically active population of 150 thousand for males but a 570 thousand increase for females between 1990 and 2000. These increases occur despite a fall of 1.3 million in the total population in the 16-24 age category over the same period. The effects of a projected decline in aggregate unemployment in the IER forecasts (IER, 1991), is to further increase the projected rise in the labour force to over 800 thousand individuals, most of whom are female (see Figure 2.2).

2.4 The spatial aspects of labour supply

The pattern of demographic change exhibits considerable spatial variation. The UK is not alone in experiencing a severe demographic downturn in the number of young people. Indeed, the position in some other European countries is much worse (e.g. West Germany). Within the UK there are significant variations across regions as indicated in Table 2.6. This illustrates projected changes in the labour force by region. The decline in the labour force of 16-24 year olds between 1988 and 1995 is expected to be most severe in Scotland, the North of England, the North West and the West Midlands. The overall impact of these supply-side changes also depends on what is happening on the demand side. Comparing the projected reductions in the labour force with recent unemployment, as shown in the final column of the table, illustrates that, as a proportion of unemployment levels, it is the southern region which may face the most severe problems. In all cases the projected decline in the labour force of 16-24 year olds exceeds current unemployment levels. The corresponding change in the total labour force of working age is also shown in the table. This also varies dramatically across regions, from quite strong growth in the South to declines in the North and North West.

The results of the analysis of the Labour Force Survey reported in Chapters 7 and 8 provides a more detailed anlaysis of the supply of those with nursing and related skills at a spatially disaggregated level.

2.5 Ethnic background

Regrettably there are no official projections of population or the labour force distinguishing ethnic origin. However, some data are available for the historical period, which provide an indication of potential labour supply from minority groups. Table 2.7 and Figure 2.3 present data from the 1986, 1987 and 1988 Labour Force Surveys combined to avoid problems of sampling error. About 5.6 per cent of the population in Great Britain were from the minority ethnic groups. Over two thirds of these were either from the West Indian/Guyanese or Indian/Pakistani ethnic groups. All minority ethnic groups have different age structures from that of the white population. About 21 per cent of the white population was aged 60 or over compared to just 7 per cent for the West Indian/Guyanese

Table 2.8
Economic status of the population of working age in Great Britain by sex and ethnic group, 1985-87

	Males Ethnic group						Females Ethnic group					
	White	West Indian or Guyanese	Indian	Pakistani Bangla-deshi	Other[a]	All males[b]	White	West Indian or Guyanese	Indian	Pakistani Bangla-deshi	Other[a]	All females[b]
Economically active (percentages)												
In employment												
- Employees	65	56	52	41	49	64	58	59	43	8	44	57
- Self-employed	13	7	20	13	13	5	::	::	6	::	::	4
- On government scheme	2	::	::	::	::	2	1	::	::	::	5	1
All in employment	80	69	75	58	65	80	65	65	51	17	52	63
Out of employment	8	15	8	19	8	8	6	10	7	4	7	6
All economically active	89	85	84	77	74	89	70	76	58	21	59	70
Total of working age[c] (= 100%)(thousands)	16,649	168	261	151	233	17,462	15,216	173	253	138	223	16,003

Source: ED, *Employment Gazette*, (February 1991), p.62.

Notes:
(a) Includes African, Arab, Chinese, other stated, and Mixed.
(b) Includes ethnic group not stated.
(c) Males aged 16-64, females aged 16-59.
(d) The symbol .. indicates sample size too small for reliable estimates.

Table 2.9
Economically active people of working age, by gender, highest qualification, ethnic group and unemployment rate, Great Britain, 1987-89

Sex and highest qualification[2]	Ethnic group					
	White			All ethnic minority groups		
	000s	%	unemployment rate[a]	000s	%	unemployment rate[a]
Men aged 16-64						
Higher[b]	2,212	15.0	3	102	15.4	6
Other	7,633	51.8	7	300	45.3	13
None	4,751	32.2	14	246	37.2	21
All economically active[c]	14,736	100.0	9	662	100.0	15
Women aged 16-59						
Higher[b]	1,546	14.4	4	83	18.5	5
Other	5,449	50.9	8	215	47.9	15
None	3,651	34.1	11	144	32.2	15
All economically active[c]	10,714	100.0	8	448	100.0	13

Source: Office of Population Censuses and Surveys, *Labour Force Survey*, 1988 and 1989, Series LFS No.8, p.28, Table 5.36.

Notes: (a) Per 100 economically active people ILO/DECD definition
(b) Higher includes all qualifications above GCE A level.
(c) Includes those who did not state their highest qualification.

ethnic group. Young people form a smaller proportion of the white population than they do for the minority ethnic populations. The health service has traditionally drawn quite heavily on certain ethnic minorities for many of its staff. These figures cast at least a small shaft of light in an otherwise gloomy picture for employers looking to expand recruitment. However, other employers may well target such groups more intensively if serious labour shortages do emerge.

Figure 2.3 illustrates the differences in age structure between the United Kingdom-born and the overseas-born members of the ethnic minority population. Most of the overseas-born entered the UK as young adults, or as dependents, while the UK-born are the first or second generation children of these earlier immigrants. Consequently, about two thirds of the UK-born minority ethnic population were aged under 15 and less than 7 per cent were aged over 30 in 1986-1988. In contrast, less than 8 per cent of the overseas-born ethnic minority population were aged under 15 while over two thirds were aged above 30.

Table 2.8 shows that the proportion of men of working age in Great Britain who were economically active was higher among the white population and the West Indian/Guyanese group than among those from the 'other' ethnic group. The low activity rate for the latter results, at least in part, from a higher proportion of full-time students. Among women the variation between ethnic groups was greater. Only 58 and 21 per cent respectively of those from the India and Pakistani/Bangladeshi ethnic groups were economically active compared to 70 per cent in the white group and 76 per cent of those from the West Indian/Guyanese group. Unemployment rates also vary between ethnic groups, with unemployment much higher amongst West Indian/Guyanese and Indian/Pakistani/Bangladeshi groups, especially for males.

The proportion of the ethnic minorities having higher qualifications (above GCE A level) is very similar to the white group (see Table 2.9). For males, the proportion with intermediate level qualifications is however lower for other ethnic groups. There are important differences between minority groups, with the Indian/Pakistani/Bangladeshi group being much better qualified than the others.

The overall conclusion from this analysis is that the ethnic minorities, especially those who are UK-born, provide a small but potentially important source of labour supply of new entrants in the 1990s. This is a group from which the health service has traditionally drawn significant numbers of nursing staff. The problem in the 1990s is that an increasing number of other employers are likely to cast their nets in the same direction.

2.6 Qualified school leavers and the supply of new graduates

Recent and ongoing work at the IER, sponsored by the Employment Department Agency, has focused on trends in the supply of highly qualified persons (Wilson et al., 1990). The proportion of young people staying on in education after the age of 16 has been rising steadily over the last 30 years or more. The percentage leaving school with two or more 'A' levels increased rapidly from 1955 to 1970. While this proportion has continued to grow, the rate of increase, in the 1970s and 1980s has been much smaller. A variety of influences have been at work, including rising incomes, easier access, changing social class structure and, more recently, declining returns to investment in education. The increasing proportion and (until recent years) numbers of young people meeting higher education entry standards has been reflected in the growing number of students awarded first degrees.

The most rapid growth of university degrees occurred in the mid-1960s, when a number of new universities were established. Growth has continued, albeit at a somewhat slower rate, until recent years, when there has been some decline in university degree awards. Interestingly, the decline in university applications in the late 1980s centred on the sciences (particularly combined sciences and engineering, engineering and technology); business administration grew especially strongly, followed by social sciences and humanities. Since the 1970s the most rapid expansion has been in the public sector, with the numbers of graduates from polytechnics increasing almost 16 fold between 1970 and 1987 (to 46 thousand per annum). University graduates increased by around 50 per cent over the same period (to 72 thousand per annum).

The results already presented in Section 2.2 and Table 2.3 indicate that the numbers of those staying on at school in order to obtain further qualifications will fall less than the overall number of young people. The proportion of those that go on into further or higher education rose from 27 per cent in 1980/81 to 35 per cent in 1988/89 (DE, 1990). This is the latest year for which data are currently available. The official projections to the turn of the century are for a continued rise, reaching 42 per cent in the late 1990s. These revised projections may still be underestimates if educational participation rates in the UK continue to rise to levels more in line with other developed countries. As noted above, the latest indications are that staying on rates are rising much more rapidly than the earlier DES projections suggest (DES, 1990), but whether this is attributable to these institutional factors such as the introduction of GCSE and the National Curriculum (as DES have suggested) or to a return to long-term trend rates of growth in educational participation rates, as suggested by Whitfield and Wilson (1991a and 1991b), remains unclear.

The proportions of those aged 16-18 in the UK staying on at school or in formal education is currently quite low by international standards. This figure reaches almost 90 per cent in the US, Germany and Japan, compared with just over 60 per cent in the UK (over two thirds of which is part-time, see Smithers and Robinson, 1989). There is therefore considerable scope for further increases in educational participation rates by international standards. Even within the UK there are considerable variations across local education authorities, ranging from just over 30 per cent in Barking to over 70 per cent in Harrow and Brent. Such differences may reinforce the regional disparities in labour supply trends we have already highlighted.

Table 2.10
Numbers and projections of qualified leavers, Great Britain

thousands[a]

	1975	1980	1985	1990	Projections	
					1995	2000
Males	64	70	78	73	61	70
Females	52	63	71	70	59	68
All	115	133	150	142	121	138
Percentages of cohort aged 18 and 19						
Males	8.0	7.6	8.5	9.0	9.6	10.0
Females	6.8	7.2	8.1	9.1	9.7	10.1
All	7.4	7.4	8.4	9.0	9.7	10.1

Source: DES (1986), Table A3, Projection Q.
Notes: (a) Unless elsewhere specified.

In 1987 about 78 thousand youngsters entered the labour market with 5 higher grade 'O' levels but less than 2 'A' levels. There were about 30 thousand who entered the labour market who had 2 or more 'A' levels. The official projections indicate that these figures will decline by the mid-nineties to 63 and 26 thousand respectively (DE, 1986). The overall numbers of those with 2 or more 'A' levels are shown in Table 2.10 together with projections to 2000. The figures include individuals going on into higher education. Again, these may be underestimates if a larger proportion of youngsters stay on in full-time education. The numbers shown in the table are based on so called 'projection Q'. This was the higher of a range of projections produced in 1986. They form the basis for Government policy as laid out in the 1987 White Paper, 'Meeting the Challenge' (DES, 1987). More recent projections were reported in the summary report of the Interdepartmental Review on *Highly Qualified People Supply and Demand* (DES, 1990). These suggest that the numbers in home full-time higher education will rise from just under 700 thousand in 1988 to over 800 thousand by 2000 with only a minor turn down in the mid 1990s. This projection was made in 1989 and was subsequently

Table 2.11
Projections of numbers in higher education

thousands

	1987	1988	1989	1990	1991	1992	1993	1994	1995	1996	1997	1998	1999	2000
Home Full-time Equivalents														
Reference[a]	656	652	648	621	581	539	509	483	463	462	501	529	537	533
1986[b]	656	663	671	673	672	663	655	647	639	636	643	655	665	666
1989[c]	676	692	714	735	750	752	748	743	740	745	762	787	807	816
1990[d]			739	779	806	811	805							
Age Participation Indices (API)[e]														
1986	14.5	14.6	15.2	15.4	16.0	16.5	16.9	17.2	17.4	17.7	18.1	18.1	18.3	18.5
1989	14.6	15.1	16.0	17.4	18.3	19.0	19.6	20.0	20.3	21.4	21.9	22.0	22.3	22.9
1990			16.8	18.3	19.2	19.8	20.5							
Full-time and Sandwich Courses[f]														
Postgraduates	46	48	48	48	49	49	49	49	50	50	50	50	50	51
First and Sub-degree	503	515	535	555	568	570	565	560	557	562	581	606	626	636
Part-time Students[f]														
Open University	86	87	88	88	88	88	88	88	88	88	88	88	88	88
Postgraduates	54	58	60	62	63	64	65	65	65	66	65	65	64	64
First and Sub-degree	220	222	225	227	229	229	230	228	227	225	224	222	220	218

Source: DES (1990).

Notes:

(a)   Index of 18 to 19 year old population, applied to 1987 home, FTE student numbers.
(b)   Published in *Projections of Demand for Higher Education in Great Britain 1986-2000*.
(c)   Figures for 1987 are actual; those for 1988 are provisional, 1989 projections.
(d)   Incorporates provisional 1989 enrolments, 1990 projections.
(e)   The API is the number of young (under 21) home initial entrants to higher education expressed as a percentage of the 'relevant age group', being half the total number of 18 and 19 year olds in the population.
(f)   Figures relate to the 1989 projections of student numbers (see notes 1-3).

Table 2.12
Projection of home student numbers in higher education in Great Britain

thousands

Academic year beginning	Actual					Projection								
	1987	1988	1989	1990	1991	1992	1993	1994	1995	1996	1997	1998	1999	2000
Full-time and sandwich initial entrants	170	178	197	217	237	250	254	257	261	276	295	306	310	313
Age participation index[a]	14.6	15.1	17.1	19.3	22.5	25.2	26.6	27.5	28.1	29.7	30.7	30.7	31.3	32.1
Full-time and sandwich first and sub-degree students	503	517	551	598	658	710	749	770	782	804	841	886	921	940
Full-time postgraduate students	46	47	49	50	51	52	52	53	54	54	55	55	56	56
Part-time students	359	379	396	419	432	443	453	462	468	474	479	485	490	495
Full-time equivalent students[b]	677	697	739	795	860	918	960	984	999	1024	1064	1110	1148	1170

Source: DES (1991).

Notes: (a) The number of young home initial entrants to full-time educatin expressed as a proportion of the averaged 18-19 year old population.
(b) A factor of 0.35 has been used to convert part-time students to their full-time equivalent.

37

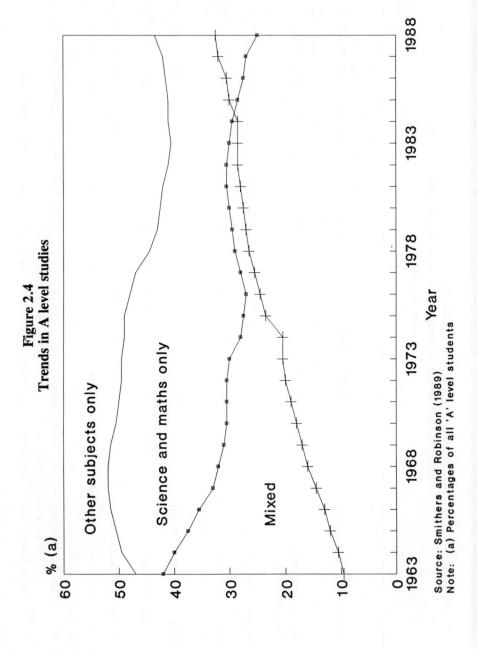

Figure 2.4
Trends in A level studies

% (a)

Other subjects only

Science and maths only

Mixed

Year

Source: Smithers and Robinson (1989)
Note: (a) Percentages of all 'A' level students

38

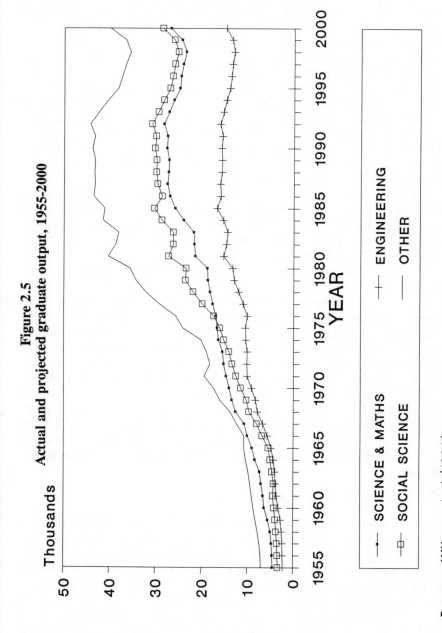

Figure 2.5

Actual and projected graduate output, 1955-2000

Thousands

YEAR

—•— SCIENCE & MATHS   —+— ENGINEERING

—□— SOCIAL SCIENCE   —— OTHER

Source: Wilson et al (1990)

revised upwards, although the revision only went up to 1993. The revised estimate for that year was 805 as opposed to 748 thousand. These projections are summarised in Table 2.11. The latest DES forecast (Table 2.12) suggest an even greater rise in educational participation rates, with the proportion of those going into higher and further education doubling to over 30 per cent by 2000. These figures do not however, appear to be based on a rigourous analysis of the causes of recent increases in educational participation but simply extrapolate the latest increases forward. They may prove to be exaggerated.

Detailed projections are not available of those with certain types of 'A' level (e.g. science, or particular grades). However, as a rough rule of thumb one would expect the numbers of people emerging with particular types of 'A' level to follow a similar profile to that shown in Table 2.10. The current trends are for the numbers of those taking pure science and mathematics at 'A' level to decline (see Figure 2.4). The big growth area has been 'mixed' 'A' levels, that is, science subjects, including mathematics, mixed with others. Smithers and Robinson (1989) attribute this to the growth in popularity of economics. Only about 20 per cent of those taking mixed 'A' levels were planning to continue in their science specialism. Most were hoping to move into accountancy, business studies, finance, etc. These trends seem likely to continue.

The DES does not make projections of graduate numbers over the medium term. Nevertheless, projections are available from two other sources. Those produced by IMS (1989) show a further growth in the number of first degree graduates up to 1992/3, after which time the demographic effects outlined earlier take effect. These reduce the numbers modestly up to 1998, before eventually recovering to just under 130 thousand at the turn of the century. An independent set of projections have been made by IER, based upon a very different methodology (Wilson *et al.*, 1990). The overall results, for first degree graduates only, are summarised in Figure 2.5. They exhibit a similar profile, in total, to the IMS projections. Neither of these projections takes on board recent increases in educational participation rates for 16 year olds. The actual outflow of graduates may therefore be rather higher than these figures suggest.

2.7 The total stock of qualified persons

The implications of these projections for total stocks of highly qualified persons are summarised in Table 2.13. The number of economically active graduates and postgraduates is projected to rise by over 0.8 million between 1990 and 2000, an increase of almost 30 per cent. This reflects a steady inflow of newly qualified graduates which is only partially offset by losses due to deaths, retirements and net migration. Even if the proportion of young people obtaining degree level qualifications stabilised at current levels it would take many decades before the total stock would cease to grow because of the much smaller proportion of qualified persons in older age groups.

The table also illustrates the breakdown by discipline. Engineering and technology graduates and postgraduates are expected to increase by about 85 thousand from the 1990 value of 396 thousand. The science numbers show an even more rapid rate of growth, with an increase of 180 thousand from a level of 413 thousand in 1990. The largest absolute increases are for those qualified in the social sciences however, with a rise of 250 thousand. The most rapid rates of increase are projected for postgraduates rather than those with first degrees.

The implications of these projections for NHS recruitment and retention depend, of course, on whether the demand for such persons from other employers will keep pace with this quite dramatic growth. This forms the main topic of discussion in Chapters 3 and 4.

Table 2.13
Total supply of persons with degrees

thousands

	1981	1990	2000
Postgraduates	189	540	791
First degree graduates	1,708	2,262	2,833
All graduates	1,898	2,802	3,624
or which:			
Education	326	391	458
Health	153	182	231
Technology	327	396	481
Agriculture	21	23	31
Science	259	413	595
Social Science	441	678	929
Vocational	79	100	135
Language	136	164	233
Arts (not elsewhere specified)	83	196	239
Music & other	72	258	291

Source: Wilson (1991).

3 The demand for skills from other employers

3.1 Macroeconomic scenario

The objective of this chapter is to set the general labour market scene against which future developments in the NHS need to be considered. In contrast to the previous chapter, it focuses on the demand side of the picture. The chapter draws very heavily on the *Review of the Economy and Employment, 1991, Occupational Assessment*, IER (1991). This provides a detailed assessment of the changing occupational structure of employment in the UK economy, with projections up to the year 2000.

At the time of writing, the main preoccupation of macroeconomic pundits was the recession of 1990/91, which had been deeper and more sustained than was orginally anticipated. The time scale for the recovery from the 1990/91 recession remains uncertain but the economy is expected to be back on its long-term growth path by the early to mid 1990s. However, the very rapid rate of growth in GDP achieved during the late 1980s is not expected to be repeated over the medium term. Nevertheless, performance is expected to compare quite favourably with that during the 1970s and early 1980s, with the economy settling down to a modest rate of growth of around 2 per cent per annum. This is still a relatively rapid rate of growth (at least in historical terms), which is likely to maintain inflationary pressures. Over the period to the year 2000, price inflation is projected to average around 4 per cent per annum. Earnings are expected to grow more rapidly, reflecting continuing improvements in productivity. As a consequence, real incomes are expected to grow steadily by some 2¼ per cent per annum over the period. The latter is primarily responsible for the continued growth in consumers' expenditure, which, together with gross fixed capital formation, provides the main source of growth in domestic demand. In the medium term the central problem will remain the balance of payments and the need to compete in world markets.

Productivity growth is expected to slow significantly in most sectors compared with the very large gains observed during the 1980s. The rates of increase observed in the mid 1980s are not expected to be repeated over the medium term, although some improvement in the long-term trend rate of growth is expected compared with the 1970s, reflecting changed attitudes, improved working practices and continuing technological, institutional and organizational changes.

3.2 Labour demand by sector

Although the early 1990s has seen a sharp decline in employment, the prospects for the medium term are for substantial increases. In total, 0.73 million more jobs are projected by the turn of the century (compared with 1990). The industrial structure of employment is expected to continue to alter in favour of the service sector and away from primary and manufacturing industries. The fastest increases are projected for business and miscellaneous services which gain over 600 thousand jobs. (See Figure 3.1 for details.) The competition for labour from other employers is therefore likely to intensify over the decade.

It is important to note however that these projections focus upon the demand for labour. Restrictions from the supply side (e.g. the fall in the number of school leavers or regional imbalances) may mean that these demands cannot always be met and that skill shortages rather than increased employment could occur for high growth areas.

Primary industries and utilities are expected to lose a further 200 thousand jobs by the end of the century. This represents a continuation of long term downward trends in employment, in agriculture and coal mining in particular, coupled with continuing improvements in productivity in all these industries, resulting in reduced labour demand per unit of output.

The manufacturing sector is also expected to see further losses, albeit at a much slower rate than in the 1980s. About a million jobs are likely to disappear by the year 2000. While job losses in the early 1980s were attributable to falling demand for the sector's products, the job losses in the 1990s take place against a background of significant productivity improvements, with growing output but falling employment (although in the short term the falling demand for output will be a major factor). The best performance is expected in those industries which have invested heavily in the 1980s and where productivity growth is expected to maintain the competitive edge gained then. Even here job gains are expected to be minimal (e.g. motor vehicles). In other cases, such as mechanical engineering, motor vehicles, food, drink and tobacco and textiles and clothing, substantial job losses are likely, as foreign competition maintains

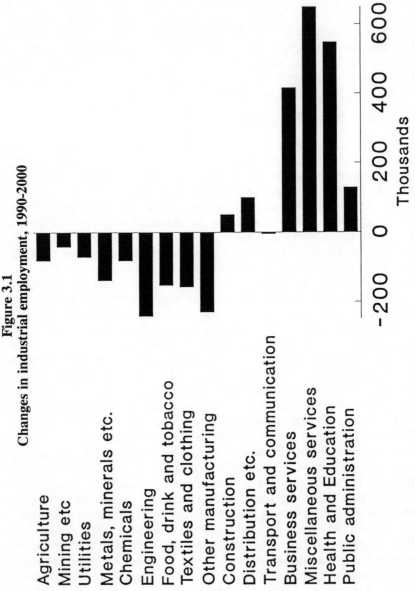

Figure 3.1
Changes in industrial employment, 1990-2000

Agriculture
Mining etc
Utilities
Metals, minerals etc.
Chemicals
Engineering
Food, drink and tobacco
Textiles and clothing
Other manufacturing
Construction
Distribution etc.
Transport and communication
Business services
Miscellaneous services
Health and Education
Public administration

-200   0   200   400   600
Thousands

Source: IER Review of the Economy and Employment, 1991: Occupational Assessment

pressure on UK market share, while continuing technological and organizational changes result in falling labour requirements.

Construction is expected to remain a relatively depressed area in the medium term as far as employment is concerned. The continuing difficulties in the housing market, together with the downturn in the pattern of demand for substantial infrastructure projects financed by both public and private sectors, are expected to lead to further job losses over the medium as well as the short-term. Regional imbalances are however likely to continue, with some shortages in, for example, the South East once the economy picks up.

Within the service sector, distribution and transport and communication are also expected to experience growth in employment over the medium term, reflecting increasing demand for such services from both consumers and producers. However, technological and organizational changes, such as computerisation of retail operations, larger store sizes etc., are likely to moderate the number of additional jobs created. Many of the new jobs will be part-time.

Business services (banking, insurance and other business services) are also expected to experience substantial increases in employment, although at less than half the rate that occurred during the 1980s. These sectors have been hard hit by the current recession and have cut back employment. This is expected to be reversed once the economy recovers. But the rates of growth are unlikely to match those of the 1980s. The continuing process of innovations in new products and services for both individuals and companies seems likely to maintain recent trends in output levels during the 1990s. However, the progress of information technology and increased levels of competition seem certain to result in these increases being achieved with a much smaller increase in labour demand than during the 1980s. This group of industries has in the past been a prime competitor to the NHS for young female labour market entrants.

The areas of really significant employment growth over the medium term are expected to be those service industries concerned with leisure and tourism, although again, these sectors may also experience problems in the short-run. Hotels and catering is expected to see substantial further growth in employment, although many of the projected 240 thousand additional jobs are likely to be part-time and rather poorly paid. Miscellaneous services, which includes a broad range of private and personal services is expected to see even more substantial growth, with more than half a million additional jobs by the year 2000. This sector includes private health and education services, which, if current government policy continues, also seem to be likely areas of employment growth. Many of these areas are of course in direct competition for labour with the NHS.

Finally, some medium-term increases in employment are expected amongst non-marketed services, which includes public health and education services as well as public administration and defence.

Figure 3.2
Changes in employment status, 1990-2000

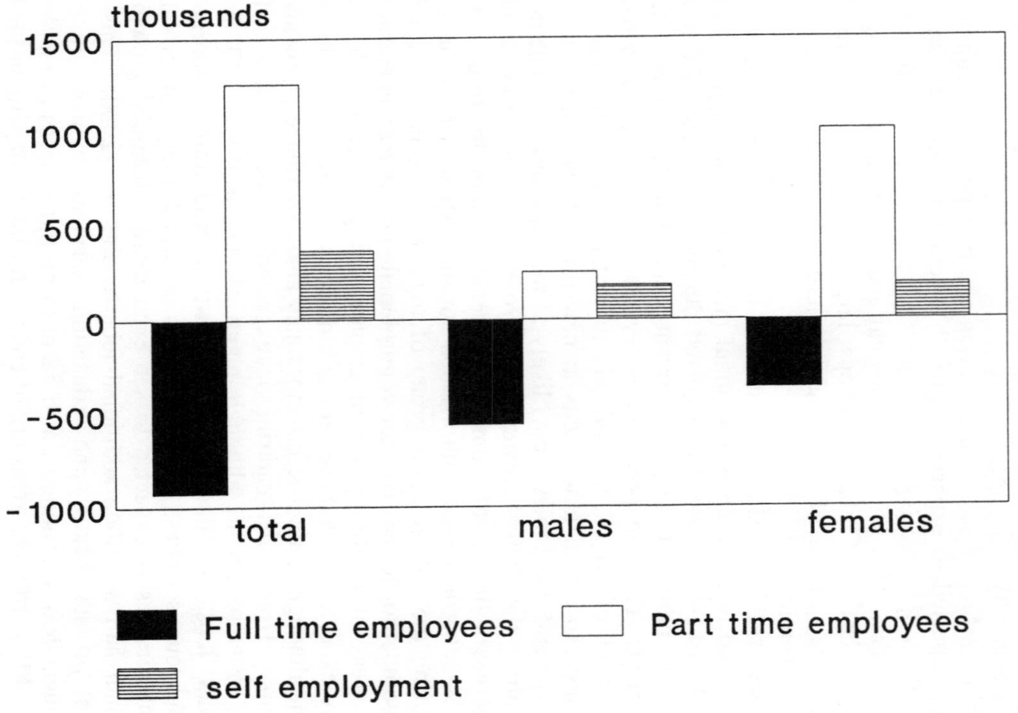
thousands
1500
1000
500
0
-500
-1000
total
males
females
Full time employees
Part time employees
self employment

Source: IER Review of the Economy and Employment, 1991: Occupational Assessment

The former, of course, includes the NHS. Government current expenditure on goods and services is expected to grow more in line with GDP during the mid to late 1990s than was the case during the 1980s. As a consequence, some 550 thousand additional jobs are expected by the end of the century. This is considerably faster growth than has been seen since 1975 but modest compared with the experience of the 1960s.

3.3 Changing patterns of employment status

The changing patterns of employment status expected are closely related to these developments in industrial structure. Self employment is projected to continue to increase its share of total employment, with a further rise of 370 between 1990 and 2000. Part-time employment is also expected to rise substantially (by over 1¼ million jobs). The number of full-time employees is projected to decline. Females are expected to be the main beneficiaries of these changes. They are expected to account for nearly all of the net increase in employment. Details are shown in Figure 3.2.

Self employment

In 1979 there were 2 million persons in self employment. This was little different from the corresponding figure 30 years earlier. During the 1950s self employment was concentrated heavily in distribution etc. (small retail establishments, restaurants and hotels) and agriculture with much smaller numbers in construction and business and miscellaneous services. By 1980 the numbers in agriculture had fallen substantially (reflecting the general decline in employment in this industry). Numbers in distribution etc. had also fallen. In contrast, the construction industry and various service sector industries had experienced substantial growth.

Over the next 10 years much more dramatic changes occurred. During the 1980s over a million persons have been added to this category, which now accounts for almost 12 per cent of total employment. The composition of the total has also changed dramatically. Self employment in construction continued to grow very rapidly, mainly at the expense of employees. Agriculture and distribution etc. also saw a reversal of previous declines. There was however, a much sharper rise in most other sectors, including manufacturing. The largest absolute increase occurred amongst business and miscellaneous services.

The causes of these developments have been the subject of considerable research. In part the changes observed can be regarded as simply reflecting the changing industrial structure of employment and the growth of demand for services among both businesses and final consumers. Such services are often provided in very competitive markets and this has tended to favour small enterprises. These structural changes have been reinforced by the continuing process of specialisation, which has been associated with the subcontracting of many tasks previously carried out 'in house' to other businesses or to individuals. This has encompassed a

47

broad range of services from catering and cleaning through to many specialist business and professional services. The worker may gain independence and a chance to earn more in self employment, while the firm gains in terms of enhanced flexibility and reduced costs. In terms of preferred options for maximising flexibility however, most firms emphasise the use of permanent part-time workers and temporary workers.

Some have attributed the recent growth of self employment to an entrepreneurial revolution associated with the current government's policy of encouraging enterprise, including the introduction of schemes such as EAS. Others have argued that self employment represents a reaction to high levels of unemployment. However, the link between the two is far from clear cut. Undoubtedly the factors behind the recent trends are quite complex and the relative importance of these, and various other influences, has varied for different industries and for different time periods. From the point of view of NHS recruitment and retention, the most important aspect is the tendency of individuals to want to have more control over their own working lives. This is a point to which we return in greater detail in Chapter 5.

In total, IER is projecting a further increase of about 370 thousand self employed by the turn of the century. The share of self employment is projected to rise in all parts of the economy. The most substantial increases are expected to occur in the service sector, with miscellaneous services exhibiting the fastest rate of growth and the largest absolute increase of 150 thousand. The largest increase outside the service sector is expected in construction where the rise of almost 130 thousand contrasts with the modest 50 thousand increase in total employment projected in that industry between 1990 and 2000.

Part-time working

Simultaneous with the shift towards self employment has been the move towards a greater proportion of part-time working, with more than one in five of today's workforce in part-time employment. The 1980s saw a substantial loss of both male and female full-time jobs; female part-time jobs, on the other hand, grew by over 600,000, equivalent to the loss of male jobs. The majority of these jobs were in the service sector: non-marketed services, business and miscellaneous services and distribution and transport. All these sectors had around 30 per cent of their total employment as part-time by 1990. Together, these three sectors account for over 90 per cent of all part-time employment. In contrast, part-time employment in manufacturing started to decline recently.

The trends in part-time working have also been the subject of much recent research. Part-time working has been found to be greatest where the demand for a company's product or service fluctuates and a female labour supply is preferred. Examples include hotels and catering. Research has shown that, in some industries, employers look to reduce labour costs by ensuring that part-time earnings fall below the lower earnings limit at which the employer starts to pay tax. Evidence from case study work has linked these changes to the decline of semi-skilled assembly workers in the electrical engineering industry and the increase in waiting, servicing and cleaning staff in the hotels and catering industry. That is, changes in industrial and occupational structure have affected the extent of part-time working.

Such demand side influences have been reinforced by pressures from the supply side. Recent Labour Force Survey evidence indicates that two-thirds of females took part-time work because they 'didn't want a full-time job'. When the category 'part-time workers' is examined, one finds it comprises married women with young children, young people in higher education or older workers. Their inferior pay and conditions, however, have led researchers to conclude that the women prepared to accept such conditions are mostly those returning to work after beginning the family formation stage of their life (i.e. when they are willing to substitute the salary and fringe benefits of a full-time job for a lower workload and convenient hours).

The proportion of part-time employment for males and females has increased in most sectors of the economy in the last few years. The IER projections are for a continuation of the trend towards a greater share of part-time employment in total employment, rising to over one quarter by 2000. Part-time employees are expected to more than account for the three quarters of a million increase in employment projected between 1990 and 2000. This growth reflects a combination of both changing industrial structure in favour of those sectors which employ large proportions of part-timers as well as rising shares of part-time employment within most sectors.

It is probably the supply side of the picture that is most relevant from the point of view of NHS recruitment and retention. The trends towards shorter hours are in fact more general than just a move towards a greater proportion of part-time jobs. Shorter working weeks, longer holidays and earlier retirement are other important aspects. Much of the fruit of economic growth has in fact been consumed as greater leisure time rather than in the form of more goods. Again, these issues are discussed in greater detail in Chapter 5.

Pool of female workers

Changes in the industrial structure of employment, away from the primary and manufacturing sectors towards services, has especially benefited females. The same factors, in conjunction with changes in working practices towards more flexibility and in particular the greater use of part-time working, have also tended to favour the employment of women. This reflects the greater willingness of women to work part-time. The increase in female labour market participation, especially amongst those aged 25-54, has facilitated the changing patterns of labour demand. These trends are expected to continue as an increasing proportion of females seek to

49

combine formal employment in the labour market with duties connected with family formation and childcare.

Females have accounted for the bulk of the increases in employment observed during the 1980s. Between 1981 and 1990 women took over two thirds of the net increase in employment. More than three quarters of women in 1990 were employed in service industries; females account for approximately half of total employment in non-marketed services, business and miscellaneous services and distribution and transport. These three sectors contain the largest numbers and proportions of female workers. Manufacturing and construction still contain relatively few women. However, all industries have seen a rise in the female share of total employment in the last decade. Female employment is projected to account for the bulk of the three quarters of a million new jobs forecast by 2000. Women are expected to benefit disproportionately from the tightening labour market for young new entrants. Females in the 25-54 age group, especially women-returners, will provide employers with the greatest potential for meeting their additional demands in the next decade, given their still relatively low activity rates. Success in this will depend on factors such as the level of retraining, child care provision, career break schemes and flexible hours for women in the workplace in the future.

The changes in industrial structure and work patterns that are expected to favour the employment of females are facilitated by developments on the supply side, outlined in Chapters 2 and 6 which mean that the numbers of 'prime age' females entering the labour force is expected to grow steadily. This will in fact more than offset the much publicised decline in the numbers of young entrants. In total the labour force is projected to have grown by around 700 thousand by the turn of the century. Most of the net additions will be women between the ages 25-54. The growth in labour supply of both men and women over the medium term means that, despite the increased demand for labour, total unemployment will rise modestly from 1990 levels.

3.4 The pattern of demand for skills

The pattern of demand for skills has altered dramatically over the last 20 years and further substantial changes are expected by the turn of the century. Between 1971 and 1981 civilian employment declined by 150 thousand. This decline was not evenly spread across all occupations. The fastest rate of decline was for plant and machine operatives. Over 700 thousand jobs disappeared for this group. Craft and skilled manual occupations lost almost 600 thousand jobs while other occupations (primarily unskilled labourers) lost about 350 thousand. In contrast there was very rapid growth in employment opportunities for professional (including doctors) and associate professional occupations (which includes nurses). The former experienced an increase in employment of almost 500 thousand and the latter an increase of about 300 thousand. Managers and

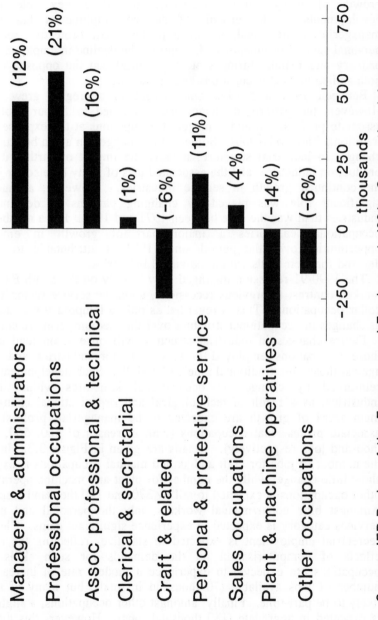

Figure 3.3
Changes in occupational employment, 1990-2000

Managers & administrators (12%)
Professional occupations (21%)
Assoc professional & technical (16%)
Clerical & secretarial (1%)
Craft & related (-6%)
Personal & protective service (11%)
Sales occupations (4%)
Plant & machine operatives (-14%)
Other occupations (-6%)

-250   0   250   500   750
thousands

Source: IER Review of the Economy and Employment, 1991: Occupational Assessment

administrators and personal and protective service occupations also experienced substantial growth.

It is clear from detailed analysis that an important part of this change can be attributed to changes in industrial structure. In particular the decline in the UK manufacturing sector in 1980 and 1981 and the steady growth of many service industries played a key role in these developments. The growth of service employment has benefited managerial, professional, associate professional, protective service and personal service occupations. In contrast the decline in employment in the primary and manufacturing sectors has produced the opposite effect for both skilled manual occupations and operatives.

Between 1981 and 1990 employment in aggregate grew strongly. However, the pattern of change has continued to favour professional, associate professional and managerial occupations at the expense of more traditional blue collar jobs. Some of this change can again be attributed to changes in industrial structure, notably the impact of further decline in production industries (and the associated loss of many blue collar jobs) and the continued growth in service industries. However, a much more significant role was played by changing patterns of demand within industries than was the case between 1971 and 1981. For a number of key occupational categories a major part of growth in employment opportunities over the period since 1981 is attributable to increased demand for their skills within individual industries.

The 1990/91 recession impinged very heavily on the South East and, in marked contrast to previous recessions, upon the service sector and white collar occupations. This is regarded as only a temporary set back, as far as changes in occupational structure over the medium-term are concerned.

Future changes in industrial structure will once again tend to favour those occupations employed in service sector industries and to work against those with traditional blue collar skills. Such developments will be reinforced by changes in occupational structures within individual industries, as a result of technological and organizational change. The main areas of growth are expected to be managerial, professional and associate professional occupations (with increases of 460, 560, and 340 thousand jobs respectively). Details are given in Figure 3.3. In contrast the number of jobs for craft and skilled manual occupations is expected to show little change, while the number for plant and machine operatives and other occupations is expected to fall by 370 and 180 thousand respectively. Amongst blue collar/manual workers only the personal and protective services category is expected to experience significant gains. Clerical and secretarial employment is expected to stabilize, reflecting the continued effects of computerisation on the demands for such skills. Sales occupations are expected to experience a modest rate of increase in the number of jobs available (70 thousand in total), but many of these are likely to be part-time. Finally, amongst other occupations, a slight decline is expected in aggregate (180 thousand jobs). However, this disguises a continuing shift away from male, full-time jobs in primary and manufacturing industries towards female part-time workers, employed in services (mainly as cleaners and domestics).

3.5 The demand for qualifications

Another major change to highlight is the very rapid growth in the proportion of those holding qualifications. Between 1979 and 1989 the numbers holding no formal qualifications fell in every occupational group, while the numbers with some form of qualification (ranging from CSEs to higher degrees) rose substantially. The reasons for these changes are manifold. In many cases it is argued that it reflects changing demand patterns which are leading to increasingly complex jobs, which require considerable amounts of formal education and training. It is also argued however that in other cases this phenomenon may represent 'qualification inflation' as an over supply has resulted in people competing for jobs by bidding up entry requirements. This trend seems likely to be reversed if labour markets for young new entrants tighten as the 1990s unfold.

Some evidence in support of both phenomena is found in the information on movements in pay differentials. The results suggest that while professional and other more highly qualified occupations have benefited from increasing demand, reversing the previous long-term decline in relative pay, groups at the opposite end of the occupational spectrum have lost ground relative to the all worker average in recent years, despite becoming increasingly well qualified. Thus, for professional people, the increasing proportion holding qualifications may reflect a real increase in the demand for more qualifications, while for those at the lower end of the occupational spectrum, the same change may reflect qualifications inflation.

Highly qualified persons include all individuals who hold a specific degree or an equivalent professional qualification. The term is often also used to include non-graduate level qualifications which are rated above 'A' levels including HNC, HND and nursing qualifications. Many such individuals work in professional occupations although an increasing number can also be found in the managerial and associate professional groups. The labour markets for highly qualified persons have a number of special features. Long periods of investment in human capital are required which give rise to major private and social outlays and cause important lags in supply. Education and training at this level tends to be concentrated amongst younger individuals, although there is an increasing proportion of mature graduates. Associated labour markets are frequently national (rather than local) and sometimes international. Qualified individuals tend to work in activities involving high levels of technical and/or organizational skills, often associated with the dynamic performance of the economy. However, not all individuals with a degree (or equivalent) make direct use of the level or type of qualification which they hold, and not all managerial and professional jobs are undertaken by highly qualified persons.

The NHS demand for labour in the 1990s is likely to focus quite heavily on the more highly qualified. Comparing the health service with other industries the proportion of higher level occupations is much greater. The IER's data base indicates that just under 14 per cent of NHS staff fall into the 'professional' category (excluding management), while the associate professional group (which includes all nurses) accounts for over 40 per cent. These shares compare with the situation for all industries and services other than health services where some 9 per cent fall into the professional category and only 6 per cent into the associate professional group.

The demand for highly qualified persons in most discipline areas was severely affected by the recession of 1980/81. The number of graduates, whose first destination on graduating was employment, fell between 1979 and 1981, with sharp increases in graduate unemployment. Nevertheless, the graduate labour market was by no means so badly hit as those associated with lower levels of formal educational qualifications, such as craft skills. Some disciplines experienced a relatively buoyant market despite the recession, particularly those linked with the new technologies, such as microelectronics. Others have benefited as the economy has grown in the 1980s and as special projects, such as the Channel Tunnel, have been commissioned. There have been significant regional disparities in both the level and rate of recovery of activity. The strength of demand has been greatest in the South East.

The period of persistent growth since the 1981 recession has resulted in marked increases in recruitment levels. First destination statistics show that, during the 1980s, recruitment increased steadily in banking and insurance, law and other commerce, although over this period as a whole, recruitment fell in engineering and teacher training. Teacher training has been influenced by reductions in government spending, linked with the demographic trends outlined above. The current recession is likely to result in at least a temporary slowdown in graduate recruitment by many companies. But this is expected to soon be reversed.

It is important to distinguish between the labour market for **newly** qualified graduates (or other equivalently qualified new entrants to the labour market) and the labour market for highly qualified persons generally who have been in the labour market for, in some cases, many years. The former is a much more open and external market than the latter, which tends to depend very much more on internal developments within employing organizations. The supply of and demand for newly qualified persons operates on the margin of the more general labour market for qualified persons. It is concerned primarily with the flows of new entrants rather than the total stock of both past and present entrants. This market is much more volatile than that for all qualified persons. Fluctuations in the latter tend to be amplified in terms of the impact on the balance of supply and demand for newly qualified persons. Research conducted within the IER (partly in collaboration with the Policy Studies Institute (PSI)), focused on both aspects.

The results of a large telephone survey of employers by Rigg, *et al.* (1990) suggested that, although there were some problems of graduate shortages in 1988, these were not a major problem for most employers. Most employers appeared to be anticipating a continued trend towards the use of graduates in jobs previously undertaken by non-graduates. This, together with general expansion of activity levels over the medium term, particularly amongst smaller firms, meant that very substantial growth in demand was expected over the medium term although such expansion has clearly been, at least temporarily, postponed as a result of the recession. In total, an increase of 30 per cent in the demand for new graduates between 1988 and 1992 seemed possible. This was of course before the depth of the current recession became apparent.

The demographic downturn, discussed in Chapter 2, was anticipated by many employers to have a significant impact on graduate availability. Indeed many believed that this would be exacerbated by negative effects on the proportion of young people deciding to go on into higher education. These will arise due to the introduction of student loans and the possible increase in relative pay, as a result of intensified competition by employers, for those who do not stay on in school beyond the minimum school leaving age. Quite severe problems in recruitment were therefore expected by many employers, particularly for those disciplines already in short supply.

These results were confirmed in the more intensive inquiry reported in Elias *et al.* (1990) This provided further evidence of current shortages, especially in science and engineering disciplines. Again, substantial increases in demand were expected in the medium-term, a period when the level of graduate output was likely to be flattening out. General growth in demand for graduate level labour, as well as the need to upgrade management cadres were emphasised as the underlying causes of increased demand.

The deep recession of 1990/91 has, temporarily at least, caused these influences to moderate. Depressed demand conditions have meant that most employers have had few problems in recruitment over this period. However, the basic arithmetic of long-term decline in numbers available because of demographic change, coupled with long-term growth in demand for qualified personnel, means that the problems of serious labour shortages merely lie dormant rather than having been cured. Taking a longer-term view therefore suggests that the difficulties of the late 1980s could soon be repeated once the economy does recover from recession.

Examination of the medium-term prospects, suggest substantial increases in demand for **newly** qualified graduates, and for highly qualified persons generally (Wilson *et al.*, 1990; and Wilson, 1991). This work examines the implications of the general labour market assessment outlined

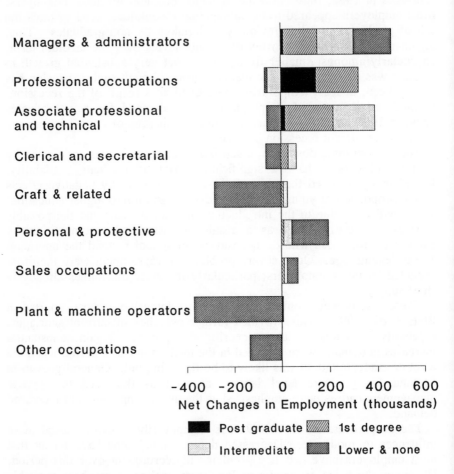

Figure 3.4
Changes in qualification held by occupation, 1990-2000

Managers & administrators

Professional occupations

Associate professional
and technical

Clerical and secretarial

Craft & related

Personal & protective

Sales occupations

Plant & machine operators

Other occupations

-400 -200   0   200   400   600
Net Changes in Employment (thousands)

■ Post graduate ▨ 1st degree
□ Intermediate ▨ Lower & none

Source : Wilson (1991)

in Section 3.4 for the demand for persons of all ages with different higher qualifications. The results are summarised in Table 3.1 and Figure 3.4. In total, an increase of over a million is projected in the demand for all graduates. The demand for post-graduates is expected to grow by almost 170 thousand and that for first degree graduates by over 800 thousand. Although substantial growth is projected for the demand for those qualified in science, engineering and technology, the growth is most rapid for those with social science qualifications (most notably business and related studies). The implications for the balance between supply and demand is considered in Chapter 4.

Table 3.1
Demand for graduates by subject

thousands

	1971	1981	1990	2000
Postgraduates	92	186	340	315
First degree graduates	951	1,613	2,281	3,150
All graduates	1,043	1,799	2,622	3,663
of which:				
Education	26	316	422	473
Health	125	148	178	212
Technology	247	313	367	520
Agriculture	14	20	26	40
Science	160	247	350	532
Social science	238	422	607	964
Vocational	44	66	88	124
Language	99	120	135	213
Arts (not elsewhere specified)	52	76	176	252
Music & other	37	71	273	334

Source: Wilson *et al.* (1990).

4 The balance of labour supply and demand in the 1990s

The discussion in Chapters 2 and 3 has outlined likely developments in labour supply and demand, both for new entrants to the labour market and in more general terms. This chapter assesses the likely balance between supply and demand for different skills and different types of qualified person. It considers the labour market as a whole, rather than focusing on the NHS in particular, but any significant implications for the health service are highlighted as appropriate. The chapter begins with the prospect for the labour market generally and the likelihood of skill shortages for particular occupations. The emphasis is on the medium-term prospects beyond the next year or two rather than the effects of the 1990/91 recession. The discussion then turns to the labour market for the highly qualified. Consideration is given to the impact of the completion of the internal market in Europe. Finally, the reactions of other employers to skill shortages are discussed.

4.1 The prospects for skills

The forecasts of demand for skills outlined in Section 3.4 are based upon applying projections of occupational employment shares within industries to projected industrial employment levels produced using a detailed multisectoral macroeconomic model. Past values of these coefficients are obviously the outcome of both supply and demand influences on employment structure. However, assuming employers have not been unduly constrained from the supply side, (and this does not seem an unreasonable assumption given the generally high levels of unemployment in the 1970s and 1980s) these coefficients can probably be regarded as primarily reflecting changing demand patterns.

There is regrettably little corresponding information which can currently be drawn upon to reflect the supply side of the picture. However, some tentative conclusions can still be drawn on the basis of the *ad hoc* information that is currently available. The key points identified for each of the main occupational groups regarded as being of relevance in terms of NHS recruitment and retention are summarised in the remaining discussion in this section. Occupations are defined according to the new Standard Occupational Classification, (OPCS, 1990).

In the case of managers and administrators, it seems likely that the demand for 'high fliers' will continue to grow over the medium term and that some shortages may arise, especially for corporate managers and administrators. The possibility of declining numbers of graduates caused by demographic changes, coupled with the general growth in demand for such personnel, seems likely to cause a number of recruitment problems. About 5 per cent of health service employment falls into this occupational category compared to 7½ per cent for the economy generally (belying the oft quoted criticism about the growth of bureaucracy!)

Amongst the professional occupations, demand is also expected to grow substantially over the medium term. All groups other than health professionals are expected to see employment grow by more than 1½ per cent per annum. The projection for health professionals is based on government plans for expenditure on health services. The projected growth in demand for professionals is in contrast to the supply side, where the prospective decline in the flow of new graduates promises a sharp tightening of the labour market in many cases. The most likely areas where shortages will be a problem are those such as electronic engineering, business studies and economics and computing which are already facing severe difficulties. Because of the general tightening of the labour market for graduates, even those areas where smaller increases in demand are anticipated may experience problems, especially if relative pay levels are such that young entrants are not attracted into the profession. This could, for example, cause acute difficulties in some teaching professions. There are already problems in finding secondary teachers in subjects such as languages, mathematics, etc., while universities are finding it increasingly difficult to recruit and retain top quality personnel for many scientific and business related disciplines. Given the influence of the Review Body on Doctors Remuneration it seems unlikely that the NHS will face such severe problems in recruiting sufficient doctors.

The situation for associate professional and technical occupations is in many ways similar to that for professionals. Demand is projected to rise while the number of new entrants is likely to fall sharply. In this context it is likely that recruitment and retention problems will increase, especially in those areas where employers have failed to properly address problems of declining relative pay and conditions of employment. At the present time there are high rates of turnover in many occupations, notably nursing, particularly in the more buoyant local labour markets. With the onset of a demographic downturn in numbers of young people, more attention will have to be devoted to considering new recruitment channels. Greater emphasis on computing skills is likely to be a feature across a wide range of occupations, and particularly in the more specialist occupations there may be growing pressures, including some parts of nursing, to concede professional status. The general demand for persons with intermediate and higher level qualifications seems likely to place increasing pressure on the NHS, which has traditionally accounted for a very large proportion of such persons, especially females qualified at intermediate level.

Skill shortages seem unlikely to be very important over the medium term amongst clerical and secretarial occupations generally. The overall numbers are expected to grow slightly but it seems likely that increases in the supply of labour, particularly by women wanting part-time work, will at least keep pace with demand. Again, the health service share of employment in such categories is below average at 14 per cent (compared with 17 per cent for the economy generally). Sales occupations as a whole also seem unlikely to face significant shortages. Demand is only expected to grow slightly and will mainly affect part-time females. The health service employs insignificant numbers of people in such categories at present.

Amongst craft and skilled manual occupations employment has been in decline for many years, yet apparently shortages still persist. This seems to reflect the failure to train sufficient numbers of new entrants into such occupations, together with the loss of skilled persons as they have been attracted to other jobs as a result of falling relative pay. It is likely that recruitment problems and skill shortages encountered currently will increase. The NHS only employs a relatively small number of such personnel, however, so it is unlikely to prove an area of major concern, assuming some flexibility in wage structures is allowed.

Demand for personal and protective service occupations is expected to continue to rise during the 1990s especially for females in personal service occupations. Given the anticipated growth in female labour supply, employers are not however expected to face serious problems in meeting their labour requirements. There may be particular problems for employers trying to maintain, or even raise, entry standards of new entrants (as measured by the possession of formal qualifications). This seems more likely to be a problem for protective service occupations than for personal service occupations. The NHS accounts for around 200 thousand of the 1½ million persons in these occupations (primarily at the 'personal' service end of the spectrum). Its main competitors in this area are in distribution, hotels and catering and miscellaneous services.

The only other group which is significant for the health service is 'other occupations'. This group comprises 'other occupations in agriculture' (mainly farm workers) and 'other occupations excluding agriculture' (which includes labourers and cleaners working in all other industries). The NHS employment falls into the last category (cleaners and porters). Few problems are anticipated in this area.

4.2 Labour market issues in the 1990s

The earlier discussion has already hinted at a number of important developments that will affect the future market for more highly qualified persons:

· the demographic downturn
· changes in the system of student grants and loans
· the general economic climate
· the level of commitment to dynamic activities, such as R&D
· continued technological change and the emergence of new and largely unknown technologies
· continued organizational change
· changes in the nature of graduate recruitment
· the effects of movement to the single European market in 1992.

As argued in Chapter 2 the demographic downturn will have significant effects on the numbers flowing through higher education, even though the decline is somewhat less for social classes I and II, from which new entrants have usually been drawn. The effects will be further cushioned by the efforts of higher education institutions to spread their net more widely, continuing to attract more mature students. The impact of the demographic downturn on higher education will also be reduced by increased participation rates.

On the demand side, the economy is forecast to continue to grow over the medium-term (once the current recession is past), albeit at a somewhat slower pace than that observed in the middle and late 1980s. However, the medium term rate of productivity growth will be high, at least by the standards of the 1970s (although not as high as during the 1980s). This will affect the number of job opportunities for graduates, particularly in the manufacturing sector. Demand for both management and associate professional occupations are also forecast to be very buoyant, the latter perhaps more so than the professional group. Entry to these occupations is not limited to persons with degrees, and this may attract potential students away from higher education. Certain dynamic activities, such as investment in physical plant and machinery recovered strongly during the 1980s, increasing the demand for highly qualified persons to install and operate the new units. Other activities, such as R&D also recovered during the 1980s, but not strongly, and here, UK performance is well down on many of our major industrial competitors. A major growth of R&D would produce a significant boost in the demand for science and engineering specialisms, which might well accentuate the skill shortages which are already apparent.

Table 4.1
Balance of supply-demand for persons with a degree

thousands

	1981	1990	2000
Postgraduates	3	200	278
First degree graduates	95	-19	-317
All graduates	98	180	-39
of which:			
Education	10	-31	-14
Health	5	4	19
Technology	14	29	-39
Agriculture	1	-3	-9
Science	12	63	63
Social Science	20	71	-35
Vocational	13	12	11
Language	16	30	20
Arts (not elsewhere specified)	7	20	-13
Music & other	1	-15	-43

Source: Wilson (1991)

Note: A negative sign indicates excess demand

Recruitment and utilisation policies seem likely to be increasingly re-evaluated if as expected, once the present recession is over, skill shortages reappear. Employers will be attempting to ensure that jobs are designed which fully exploit the skills of qualified persons, leaving less demanding tasks to other, less qualified members of their workforce. Recruitment is becoming more targetted, linked more closely to firm goals and objectives. Older style practices of recruiting staff 'in their own image' will come under increasing pressure and the recruitment net will be spread wider. The ease of substitution between graduates and non-graduates, the growth of credentialism and the barriers created by professional institutes will also come under increasing scrutiny.

As noted in the next section, the movement to a single market appears to make Europe a potential source of graduates during periods of increasing shortage. In practice, the more advanced European countries have similar demographic trends to our own. The likelihood that they might be an alternative source of graduates is further reduced by their longer periods of investment in higher education and by their relatively high salary levels for graduates (as the UK has slipped down the international ranking of industrial countries). If anything these factors appear to suggest that the balance of flows might prove to be in the other direction. These issues are discussed in more detail in the next sub-section.

All of these factors appear to indicate that the kind of shortages experienced in the 1980s could reappear over the medium term. This will pose very real problems for many employers (including the NHS), as well as those concerned with the provision of education and training in order to ensure that Britain has the skilled people that will be needed for future prosperity.

The analysis by Wilson *et al.* (1990) and Wilson (1991) confirms that the balance between demand and supply for more qualified people is likely to tighten rather than weaken over the medium term. This is illustrated in Table 4.1. However, the main problem areas are likely to be in non-scientific disciplines, such as business studies rather than those disciplines particular to health services.

As noted in Chapters 1 and 13, there is a tendency amongst some personnel managers within the NHS to regard the, so called, demographic timebomb as something of a damp squib. There is a danger however that the bomb has not been defused but remains ticking. The depth of the 1990/91 recession, combined with a change in the pattern of recruitment away from the traditional young, female, school leaver have meant that thus far the NHS has not faced major recruitment difficulties. This picture could alter very quickly (if and) when the economy does recover.

4.3 1992 and the completion of the internal market

The completion of the European internal market will have effects on both the demand and supply situation in the labour market. From the demand side, the restructuring of economic activity that may follow from the completion of the market, the possible positive impact on overall demand, and the reorientation of demand for labour (for example towards greater emphasis on languages) may all have an effect on the domestic labour market. Competition for UK graduates and other qualified persons from mainland employers may also accentuate any domestic pressures in UK labour markets.

On the supply side, the opening up of the labour market may lead some individuals to migrate to the continent to a much greater degree than has happened in the past. This of course may be offset by continental Europeans who want to work in the UK. It seems likely that professional labour markets, which already operate at a national level, will tend to expand across national borders. Disparities in pay and terms and conditions of employment in the member countries of the EEC, can in the long term, be expected to be gradually eroded. This will mean that all employers, including the NHS, will need, increasingly, to consider not just domestic but also international competitors for their staff.

The mobility of individuals, such as health service staff between countries depends on relative costs and benefits (pecuniary and other); growth in new job opportunities in different countries; language barriers and differences in language abilities; restrictions relating to the recognition of qualifications; and finally demographic considerations.

Examples of the effects of relative wages on the movement of individuals between the UK and the USA have been relatively well documented. Similar effects may emerge between EEC countries after 1992. The UK now has one of the lowest incomes per head of the main European countries and there is some evidence that medical staff are relatively poorly paid, suggesting that the direction of UK net migration will be outwards.

Job opportunities may be as important as relative wages. A recent example has been the small number of newly qualified teachers leaving West Germany (where there is a surplus of such people) to find posts in the UK where there are specific skill shortages (particularly in science and mathematics). In the main, however, it seems likely that countries with more rapid growth, other things being equal (i.e. labour force growth and productivity growth), will have more new job opportunities.

The UK has been notorious for its lack of emphasis on languages. This suggests that many of our European neighbours may be better equipped to compete in the UK than UK citizens are able to compete abroad (although from the point of view of recruitment or retention, this could be a blessing in disguise). English is often studied as the primary second language in other countries. However, things may have improved somewhat in the UK in recent years. The EC LINGUA programme which began in 1990, was aimed at promoting language training for members of the professions, so any advantage the language barrier may provide to mobility could be shortlived.

The ease of flow between countries will be increased by the removal of restriction on the recognition of professional qualifications. The general Directive on professional qualifications, which has been agreed by Ministers, will enable fully qualified professionals in one Member State to practise in another EEC country without the need to requalify.

The mobility of individuals is influenced strongly by age. It seems fairly clear from the demographic trends that the decline in the size of the youth cohort and the general ageing of the population will reduce UK outflows. However, this is also true of a number of other European countries, and some, such as West Germany, have even stronger trends towards older populations. Often less well developed EEC countries are not experiencing such dramatic changes and may, therefore, exhibit higher outflows.

The results reported by Elias et al. (1990), in research conducted as part of an Interdepartmental Review of the labour market for the highly qualified (DES, 1990), suggest that although many employers did not expect '1992' to have much impact, a roughly similar proportion (one-third) thought it would cause difficulty for both supply and demand reasons (as outlined above). About 20 per cent of the sample felt unable to answer such questions. Those in the service sector were more concerned about the effects of 1992 on recruitment. The study concludes that in many respects the UK graduate labour market is more predictable, homogeneous and open than those in European countries. For example, direct recruitment on the campus, often organized by careers advisors in the UK, is in many cases banned in Europe. Personal and local contacts are often much more important on the continent. This may make it easier for foreign employers to recruit UK personnel than *vice versa*. However, as noted above, this may be offset to some extent by the greater propensity of those in Europe to speak English than for those in the UK to speak other languages (the obvious exception here being Ireland).

As noted in earlier discussion, the demographic downturn is even more dramatic in some mainland countries than in the UK. On the demand side, although there are serious problems of comparability, studies such as Lindley (1987) and Wilson and Bosworth (1987) suggest that there is a convergence in demand trends (in terms of changing industrial and occupational employment structures). These changes have been discussed in detail for the UK in Chapter 3. They imply a growing requirement for highly educated personnel to sustain future economic prosperity.

The increasing internationalisation of both business activity and labour markets seems likely to continue. Migration from the UK has already increased sharply (IMS, 1989 p. 38). From a small imbalance in 1976 (an outflow of 5,700 compared with an inflow of 4,100 managerial/professional people), the situation changed in 1986 to a major net loss (an inflow of 5,200 dwarfed by an outflow of 17,700). Nevertheless, despite these changes, migration remains a relatively small factor in the context of projected annual growth in demand for all managerial and professional occupations of over 80 thousand per annum (IER, 1991). However, the effects of '1992' are unlikely to ease problems of recruitment and retention for UK employers, including the NHS, over the medium term.

4.4   Reaction of other employers to expected shortages

The scenario outlined above is one of a significant decline in the number of well qualified new entrants to the labour market and rising demand for such people, coupled with a general trend towards increased requirements for well qualified persons of all ages, as a consequence of continuing technological, organizational and structural change within the economy. This section addresses the reactions of those employers outside the NHS who are anticipating serious shortages over the medium term.

Atkinson (1989) has analysed the possible response to shortages in terms of measures designed to influence supply and those aimed at altering demand. We can also distinguish tactical from strategic policies. In the first instance employers may react rather passively, allowing hiring standards or activity levels to fall or overtime working to increase, etc.

The second round of responses may still be tactical rather than strategic, but aimed at improving recruitment by intensifying effort in this area. Such policies could include improving liaison with educational establishments, improving the image of the organization, competing more aggressively by raising pay, etc. Such initiatives are essentially aimed at influencing the supply of labour to the organization. Some authors, including Atkinson, appear to regard the pay option as self-defeating. Barring dramatic changes in migration, the overall numbers of young people are of course basically fixed. In raising pay, employers will only bid up the price of labour and increase their labour costs. However, this price rise is a crucial part of the adjustment process. The increase in wage costs effectively rations out the limited supply to those that value it most highly. It also signals to prospective entrants the benefits of undertaking certain courses of education or training.

The third phase of response is a more strategic one. This also concentrates upon the supply side of the equation, exploring new sources of supply such as mature females, older workers, those currently unemployed, etc. It also concentrates on the factors influencing retention/wastage rates and attempts to improve them from the organization's viewpoint.

The surveys, conducted as part of the Interdepartmental Review, suggest that employers who were aware of the forthcoming problems, were planning to adopt a number of different strategies and tactics in order to attempt to avoid or overcome problems. These included reorientating recruitment towards groups which were likely to be more readily available, such as mature or experienced persons (e.g. postponing retirement), women and ethnic minorities. The results in Chapter 2 have highlighted the potential that such groups may offer. These groups may of course be targeted by many employers and so, although it may be easier to find such people than the traditional young female recruit, employers are still likely to face a seller's market, especially for the above average candidates.

The final phase continues the more strategic theme, but concentrates more on the demand side. Improvements in internal labour market deployment, and mobility, training and retraining are the key elements here.

Training of existing staff is another avenue stressed in responses to both the telephone survey (Rigg et al., 1990) and the more intensive survey (Elias et al., 1990) conducted as part of the Interdepartmental Review. This offers the joint advantage of raising the average quality of the existing workforce, as well as providing an incentive for staff to remain with the organization. The downside however, is that, once retrained, such individuals may be even better equipped to look for employment outside the organization.

In recognition of this, many employers are aware of the need to improve the attractiveness of the overall career package on offer. This does not simply concern pay, but also promotion prospects, non-wage benefits and the general image of the organization.

In order to compete more effectively in recruitment of newly qualified persons, sponsorship including, in the future, paying-off student loans, is seen as an important weapon in the armoury. However, few employers expect to be able to enforce a binding contract. Some discussion of the problems of developing and enforcing 'Training cost recovery contracts' is given in Brinkworth and Snape (1989). This paper outlines the pros and cons of such contracts and some of the pitfalls to be avoided.

5 Conditions of employment and career aspirations

5.1 Introduction

The pay and conditions of individuals in the NHS have been regularly reviewed on a number of occasions (see, for example, the pay review bodies for both doctors and nurses). This chapter presents general trends throughout the economy, against which developments within the NHS can be judged, concentrating on non-pay aspects. Conditions of employment are broadly interpreted, to include: pay, hours of work, length of contract, promotion prospects, pensions and other fringe benefits. The period of the 1970s and 1980s, in particular, has seen major changes in most of these conditions of employment.

Pay levels have increased dramatically throughout the economy over the last 20 years (see Figure 5.1). In part this, of course, simply reflects inflation. However, real pay levels have also risen substantially. The review bodies covering both nurses and doctors have from time to time focused on various aspects of both pay and conditions of employment. However, valuable though these have been, there seems to be a lack of emphasis on other aspects of changing conditions of employment. This chapter aims to summarise general developments in this area thus setting the backdrop against which changes within the NHS can be considered.

Developments in pay could form a report in their own right. However, it was not deemed appropriate to devote much of the present review to this subject. This is not meant to reflect the importance of the topic, which, as noted below, is crucial in terms of perceptions of what is good or bad about employment in the health service. Rather it reflects the view that

Figure 5.1
Weekly earnings, 1972-1990

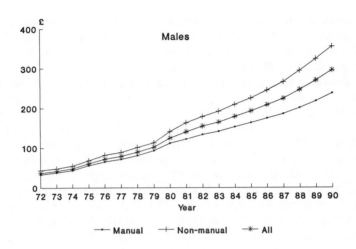

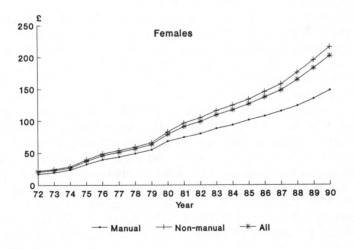

Source: DE Gazette

69

such a topic has been well covered by the various review bodies and that there is little point, therefore, in duplicating their effort here. Nevertheless, a brief overview is given, based on independent sources. The emphasis is on examining general trends outside the NHS, against which developments within the service need to be considered.

5.2   Pay, fringe benefits and pensions

An enormous amount of information is available with which to address these questions. The Department of Employment publishes regular series on earnings in the *Employment Gazette*, including material from the *New Earnings Survey*, (NES). The NES, which has been in existence since 1968, provides very detailed data on earnings by industry, occupation and region. Data on professional groups are available from surveys conducted by the professional institutes (PIs). These cover a broad range of different professions from engineers to teachers. (See Wilson, 1986; and Bosworth and Wilson, 1989; for further details.) Another important source of pay information is the series of reports produced by *Incomes Data Services* (IDS). IDS collects data from many primary sources, including the NES and PI surveys noted above. It also publishes articles on developments in pay and conditions of employment. Detailed study of relative pay in the NHS compared with other employers is obviously a crucial element in assessing whether such conditions of employment are set at appropriate levels to compensate for some of the negative elements of service employment highlighted below, but as noted above, this is regarded as lying outside the scope of the present report.

Information on fringe benefits, as well as data on pensions, is also included in many of the surveys by the professional institutes. As for basic pay, the developments in this area could easily form the subject of a separate report. The discussion here is confined to noting the growing importance of fringe benefits for many professionals. These include such things as a company car (most senior executives, and many not so senior ones, now have access to a company provided car) and non-contributable pension schemes. As for pay generally, the provision of these and other perks varies across different groups and detailed analysis would be needed to compare different grades within the NHS with the most appropriate comparator in the private sector. Such comparisons need to be conducted on a regular basis if the NHS is to keep up to date with the rapid pace of change in the private sector. A particularly important item here could be the provision of childcare facilities or assistance towards such costs.

IDS and PI sources also contain some information on other aspects of conditions of employment including the length and nature of the employment contract and promotion prospects. Demands by employers for more flexible work contracts have been noted in Chapter 3. Pressure for contracts to enable retrieval of training costs (by employers of employees who subsequently leave) is also an important recent development (see Section 4.4 above). Finally, information on perceptions

Figure 5.2
Trends in hours of work

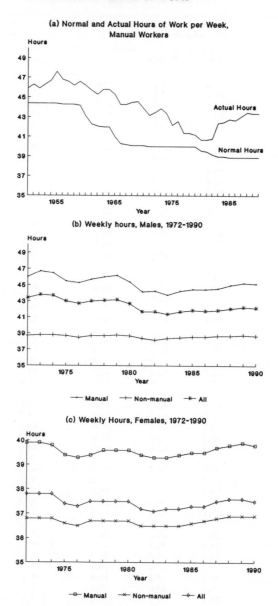

(a) Normal and Actual Hours of Work per Week, Manual Workers

(b) Weekly hours, Males, 1972-1990

(c) Weekly Hours, Females, 1972-1990

Source : DE Gazette, New Earnings Survey

Table 5.1
Normal and actual hours of work

Year	Normal weekly hours of manual workers			Actual weekly hours of manual workers		
	Men	Women	All	Men	Women	All
1950	44.4	44.5	44.4	47.3	41.7	45.9
1951	44.4	44.5	44.4	47.9	41.6	46.3
1952	44.4	44.5	44.4	47.5	41.2	45.9
1953	44.3	44.5	44.4	47.9	41.8	46.3
1954	44.3	44.4	44.4	48.4	41.8	46.7
1955	44.3	44.4	44.4	48.9	41.7	47.6
1956	44.3	44.4	44.3	48.6	41.3	46.8
1957	44.2	44.4	44.3	48.4	41.2	46.6
1958	44.2	44.3	44.3	47.9	41.0	46.2
1959	44.2	44.3	44.2	48.3	41.4	46.6
1960	43.0	43.4	43.1	48.0	40.7	46.2
1961	42.3	42.3	42.3	47.7	39.8	45.7
1962	42.1	42.2	42.1	47.2	39.5	45.3
1963	42.0	42.1	42.0	47.8	39.7	45.8
1964	41.9	42.1	42.0	47.8	39.7	45.8
1965	41.0	41.2	41.0	47.3	38.9	45.3
1966	40.3	40.5	40.3	46.2	38.3	44.3
1967	40.2	40.4	40.2	46.2	38.2	44.3
1968	40.1	40.2	40.1	46.3	38.4	44.5
1969[a]	40.1	40.1	40.1	46.5	38.1	44.6
1970	40.1	40.0	40.1	45.7	37.9	43.9
1971	40.0	40.0	40.0	44.7	37.7	43.2
1972	40.0	40.0	40.0	45.0	37.9	43.5
1973	40.0	40.0	40.0	45.6	37.7	43.9
1974	40.0	40.0	40.0	45.1	37.4	43.4
1975	40.0	40.0	40.0	43.6	37.0	42.2
1976	40.0	40.0	40.0	44.0	37.4	42.6
1977	40.0	40.0	40.0	44.2	37.4	41.4
1978	40.0	40.0	40.0	44.2	37.4	41.4
1979	40.0	40.0	40.0	44.0	37.4	41.2
1980	39.8	38.5	39.6	43.0	37.5	40.7
1981	39.7	38.4	39.5	43.0	37.7	40.7
1982	39.4	38.3	39.2	42.9	38.0	40.8
1983	39.2	38.3	39.0	43.3	38.2	42.4
1984	39.1	38.1	39.0	43.4	38.2	42.5
1985[b]	39.1	38.0	38.9	*	*	42.8
1986	39.1	38.1	38.9	*	*	42.7
1987	39.1	38.0	38.9	*	*	43.1
1988	39.1	38.1	38.9	*	*	43.5
1989	39.1	38.1	38.9	*	*	43.4
1990	39.1	38.0	38.9	*	*	42.9
1991	39.1	39.7	38.9	*	*	42.9

Source: British Labour Statistics: Historical Abstract, Department of Employment
Gazette (e.g. Table 5.4) and *New Earnings Survey*, Tables D86 and D87.
Notes: (a) Change in series.
(b) Data on actual weekly hours are in some cases not available after 1985.
See Table 17 for alternative estimates.

Table 5.2
Overtime and short-time working in manufacturing industry

Year	Overtime % of all operatives	Overtime Average hours/week per operative on overtime	Short-time % of all operatives	Short-time Average hours/week per operative on short-time
1950	n.a	7.3	n.a	14.8
1951	n.a	7.5	n.a	13.0
1952	20.7	7.7	3.8	15.0
1953	24.0	7.8	1.0	11.1
1954	26.5	8.0	0.7	11.4
1955	27.5	8.0	0.8	13.3
1956	25.7	7.9	1.5	10.9
1957	26.1	7.8	1.1	10.5
1958	23.1	7.6	2.8	14.0
1959	26.4	7.6	1.3	11.9
1960	30.5	7.9	1.0	10.5
1961	29.1	7.9	1.2	12.4
1962	28.1	7.8	1.7	10.4
1963	29.3	7.9	1.3	10.9
1964	33.0	8.2	0.4	10.3
1965	34.6	8.5	0.5	12.4
1966	33.9	8.5	1.2	9.8
1967	32.4	8.4	1.6	10.8
1968	35.1	8.5	0.5	11.2
1969	35.7	8.5	0.5	13.0
1970	34.4	8.5	0.6	12.4
1971	29.8	8.1	1.6	11.8
1972	29.9	8.2	2.6	12.2
1973	35.0	8.5	0.4	15.0
1974	33.0	8.4	4.5	14.5
1975	30.3	8.3	3.2	15.6
1976	32.2	8.4	1.6	11.7
1977	34.6	8.7	0.9	17.4
1978	34.8	8.6	0.7	15.1
1979	35.6	8.6	0.9	15.9
1980	29.5	8.3	5.9	14.3
1981	26.6	8.2	7.8	12.6
1982	29.8	8.3	3.5	12.4
1983	31.5	8.5	2.0	12.9
1984	34.3	8.9	1.5	14.4
1985	34.9	9.0	0.7	14.9
1986	34.2	9.0	0.9	14.4
1987	36.0	9.4	0.6	14.6
1988	37.9	9.5	0.5	14.4
1989	37.6	9.6	0.6	13.7
1990	37.5	9.5	0.7	15.7
1991[a]	33.0	9.2	2.3	12.4

Source: Department of Employment, *Employment Gazette*, various issues
(1950-91) (e.g. Table 1.11) in Dec. 1991 issue.
Notes: (a) Average of 9 months (Jan.-Sept.).

of promotion prospects is contained in some PI surveys (see Section 5.6, below).

In all these cases there may be further scope for research to compare developments in the NHS in recent years with what has happened in the private sector. If this is to inform discussion about shortages it would clearly need to be undertaken at a detailed level, distinguishing grade, occupation and possibly region. This could complement the existing work by the review bodies.

5.3 Hours of work

Changes in the number of normal and actual weekly hours of work of manual workers are set out, separately for males and females, in Table 5.1 and Figure 5.2[1]. The first three columns of data indicate the significant reduction in normal weekly hours which took place between 1950 and 1990, a decline of just over 5 hours (about 12 per cent). While most of this change took place in the period 1959 to 1966, there was a further downward movement around 1979 to 1985. Further reductions in the normal working week are currently under negotiation.

Average actual hours of work have also shown a secular decline, broadly following changes in normal hours, although it is clear from Table 5.1 and Figure 5.2 that they also vary significantly over the business cycle. The difference between normal and actual hours is caused by overtime (and short-time working). On balance, overtime outweighs short-time working. Overtime is much more closely associated with male employees than with females. It is an important phenomenon because any hours above normal are generally paid at a premium, often 25-33 per cent above basic rates (Bosworth and Wilson, 1990). While long hours are associated with increasing disutility, the disproportionate increases in pay often compensate. This form of compensation does not apply for certain non-manual jobs where longer hours may result in no compensating increases in pay. Although many of the more routine non-manual occupations receive premia (or pay in lieu) for overtime working, most professionals do not receive overtime payments. However, in general, the relative attractiveness of alternative jobs will in part depend on perceptions of the extent of regular paid overtime (Bosworth and Warren, 1990a).

The importance of the level and variations in overtime and short time amongst operatives are confirmed by Table 5.2[2]. The percentages of operatives on overtime and short time vary cyclically, as do the average hours per week lost on short time. However, while there has been some variation over time in the average hours of overtime per operative working overtime, this measure has remained remarkably stable over the cycle, if anything, growing secularly.

Evidence on the hours of non-manual workers is available from the DE, New Earnings Survey and the Labour Force Survey. As noted above, there are clearly problems with both sources concerning the measurement of the hours of non-manual workers. With regard to normal hours, the

74

Table 5.3
Paid hours: manual and non-manual workers

	Males						Females					
	Manual		Non-manual		All		Manual		Non-manual		All	
	Weekly earnings	Hours	Weekly earnings	Hours	Weekly earnings	Hours	Weekly earnings	Hours	Weekly earnings	Hours	Weekly earnings	Hours
1972	32.8	46.0	43.5	38.7	36.7	43.4	17.1	39.9	22.2	36.8	20.5	37.8
1973	38.1	46.7	48.1	38.8	41.9	43.8	19.7	39.9	24.7	36.8	23.1	37.8
1974	43.6	46.5	54.4	38.8	47.7	43.7	23.6	39.8	28.6	36.8	26.9	37.8
1975	55.7	45.5	68.4	38.7	60.8	43.0	32.1	39.4	39.6	36.6	37.4	37.4
1976	65.1	45.3	81.6	38.5	71.8	42.7	39.4	39.3	48.8	36.5	46.2	37.3
1977	71.5	45.7	88.9	38.7	78.6	43.0	43.7	39.4	53.8	36.7	51.0	37.5
1978	80.7	46.0	100.7	38.7	89.1	43.1	49.4	39.6	59.1	36.7	56.4	37.5
1979	93.0	46.2	113.0	38.8	101.4	43.2	55.2	39.6	66.0	36.7	63.0	37.5
1980	111.7	45.4	141.3	38.7	124.5	42.7	68.0	39.6	82.7	36.7	78.8	37.5
1981	121.9	44.2	163.1	38.4	140.5	41.7	74.5	39.4	96.7	36.5	91.4	37.2
1982	133.8	44.3	178.9	38.2	154.5	41.7	80.1	39.3	104.9	36.5	99.0	37.1
1983b	143.6	43.9	194.9	38.4	167.5	41.5	87.9	39.3	115.1	36.5	108.8	37.2
1983	141.6	43.8	191.8	38.4	164.7	41.4	88.1	39.3	116.1	36.5	109.5	37.2
1984c	152.7	44.3	209.0	38.5	178.8	41.7	93.5	39.4	124.3	36.5	117.2	37.2
1985	163.6	44.5	225.0	38.6	192.4	41.9	101.3	39.5	133.8	36.6	126.4	37.3
1986	174.4	44.5	244.9	38.6	207.5	41.8	107.5	39.5	145.7	36.7	137.2	37.3
1987	185.5	44.6	265.9	38.7	224.0	41.9	115.3	39.7	157.2	36.8	148.1	37.5
1988	200.6	45.0	294.1	38.7	245.8	42.1	123.6	39.8	175.5	36.9	164.2	37.6
1989	217.8	54.3	323.6	38.8	269.5	42.3	134.9	39.9	195.0	36.9	182.3	37.6
1990	237.2	45.2	354.9	38.7	295.6	42.2	148.0	39.8	215.5	36.9	201.5	37.5
1991	253.1	44.4	375.7	38.7	318.9	41.5	159.2	39.7	236.8	36.8	222.4	37.4

Source: DE *Gazette*, *New Earnings Survey*, Tables D86 and D87.

Notes: (a) All figures exclude those whose pay was affected by absence.
(b) Results for 1982 and the first row of figures for 1983 relate to men aged 21 and over or women aged 18 and over.
(c) Results for 1984 and the second row of 1983 relate to males or females on adult rates.

75

Table 5.4
Basic holiday entitlements

	Percentage of manual workers who have a basic holiday with pay of:										Percentage with extra service entitlement
	1 week	1-2 weeks	2 weeks	2-3 weeks	3 weeks	3-4 weeks	4 weeks	4-5 weeks	5 weeks +	Average	
1951	28	3	66	2	1					1.7	4
1955		1	96	2	1					2.0	9
1960			97	1	2					2.0	9
1962			97	2	1					2.0	10
1963			97	2	1					2.1	10
1964			92	7	3					2.2	20
1965			75	22	4					2.2	22
1966			63	33	6					2.3	22
1967			60	34	10					2.3	27
1968			56	34	14	1				2.6	27
1969			50	35	49	3				2.7	27
1970			41	7	63	4				3.0	30
1971			28	5	39	33				3.2	25
1972			8	16	36	45	4			3.5	17
1973			6	9	30	40	4			3.5	12
1974			1	1	17	51	28			3.6	14
1975			1	1	18	47	30			3.6	20
1976				1	18	47	34			3.6	26
1977				1	17	47	34			3.7	32
1978				1	7	42	35			4.1	32
1979					7	24	50			4.2	36
1980					2	11	19	55		4.4	38
1981					2	5	25	61	1	4.5	40
1982						5	21	53	19	4.6	37[a]
1983						1	17	60	18	4.6	35[a]
1984							15	61	19	4.6	36[a]
1985							16	63	20	4.6	35[a]
1986							14	63	23	4.6	32[a]
1987											32[a]
1988							10[b]	65	25	4.6	33.3[c]
1989							9[b]	64	27	4.6	33.3[c]
1990							10[b]	63	27	4.6	33.3[c]

Source: DE, *British Labour Statistics Yearbook* and *Gazette*, various issues, (1951-1991).

Notes: (a) Decline caused by alteration in Wages Council Orders. Figures for 1988 onwards are not published but are greater than one third.
(b) Employees covered by national agreements had paid holidays of four weeks or less.
(c) Employees covered by national agreements had paid holidays of five weeks or more.

76

Table 5.5
Trends in the incidence of shiftworking

Percentages working shifts

	All industries and services					Non-manufacturing	Manufacturing	
	Manual	Non-manual	Male	Female	All	All	All	Manual
1970[a]	(19.6)	(4.7)	(15.1)	(7.4)	(12.9)	(10.4)	(16.4)	(22.8)
1973	16.6	4.9	12.9	7.0	11.2	9.5	13.9	19.0
1974	17.9	5.3	14.0	7.1	12.0	10.2	14.6	19.8
1975	20.6	6.4	15.9	8.0	13.6	12.8	14.9	20.4
1976	21.2	6.9	16.1	9.3	14.1	13.5	15.1	20.9
1977	20.4	6.7	15.4	9.2	13.5	12.7	14.9	20.3
1978	22.1	7.6	15.9	9.2	13.9	12.6	16.0	21.7
1979	21.5	7.3	16.1	10.0	14.2	13.1	16.2	21.9
1980	21.0	7.3	15.5	9.9	13.8	12.9	15.4	21.3
1981	21.1	7.4	15.1	10.3	13.6	13.1	14.5	20.9
1982	21.2	7.7	15.0	10.9	13.7	13.5	14.1	20.3
1983	23.2	9.3	16.8	12.3	15.3	15.1	15.9	22.5
1984	22.0	8.9	15.8	12.2	14.7	14.4	15.4	21.5
1985	22.4	9.2	16.2	12.3	14.9	14.7	15.5	22.1
1986	22.0	9.2	16.0	12.2	14.8	15.5	15.3	21.7
1987	21.3	8.7	15.1	11.7	14.0	13.3	15.6	22.4
1988	20.6	8.3	14.7	10.9	13.4	12.6	15.8	22.6
1989	21.4	8.0	14.9	10.9	13.5	12.5	16.5	23.7
1990	20.8	7.9	14.3	10.8	13.1	11.7	16.4	23.8
1991	22.4	8.1	14.6	10.9	13.3	13.6	16.0	24.3

Source: *New Earnings Survey* various issues part D Analysis by Occupation (Tables D99-D100) and Part C Analysis by Industry (Tables C79-C82) 1970-1991.

Note: (a)   Estimates for 1970 are not directly comparable with those for later years.

77

Figure 5.3
Trends in holiday entitlements

(a)Basic holiday entitlements 1951,1971 and 1990

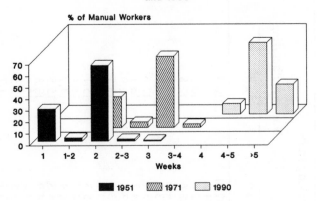

(b) Average Holiday Entitlement 1962-1990

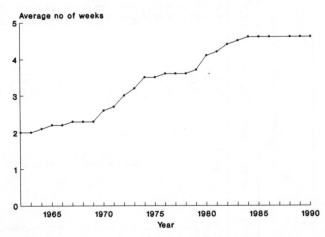

Source: DE British Labour Statistics Yearbook and Gazette

Figure 5.4
Trends in shiftworking

(a) All industries and services

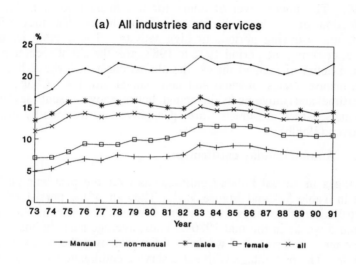

(b) Manufacturing and Non-manufacturing

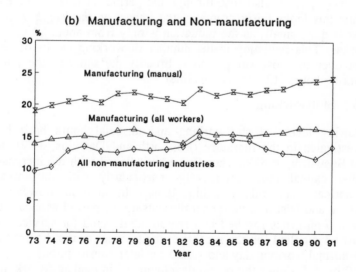

Source: DE New Earnings Survey & Wilson and Bosworth (1986)

LFS data is probably the stronger, as the concept is based on 'usual' hours of work, rather than some collectively negotiated normal hours. Collective agreements are less widespread for non-manual workers and many non-manual people work unpaid overtime. Nevertheless, Table 5.3 shows actual, paid hours of manual and non-manual workers from the NES. The lower level of hours for non-manual workers is, in part, a reflection of the unpaid element of the hours that they often work, particularly during periods of high activity. The notable features of the table, covering the period 1972 to 1988, are: the slight secular reduction in actual hours of manual males; the almost constant level of hours amongst non-manual males, manual and non-manual females. Changes in unpaid overtime and movements in actual hours above 'usual' levels for non-manuals, which are much more speculative, are mapped by Bosworth and Warren (1990b).

5.4 Annual holiday entitlements

Changes in annual holiday entitlements over the post-war period are set out in Table 5.4 and Figure 5.3[1]. They show the persistent shift in the distribution of holidays from around 2 weeks per year in 1951, to between 4 and 5 weeks in the mid 1980s. Thus, average basic holiday entitlements have increased from 1.7 weeks to 4.6 weeks over the post-war period as a whole. The percentage with extra service entitlements (i.e. through length of service, etc.), also rose through the period, at least to the early 1980s. While this looks fairly dramatic, the impact on the length of the working year is quite small, as the reduction is only from about 52 to just over 47 weeks. This reduction in the number of working weeks of about 10 per cent over the post-war period is broadly the same as the fall in weekly working hours (12 per cent decline).

5.5 Shiftworking

Growing levels of shiftworking and unsocial hours have been widely investigated in the literature (Bosworth and Dawkins, 1980; and Wilson and Bosworth, 1987). These have been linked with the increasing need to utilise capital more intensively, particularly with the introduction of numerically controlled machine tools. In addition, however, increased income and leisure time (generally outside the period Monday to Friday, 9 am to 5 pm), has resulted in a rise in the demand for services which often must be supplied 'on the spot' (i.e. the services cannot be produced during the normal working day and stored for later consumption).

Table 5.5 shows the recent developments in paid shiftworking[2]. Trends are also highlighted in Figure 5.4. Questions on shiftworking were introduced into the NES on an annual basis in 1973 (the 'one off' figure for 1970 appears to be inconsistent with the results for later years). Again, the results for non-manual employees in particular may be an under-estimate of the true position because such workers are not always

80

paid an explicit premium[3]. The results indicate a significant growth in shiftworking for each sub-group distinguished. The figure for all non-manual workers rises from around 5 per cent in 1973 to over 9 per cent by the mid-1980s. A similarly steep rise occurs for female workers in all industries and services.

It should be noted that these individuals are receiving an explicit premium for working shifts or unsocial hours. This premium is generally at least 20 per cent (say on a double day system) and often 50 per cent or higher for more unsocial shifts. Nevertheless, it should be added that many other workers, particularly in the service sector, work unsocial hours without any explicit premium. According to data from the Department of Employment's *New Earnings Survey* (1989 Part B) there are no other major groups of female workers who record the same degree of unsocial hours activity as those in nursing and related occupations. Approximately seven in every ten full-time nursing and midwifery staff received some amount of special duty payments in April 1989, (Buchan, 1989). There has always been a trade-off between the desire on the part of the individual to work unsocial hours for their own reasons and the need for the employer to pay a shift premium (i.e. as in the case of female workers on the twilight shift). In the case of the NHS, there is clearly a need to staff hospitals 24 hours per day but it is a moot point whether the allowance currently paid for such work represents adequate compensation compared with those paid in other sectors.

5.6 Work patterns and aspirations

The earlier discussion in Chapter 3 outlined the significant growth in part-time working and self employment. Both of these reflect, at least in part, changes in social attitudes. The former is associated with the attempt by individuals and families to secure the optimum balance of income, domestic work and leisure. The latter is linked with the growing desire on the part of individuals to take their own decisions, rather than to take orders from others. Self employment has been closely associated with the new wave of entrepreneurship, which has coincided with the period of Conservative government. Clearly, the conditions of employment for most NHS employees may be out of step with these developments in civilian labour markets. However, for many, such considerations would probably be undesirable. Nevertheless, some moves in this direction may be necessary; doctors after all are quite acceptably regarded as self employed. The changes in hours of work, holiday entitlements, etc. outlined in this section also highlight areas where the health service may have got out of step with conditions of employment on offer elsewhere.

The dramatic developments in all of the areas highlighted in the previous discussion, such as pay, fringe benefits, hours of work, holiday entitlements and shiftworking, suggest that the NHS may need to reassess whether the terms and conditions of employment on offer match up with

81

those in the private sector. More detailed research may be necessary to identify the scale of such possible discrepancies.

Notes

1 Data from Wilson and Bosworth (1987), up-dated from the DE *Gazette*.

2 Data from Wilson and Bosworth (1987), up-dated from the DE *New Earnings Survey*.

3 The figures for manual workers may also prove to be under-estimates because individuals on the day-shift of a multiple shift system may not be in receipt of a shift premium on the day of the survey. For a detailed discussion of the issues surrounding the measurement of shiftworking and the comparison of different sources of data, see Bosworth and Dawkins (1980).

6 Labour supply and the NHS in the 1990s

6.1 Introduction

This chapter focuses on the changing role of women in society and at work. It complements the general review on labour supply in Chapter 2 by concentrating on the factors that are likely to influence nursing labour supply. Early economic theories of labour supply focused on the individual. However, it soon became clear that the decision was taken in a household context and that the labour supply of household partners, notably husband and wife, were jointly determined. Much of the early literature in this area concentrated on the added and discouraged worker hypotheses: the former suggests that women may be induced into the workforce when the male partner is unemployed and is experiencing difficulty in obtaining a job; the latter suggests that, when jobs are scarce, one of the individuals in the household may become marginalised (i.e. would like a job but does not actively search because of the low probability of being made a job offer) and moves outside the labour force. More recently, however, changes in a variety of influences, including social attitudes to women at work, have broadened the focus of interest on women at work.

A more recent contribution of the household labour supply literature, however, has been to recognise the effects of family life on the costs of running a household and the impact of family responsibilities on the allocation of time between household members. This theory examines the joint determination of male and female household work, paid work and leisure activities. The conceptual framework is able to deal with situations

83

in which women take primary responsibility for the 'caring' activities of the household, as well as instances in which these are allocated to the male partner or equally between both spouses. The relative mix of tasks for males and females depends on the male and female (household) utility function, their relative productivity in each area and the wage rates that they can command.

It is evident that demographic changes over the 1990s will produce a general reduction in the number of potential recruits to the NHS that can be drawn from the traditional pool of young female labour market entrants. Potentially severe problems will arise in nursing and in similar (largely female employing) occupations, because of the sheer scale of NHS recruitment from each age cohort of (female) school leavers with the relevant qualifications, unless recruitment patterns are changed. In addition, and largely because of the socioeconomic breakdown of the reduction in school leavers, recruitment of young workers will also be a problem (though much less severe) in activities that employ principally male manual staff.

There are two broad approaches to these recruitment difficulties. Firstly, changes in current labour utilisation that will **reduce the demand for new entrants** could take place. This will involve policies to reduce labour turnover (which may require fundamental changes in management 'style'), to limit premature retirement and to make more effective use of the current labour force by increases in the average hours of work or, where possible, by the accelerated introduction of labour saving technologies. It may also require changes in the job grading structure which reflect altered responsibilities, in work organization and in training provision to match. A principal objective of this should be to reduce the net demand for young women with 5 'O'levels or GCSE equivalents (and also for males who might be recruited to manual jobs).

The second approach is to focus on the means by which the potential shortfall in supply can be met by **retargeting recruitment**. There are a number of ways of doing this. The present discussion focuses on five that seem to be the most promising.

Firstly, the NHS needs to fully exploit the growth in the labour force participation of mature women that is expected in the next decade. Obviously the emphasis should be on those with previous relevant training and experience. The aim should be to reduce both their time out of employment by accelerating their return to the workforce and also to make the health service such an attractive source of employment that no alternatives are considered. Many of the means through which this objective is met will also reduce the quit rate of existing employees.

This, however, is unlikely to be enough to solve the likely labour shortage. There is a growing pool of mature applicants, without previous experience but suitable for training, on whom the NHS could also draw. This could significantly reduce the current over-reliance on young trainees. There is an obvious and important interface here with the demand reducing changes (notably in respect of grading and training) briefly referred to above. The training most suited (and most cost-effective) to this group may be less comprehensive than that appropriate for youngsters making a full working lifetime career choice although the results reported in Chapter 13 cast some doubt on this.

Thirdly, the NHS could try attracting a larger share of each school-leaving cohort with 5 or more 'O' levels (or GCSE equivalents) both female and male. This will not be easy, mainly because of the growing intensity of competition in the labour market for young recruits and also because of prevailing attitudes to health service employment, notably amongst young males. Again, many of the policies to encourage 'returnees', to retain existing employees and to attract new mature recruits may also play a part here.

Fourthly, in order to deal with the shortfall of recruits to male manual jobs, action may also be necessary to increase the NHS share of each male school leaving cohort suitable for this kind of work. Some relief might be obtained by making premature retirement of existing employees less attractive compared with continued employment or by changes (increases) in hours of work. These types of policies are likely to be essential.

Finally, apart from demand side changes to improve the utilisation of current employees, a major pool of labour on which the NHS might draw, especially in parts of the UK where the labour market is slack, is the unemployed. Especially important could be the long term unemployed who, with proper training, could alleviate the projected shortages. Recent forecasts (Gregg, 1991) have suggested that the number of long term unemployed males will increase and remain high over the next few years. As a result substantial opportunities for recruitment to the NHS from this source will exist.

Following these introductory remarks, the remainder of this chapter focuses on the implications of the large literature on labour supply for the formulation of policies which might facilitate increased recruitment rates and, as a by product, will also reduce turnover. The emphasis is principally on the policies needed to enable the NHS to draw in the 1990s on the labour reserve of women currently engaged full-time with domestic responsibilities (mainly 'married' women), including both those with and without previous NHS experience. However, such policy changes are also likely to have beneficial effects on the proportion of each school leaving cohort the NHS attracts. Note that the definition of a 'married' women used in this review reflects the nature and extent of a woman's family responsibilities and not strict legal status.

6.2   Factors affecting female supply

It has been argued that a broad range of factors have influenced female labour supply, including: (i) changing social attitudes towards women and work; (ii) increasing aspirations regarding the standard of living; (iii) the effects of tenure on career prospects; (iv) falling birth rates (in part associated with improved methods of birth control) and family commitments; (v) changes in work patterns and employer preferences.

Changing social attitudes

In recent years there have been a number of publications relating to women's attitudes to working and their jobs (Agassi, 1979; McNally, 1979; Hunt, 1980; Pollert, 1981; and Wajcman, 1983;). A comparison of the results of two surveys undertaken in 1965 and 1980 (Hunt, 1968; and Martin and Roberts, 1984) shows that women in 1980 were more likely to stress the woman's right to choose and less likely to believe that a woman's place was in the home. The developments in economic theory have, therefore, mirrored fundamental shifts in the role of women in society (see, for example, Martin and Roberts, 1984).

These developments can be traced over a long period, including the two World Wars (Employment Department, 1989a). However, the pace of change appears to have accelerated in recent years, with the introduction of equal opportunities legislation, which came into force in the UK in 1975. Witherspoon (1989) and Brook, *et al.* (1989) report data on British social attitudes for 1984 and 1987. The results indicate a significant increase in the proportion of individuals who think that a wide range of jobs, including those traditionally undertaken by males (such as car mechanics, bus drivers, etc.), are 'equally suitable for women'. Other reports indicate changing attitudes to the role of men and women in the home (Jowell and Airey, 1985).

There are a number of official and semi-official groups working to further improve the position of women, such as the Equal Opportunities Commission and the Advisory Committee on Women's Employment (Employment Department, 1989b). The latter will be discussing in particular the removal of barriers to women returning to paid employment. On balance, older women tend to have more traditional views of the role of women or their position in society, while younger and more highly qualified women hold more 'radical' attitudes. This is consistent with a continuing shift in women's attitudes.

A series of CEC reports map changes in socio-political attitudes towards the role of men and women in the family and at work (CEC, 1979, 1984, 1987 and 1988). These sources provide comparative information about attitudes and changes in attitudes across the various countries of the European Community. CEC (1988), for example, reports the results of attitudes in favour of 'equal roles in the family'. In 1987, the UK had the second highest proportion in favour of equality (only Denmark was higher). The UK also showed the greatest increase in favour of equality amongst the ten countries for which data were available in both 1983 and 1987. However, the UK did not rank so highly in terms of male willingness to do housework or with regard to their preference for women to undertake paid work.

Aspirations regarding the standard of living and the tenure of work

The Women and Employment Survey, 1980, highlights the fact that many households count on the woman's income, particularly where women are working full-time, but also that most women enjoy their work (Martin and Roberts, 1984, p. 61-2). The declining relative pay for many professional and non-manual groups, together with rising financial commitments (such as increased mortgage payments), mean that, for many families, the economic participation of the wife is now a necessity if household living standards are to be maintained.

This is reinforced by the accumulating evidence from analyses of cohort information on earnings that, while opportunistic job changes can enhance careers, career development and earnings prospects are generally better for individuals who stay with the same employer. Unplanned changes can be disruptive especially for more highly qualified and career orientated women. In addition, women, in particular, often experience a downgrading of their careers on returning to work after a prolonged period of caring for young children. Thus, there are significant gains for women and, increasingly, for the family unit as a whole, from continuity of employment and planned, rather than unplanned, changes in job and location. Involuntary changes, tend to have a negative impact. The negative effects of involuntary unemployment through redundancy have been established (Bosworth, 1989). Wives may experience a similar effect where they are 'forced' to relocate because of their husband's jobs.

Family commitments

Despite these benefits of job continuity, women's labour market activity typically still falls away during the child-caring years. This is partly because of the difficulties they face in meeting the demands of their paid and unpaid roles in the absence of adequate child care provision. Despite trends towards greater equality, most of the domestic burden appears to still be shouldered by women rather than men. The trend towards smaller families has contributed to the increased participation of women. We noted in Section 2.1 that the number of births in the UK fell by 35 per cent between 1964 and 1977, although there has been a slight increase since that time. Thus, even mothers who take on a more traditional 'caring' role in the family find that the demands placed on them decline earlier in their lifetime where there are fewer children. However, changes in the timing and size of families is, in part, endogenously determined. The desire on the part of women to enter or continue in employment may be an important factor in determining the size of families.

Changes in work patterns and employer preferences

The growth of part-time working amongst women in the UK has been one of the most significant employment phenomena of the post-War period. This has greatly enhanced job opportunities for married women. In part it reflects the growth in employment in the sectors of the labour market which tend to employ large numbers of women and where part-time working is commonplace. It is also the result of a shift in employer preferences towards part-time work. Partly this is motivated by the lower level of non-wage labour costs (like employers' labour taxes and holiday/pension payments) associated with part-time work but the desire for greater flexibility is also a factor. An examination of the proportion of females undertaking part-time work by age reveals a distinctive hump in the proportion of part-time working for women aged 35-44 (*Employment Gazette*, 1989). Thus, the growth in part-time work can be influenced by the changing age structure of the female population. However, the evidence also shows that the whole relationship has shifted outwards from 1967 to 1987. In 1985, the UK had the second highest proportion of part-time working amongst women of 10 major European countries (*op. cit.*). This indicates the scale of a change that could not have occurred without big shifts in employer preferences. In times of economic buoyancy and labour shortage, like those experienced in the late 1980s, employers are even more willing to offer women flexible work opportunities including homework and part-time work at times that allow women greater freedom to reconcile their 'caring' roles with paid employment. Again, the effect has been to allow more women to continue in employment or to allow women to re-enter the workforce at an earlier age than historically would have been possible. There is clear evidence that, on average, women are spending longer in the labour market. However, a significant proportion of women find this dual, employment and caring role quite stressful, even where the work is part-time (Martin and Roberts, 1984).

Projected growth in female labour supply

It is the cumulative effect of this variety of factors, all largely operating in the same direction, that account for the recent and forecast increases in the numbers of economically active women. This is shown by the projected rise of 2¼ million economically active women between 1980 and the year 2000 (see Table 2.5 above), compared with a growth of about 400 thousand economically active males. Confirmation of this expected trend came from a recent survey of personnel managers (Gallup, 1989). Nine out of ten respondents indicated that their company would be considering employing women returning to work after a break, in order to alleviate expected skill shortages in the 1990s. Other solutions also involved increasing the female work-force, including: introducing or increasing the number of part-time workers and improving the retention of women who have babies. While less than one in ten firms interviewed have some form of creche facility or scheme, about seven in ten employers were reported to be interested in introducing a child-care voucher scheme. However, there is, thus far, little evidence that they have acted on this, despite the fact that a number of reports suggest that nurseries were set to be the 'perk of the 1990s' (LGC, 1989).

6.3   Basic theory of labour supply

The starting point is the standard analysis of the labour supply decision made by workers who are not subject to a job offer constraint (i.e. jobs are available). This mode of analysis is entirely appropriate when a solution is thought to be one of a general labour shortage (i.e. when the supply side rules). Given the general labour market prospects outlined in Chapters 2-4, this could well be the situation facing the NHS in the 1990s. The basic economic model of labour supply states that workers participate in labour market work when the market wage exceeds the *reservation* wage. In the case of adult males, young workers and single women the reservation wage is generally thought to reflect the relative costs and benefits associated with earning income and taking leisure (technically described as the marginal rate of substitution between income and leisure). This depends on personal characteristics like age and education, non-labour income and personal tastes. In the case of married women, the reservation (or home) wage reflects the valuation (by the woman and her family) of non-market time or in more technical language the marginal rate of substitution between the returns obtainable from market and non-market (home) work. In both cases the activity rate will depend upon a variety of factors including personal characteristics and tastes, family circumstances and external market conditions. A key issue for most women will be family responsibilities. For those interested, a technical description of the model is given in Box 1.

It is evident from this type of analysis that changes in activity rates for women may occur as a result of changes in either the market or in the home wage. Policies to increase the participation of women (or men) require either increases in the market wage or decreases in the home (reservation) wage or both. The NHS could introduce policies to influence both. The next section discusses the question of what labour supply studies suggest is the best strategy.

6.4   Wage changes, labour supply and strategies for labour shortage

It is possible to breakdown the effects of changes in the market wage on labour supply into two components an 'income' effect and a substitution effect (again see Box 1 for the technical details). The substitution effect of wages on labour supply is positive because increases in the market wage raise the cost of non-market time and hence increases the supply of market time. The income effect of a wage increase is negative if non-market time (i.e. leisure) is a *normal* good (i.e. increases in income increase the worker's desire for non-market time and reduce hours of work). Hence the overall effect of wages on labour supply is theoretically indeterminate and has to be resolved by empirical enquiry.

Box 1
The economics of labour supply: technical note

The reservation wage (W*) is determined by:

$$W^*_i = w^* (Z^*_i, \Omega_i) \qquad (1)$$

where W^*_i is the reservation wage and the i subscript indicates the ith individual, Z^*_i is a vector of observed characteristics and Ω_i is a parameter reflecting personal tastes. As far as married women are concerned the Z vector contains a variety of variables which determine the non-observable 'home' wage, of which non-labour income and the number of children of differing ages are particularly important.

The market wage (W_i) for the ith individual is determined by:

$$W_i = w (Z_i, \delta_i) \qquad (2)$$

where Z_i is a vector of personal and human capital as well as job characteristics (such as industry, degree of unionisation and so on) and δ is a vector of other unobservable personal characteristics. Workers participate in market work if $W > W^*$.

Since W* is unobservable the labour supply (activity rate) model for an individual is given by

$$A_i = a (W_i, Z^*_i, \Omega_i,) \qquad (3)$$

where Wi is determined by equation 2. This is the most general version of the activity rate models which are considered in this review.

The impact on labour supply of a change in the market wage (Wi) of a worker is analysed by means of the Slutsky decomposition:

$$\frac{dA_i}{dW_i} \begin{bmatrix} \text{wage} \\ \text{effect} \end{bmatrix} = \frac{(\delta A_i)}{(\delta W_i)} \begin{bmatrix} \text{substitution} \\ \text{effect} \end{bmatrix} + H_i \frac{(\delta A_i)}{(\delta Y_i)} \begin{bmatrix} \text{income} \\ \text{effect} \end{bmatrix} \qquad (4)$$

where H_i is individual hours of work per time period and Y_i is individual income. If equation 4 is multiplied through by (W_i/H_i) it gives the decomposition in terms of elasticities.

Table 6.1
Labour supply of males: results of selected UK studies

	Wage elasticity	Income elasticity	Substitution elasticity	Data used (all individual level data)
Brown/Levin/Ulph (1976)	-0.13	-0.35	+0.22	Stirling University Studies of married men 1971
Ashworth/Ulph (1981)	-0.13	-0.36	+0.23	"
Blundell/Walker Expenditure (1982)	-0.004	-0.20	+0.20	Family Survey
Brown et al. (1983) i) single	-0.33	-0.50	+0.17	
ii) married Project	-0.14	-0.44	+0.30	HM Treasury

Note: The substitution elasticity is the wage elasticity minus the income elasticity.

In the case of men, the overwhelming conclusion from the evidence is that the wage elasticity is weakly negative (a weak substitution effect is overwhelmed by a strong income effect), so that general wage increases are unlikely to persuade male employees to work longer hours. Indeed it may do the opposite if the supply curve is indeed *backward bending* as these results imply. The evidence is summarised in Table 6.1. As far as retirement decisions are concerned, again the story is similar. Male employees are unlikely to defer voluntary retirement decisions simply as a response to higher wages. Restraints imposed directly on voluntary retirement make more sense if it is desired to influence supply in this way.

In aggregate therefore, wage increases are, on the basis of the evidence, unlikely to make a significant contribution to a general shortage of adult male employees through their impact on the behaviour of existing staff. This is not to say there is no role for wage increases.

There may be strong offsetting 'efficiency wage' effects. Efficiency wage effects may arise for a variety of reasons. Paying higher wages *ceteris paribus*, attracts more productive workers. By widening the gap between NHS pay and the market alternative it also increases the incentive to make greater effort within the service. More directly, as a symbol of goodwill, it raises morale and reduces conflict. There is a growing empirical literature (Wadhwani and Wall, 1988) which lends support to this idea. If such effects were significant in the health services, wage increases might lead to higher productivity through greater effort, improved work practices and so on. This could become of increasing importance in the 1990s if hospitals are forced to operate in a more competitive environment, competing for labour with each other as well as with other employers. On all these aspects there is little or no evidence for the NHS and this is an area where further research seems desirable.

Increases in relative pay will also aid recruitment of new staff, especially of young workers. Greenhalgh (1979) found that young males had a large positive wage elasticity in contrast with their older counterparts. More recently, Robertson and Symons (1990) use the National Child Development Study and find that the choice of occupation by young males is highly wage elastic (elasticities above 2 in each of the various estimations that are reported). This is in marked contrast with the behaviour of males once occupation is selected. The evidence suggests that the benefits of more general wage increases to attract mature males from other occupations or other sectors, is much more limited. As a consequence, this suggests that the emphasis of any wage policy should be carefully targetted to get the best results.

In respect of female employees the situation is completely different. Table 6.2 gives a selection of results obtained from several empirical studies, using different methods and employing both time series and cross-section data. They all tell the same story. The wage elasticity for women workers is strongly positive as a result of a strong substitution effect overwhelming a weak income effect. The evidence in such studies strongly suggests that, unlike males, increases in NHS pay levels will significantly help overcome shortages of female labour by attracting new recruits of all ages, by reducing the quit rate of existing employees and by accelerating the return of currently inactive past employees.

This is confirmed by a number of studies of the labour supply of nurses shown in Table 6.3. Most of these relate to the US but one UK study (Phillips 1989b) tells the same story of a strong positive wage elasticity. Like Joshi (1988), Ermisch and Wright (1989) and Perry (1990), Phillips uses data from the 1980 Women and Employment Survey (WES). The great strength of this data set is that it contains information on both currently employed and non-employed nurses. This enables the researcher to minimize the selection bias that distorts wage elasticity estimates in studies that use data on working women only. The main drawback of the data is that they contain no details of each nurse's professional qualification or of her period of service, both of which are crucial determinants of pay and hence the probability of working.

Table 6.2
Labour supply of females: results of selected UK studies

	Wage elasticity	Income elasticity	Husband's income Elasticity	Substitution elasticity	Data used
Greenhalgh (1977)	+1.35	-0.23	-0.88	+1.58	Census 1971 Town level data
Layard *et al.* (1980)	+0.49	-0.04	-0.28	+0.5 ⎫	General Household Survey
Zabalza (1983)	+0.41	0	-0.09	+0.41 ⎭	Individual data
Joshi (1988) i) married a) full-time b) all ii) non-married a) full-time b) all	+1.88 +0.59 +0.81 +0.48	-0.50 -0.36 -0.20 -0.17	n/a n/a n/a n/a	n/a n/a +1.01 +0.65	Women and Employment Survey 1980 Individual data
Sprague (1988)	+1.81	n/a	-1.84	n/a	Time Series for UK 1954-82

Note: The substitution elasticity is the wage elasticity minus the income
elasticity. For the studies by Sprague and Joshi, non-labour income
is omitted or lumped together with husband's income, hence the
substitution elasticity cannot be computed in the same manner.

On the other hand there are good data on the educational qualifications
that were used to select nurses into the three categories of professional
training that prevailed at the time the WES was conducted. However,
there are bound to be some vestigial inaccuracies in the wage equation,
especially for those not currently working. Since estimates of the expected
wage used in the activity equation are derived from this source this is

bound to affect the estimated wage elasticity but probably not significantly so.

Phillips uses quite sophisticated econometric techniques (a structural probit) to estimate the wage and the participation equations for the entire sample of 319 nurses and also separately for those of the 319 who are married. The results, as far as the wage elasticity is concerned, are clear cut and virtually identical for both groups of women. There is a strong positive wage effect on nurses willingness to work. The estimated wage elasticity is 1.4 which is larger than that found by Joshi (1988) using the entire WES sample. As a result the author concludes that 'the key to increasing participation is through wages'.

Table 6.3
Labour supply of nurses: results of selected US and UK studies

	Wage elasticity	Income elasticity	Husband's income elasticity	Substitution elasticity	Data used (all individual level data)
Sloan/Lichupan (1975)	+2.82	-0.02	-1.52	+2.84	1960 US Census
Link/Settle (1979)	+0.58	-0.03	-0.72	+0.61	1970 US Census
Phillips (1989b)	+1.4	-0.38			Women and Employment Survey (1980)

Note: The substitution elasticity is the wage elasticity minus the income elasticity. For the study by Phillips, using the Women and Employment Survey, non-labour income is lumped together, hence the substitution elasticity cannot be computed in the same manner.

In general it is difficult to dispute this view but there are some qualifications. The study by Blundell, Ham and Meghir (1987) suggests that the strong positive wage elasticity found in most research only occurs if women are unconstrained by the demand side of the labour market. Most models crudely allow for this by the addition of fairly *ad hoc* variables like the local vacancy or unemployment rate. Blundell, Ham and

Meghir are more sophisticated. They employ a 'double hurdle' model which takes explicit account of employment opportunities available to each of the women workers in their sample. When this is done they obtain rather smaller (though still positive) wage elasticities than those found in other studies. This qualification is likely to be somewhat irrelevant in designing a response to the labour shortage faced by the NHS in the 1990s. It was appropriate to the early 1980s where abundant labour (especially amongst the young) limited the ability of workers to implement their supply preferences and where the case for wage increases was consequently much weaker. That is less likely to be the situation in the 1990s in the labour market for women workers. In fact the reverse is likely to be true. The results (including the large wage elasticities for women) obtained from the majority of labour supply studies which do not explicitly model the demand constraint (which are shown in Tables 6.2 and 6.3) are therefore appropriate to the formulation of a shortage strategy.

Also relevant is the work of Joshi (1988) and Ermisch and Wright (1989) both of which use the WES survey. Joshi uses the full sample of 4,348 women and finds a much larger wage elasticity for women, who work full-time. This is notably the case for married women, for whom the wage elasticity is +1.88 compared with +0.59 for the sample as a whole. Similarly Ermisch and Wright, who use the same data set, find the wage elasticity for married women working full-time is approximately twice as large as that for part-time. The reliability of these estimates is enhanced by the fact that, unlike other studies, Ermisch and Wright employ a methodology which allows for the fact that women who work part-time receive significantly inferior wage offers than those who work full-time. As a result they are able to demonstrate that a wage increase that also widens the full-time/part-time wage differential increases both the number of women who work and the proportion who opt for full-time work.

Ermisch and Wright also show that these responses are not independent of educational qualifications and occupational status. Their estimates suggest that the rate of return to investment in formal training is 60 per cent lower for women in a part-time compared with someone in a full-time job. Since the opportunity cost of opting for part-time rather than full-time work is so high for women who possess formal qualifications (like nurses and others in the NHS) they are not only more more likely to work but also to work full-time rather than part-time. According to Perry (1990) they also return to work more quickly. Phillips (1989b) finds this to be true of nurses, especially those who possess qualifications that enable them to obtain the SRN qualification. Interestingly, the UK studies of other professions in which women with formal qualifications dominate, conform with this general pattern. For example, Dolton (1990), in a study of women teachers, shows that the wage elasticity for qualified women teachers is also large. This is precisely what the evidence reviewed above would suggest is the case for highly qualified staff in the NHS.

To summarise, the evidence from studies of female labour supply suggests that a general increase in wages in female dominated occupations can be an effective cure for any labour shortage arising from the shortfall in young recruits. If female wages generally were to rise (in real terms) in the 1990s, this could enable the NHS to draw upon the increasing supply of married women workers, many of whom will require some form of training. If such an increase doesn't happen, unless the NHS at least maintains its position in terms of relative wages, the share of this source of labour employed in the NHS could fall, thus worsening the projected labour shortage.

The case for an above average wage increase is strongest for the formally qualified women on whom the NHS depends. The evidence suggests this will evoke an especially strong response, will retain existing employees and accelerate the return to work of women who have withdrawn for family reasons. More of these qualified women will opt for full-time work compared with the unqualified if the gap between the reward for full-time compared with part-time work is widened at the same time as the differential enjoyed by the qualified compared with other female workers is increased. The Phillips (1989b) study suggests that the latter differential is already too low, especially for entrants who possess an 'A' level. For this group, nursing offers a poor financial return for their qualifications. It would clearly improve matters further if, in addition to increased wages, the NHS were to actively reduce the financial penalty (e.g. through loss of seniority) imposed on most qualified women employees when they withdraw from work to have and rear children.

There is also a dynamic impact, which prolongs the beneficial impact of these wage changes and which should be taken into account. In Britain, as in the US, women who have worked more in the past are more likely to be presently employed. Increases in the current level of female participation persist. This persistence in employment is an especially strong feature of women who possess formal qualifications. It is usually explained by the positive effect of work experience on pay for all workers, especially the qualified. Ermisch and Wright (1989) in Britain and Eckstein and Wolpin (1989) in the US both provide evidence for the existence of this effect.

The impact of such wage increases will also be stronger if other changes outside NHS control take place. It would enhance the effectiveness of wage increases in the NHS if, for example, the government chose to give favourable tax treatment to married women, especially those who work full-time.

6.4   Non-wage influences on labour supply

The evidence of the labour supply studies also suggests a case for non-wage strategies in respect of women workers and these are now considered. The first such influence is labour income from other members of the household. Although income which benefits, but is not earned by NHS employees, affects their labour supply decisions and is therefore a

96

relevant constraint on policy to cure a labour shortage, it is clearly not a matter over which the service has direct control. This section is therefore deliberately brief.

Spouse's income

Most important to the labour supply of married women is the income of their husband. Increases in a husband's income provokes the same direction of response as other forms of non-own labour income but the effect is much stronger as Table 6.2 shows. Perry's (1990) study confirms this for women returners to market work. He shows increases in family income not only decrease the probability of a wife's participation but also increase the preference for part-time as opposed to full-time work. The Phillips (1989b) study of nurses lumps together all non-own labour income. The outcome of the estimation is a very small income effect (-0.02). The effect for married women is a little larger but still very small. However, it is important to note that the level of alternative income is much higher for married women. In the entire WES sample Joshi (1988) shows it to be £90.73 for married and £16.73 for unmarried women. This fact obviously makes it less likely that a married woman who benefits from her husband's wage will work and the financial incentive needed to overcome this is commensurately higher.

The main exception to this pattern occurs for women whose husbands are unemployed. The basic theory predicts that the loss of a husband's income arising from unemployment should increase women's participation through financial necessity. However, as Kell and Wright (1990) show, this tends to be offset by the operation of the social security system in the UK, which discourages the participation of the wives of unemployed men by imposing a strong financial penalty. As a result pay increases (unless they are substantial enough to take the household out of the poverty trap) will be less effective in evoking a positive labour supply response: a) in areas where male unemployment is high, b) among lower paid female occupational groups for whom this effect is most pronounced and c) if male unemployment increases in the 1990s. Most forecasts suggest that unemployment is likely to remain high, at least in the short term (see Chapters 3 and 4). Offsetting this effect on females is that male recruitment will become easier, notably in the manual categories of employment.

Non labour income

Most studies of labour supply also find evidence of effects of non-labour income in the form of transfer payments, property income and so on. Indeed the presence of such data is indispensable to the estimation of the size of the income effect. In studies of male labour supply this is strongly negative, producing the wage elasticities shown in Table 6.1. In the studies of female labour supply shown in Table 6.2, the income effect is

97

also negative but rather small and insufficient to overcome the impact of a strong substitution effect.

The 'home' wage

The basic theory outlined in Section 6.3 suggests that the economic activity rates of married women will increase not only in response to increases in the market wage but also if the home wage falls. According to the WES data, 75 per cent of female NHS employees are married so any reduction that takes place would help reduce labour shortages. There is an extensive list of variables which have been included in labour supply studies as determinants of the home wage. Few, if any of these are subject to direct manipulation by the NHS although the effects of some could be influenced indirectly. The most widely used and the most significant are variables that reflect family composition. Children increase the value of time spent in non-market work and hence increase the home wage. This significantly reduces the labour supply of 'married' women. This effect is not independent of the children's age and is most pronounced where young children are present. Older children, in contrast can act as substitutes for time spent by mothers in the home and increase the family utility derived from consumption goods relative to time spent on child care. Hence the presence of older children in the home tends to reduce the home wage, thus removing the restraint on labour force participation that arises when they are younger. Most of the labour supply literature finds the effect to be strong. Sprague (1988), for example, using time series data, finds that the presence of children under 10 significantly reduced the growth in female labour supply over the 1954-82 period. In contrast the number of children over 10 has no significant effect. Briscoe and Wilson (1992) come to similar conclusions. Similarly Gomulka and Stern (1990), who use a series of FES cross-sections between 1970-83, find that 4 of the overall 9 percentage point increase in labour force activity can be attributed to the decline in the average number of young children per household that took place in this period.

Several cross-section studies confirm that young children restrain women's employment in Britain. Using WES data, Joshi's (1988) results are typical. She shows that mothers with babies under one year of age are 64 per cent less likely to have a paid job than otherwise similar women with no dependent children. As the age of the youngest dependent child rises, the effect diminishes. Mothers with children aged 6-10 are only 13 per cent less likely to have employment than 'child-free' women. The impact of children of secondary school age is zero. Additional children under 5 enhance the effect of one child but not proportionately so. Joshi also finds (like Blundell and Walker, 1982) that the presence of other than the youngest, additional, teenage children actually increases the chances of their mothers having jobs, reflecting the fact that the care of young children is time intensive, while that of teenage children is goods intensive.

Joshi summarises the 'lifetime direct effects' of having more children in greater detail. These results are shown in Table 6.4 and reveal the significant but non-linear character of these effects. The table also indicates that the impact of young children deters participation in full-time work more than it does part-time. This is confirmed by both Perry (1990) who shows that the return to full-time work is restricted by children to a significantly greater extent than part-time work and also by Ermisch and Wright (1989).

These very important child effects on the home wage and employment are also revealed by studies of the labour supply of nurses shown in Table 6.3. These results are surveyed in detail by Phillips (1989a and 1989b). Her own work for Britain includes three family composition variables. The presence of a child under 2 has a large negative effect on participation. A significant but smaller effect is found when children aged 2-5 are present. Similar results are obtained when the total number of children is included. On the basis of these strong estimates, Phillips concludes 'the greatest barrier to female participation are exogenous family constraints'.

This conclusion is typical of the extant literature. It implies clearly that the provision by employers or by the state of high standard childcare (especially for the under fives) is likely to be the single most effective way of decreasing the home wage and thereby increasing participation in market work. This is as true of the NHS as any other employer. Unfortunately, none of the existing econometric studies tests this directly by including a child care availability variable but there are some relevant descriptive statistics for the EC shown in Figures 6.1 and 6.2. These show quite clearly that in EC countries where state provision of under five childcare is generous the activity rate of women with young children is significantly higher. In the absence of adequate state provision, these results clearly indicate that to retain, attract and accelerate the return of female employees the NHS, which is better placed to do so than many employers, needs to provide under-five child care facilities or to subsidise childcare costs for its working parents.

There are other determinants of the home wage. The valuation of non-market time , it is often argued , depends on education and training. Sprague (1988), for example, finds that the post-war increase in the school staying-on rate of 17 year-old girls has led to decreased fertility and increased labour market activity in later life. One explanation for this is that qualified women have attitudes to work that value non-market time at a lower rate than their unqualified counterparts. They are more likely to work as a result. This effect is in addition to the financial incentive of the higher levels of market pay they receive. In fact little other evidence exists to support this view. Phillips (1989b), for example, finds the possession of an 'A' level which ensures entry to SRN status, raises nurses' pay and, as a consequence, economic activity. But when included separately in a participation equation it has an insignificantly negative

Figure 6.1
Activity rates of women with and without children in the member states

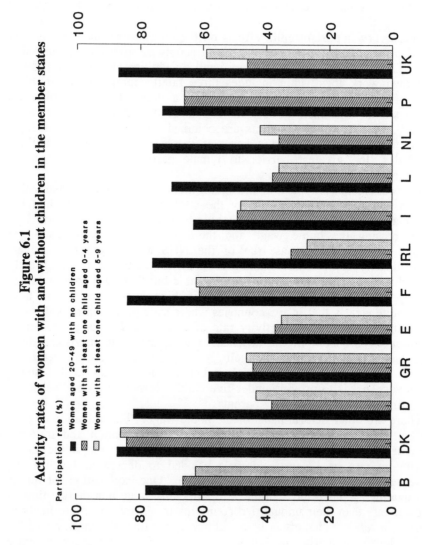

Participation rate (%)

■ Women aged 20-49 with no children

▨ Women with at least one child aged 0-4 years

▥ Women with at least one child aged 5-9 years

Source : CEC (1990)

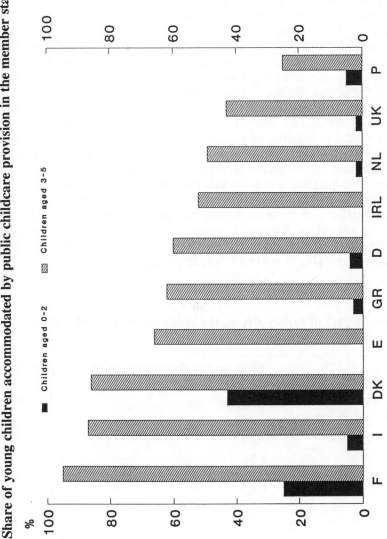

Figure 6.2
Share of young children accommodated by public childcare provision in the member states

Children aged 0-2   Children aged 3-5

Source : CEC (1990)

101

effect and not the positive one implied by the argument above. Ermisch and Wright (1989) come to a similar conclusion using a much broader sample of women workers. The implication is that, if it wants to step up the participation rate of the qualified staff it has trained, the NHS cannot rely on some exogenous fall in their home wage taking place as they become disenchanted with home work. It must offer higher pay and affect the home wage directly by the same means it would use for all staff.

A number of other variables have also been employed in empirical studies on the grounds that they are determinants of the home wage and therefore of female labour supply. Most of these variables cannot be affected by the NHS, so they are either not discussed at all here or only mentioned in terms of the way they might constrain the operation of a policy for labour shortage. One variable that has featured prominently, in the studies that use the WES data, is the possession of a mortgage. Phillips (1989b), for example, shows that household debt of this form increases the probability of participation by nurses. Ermisch and Wright (1989) find the same but they also find that it does not affect the full-time/part-time preferences of women as a whole. The time series evidence of Sprague (1988) reveals that increases in the interest rate, that intensify the burden of mortgage debt, increase the supply of women in the labour market. If home ownership continues to grow in the 1990s, this could be one of the favourable exogenous factors which leads to greater participation, creating an increased supply of labour upon which the NHS can draw especially if interest rates remain high.

Table 6.4
Effect of family size on the economic activity of women

	Reduction attributable to children in years of	
Number of children	Paid work	Full-time work
One	3.2	5.7
Two	4.9	7.5
Three	6.6	9.2
Four	8.5	10.9

Source: Joshi (1984).

6.5 Main implications

General economic studies of labour supply produce some clear implications for dealing with the demographically induced labour shortages that are likely to face the NHS in the 1990s. General wage increases which are weighted in favour of new entrants and highly qualified employees could prove a potent weapon for avoiding potential labour shortage, especially among the female staff upon whom the NHS depends.

In order to retain existing married women staff, to accelerate the speed of return of previous employees and to aid recruitment of other women the labour supply studies also imply that a variety of non-wage strategies could be appropriate, the most important of which is the provision of improved workplace childcare facilities or the subsidisation of the costs of childcare.

7 Demand and supply within the NHS: General issues

7.1 Introduction

Economics provides a framework to analyse labour shortages, and employers' responses. If an employer faces, or expects to face, a shortfall of labour, their correct 'market response' is to raise the wage rate.

This action should both increase the attractiveness of the employer's jobs to potential employees and encourage the employer himself to use the labour more efficiently. This indeed is the line taken by Maynard in a short and decidedly pithy piece on nursing shortages (Maynard, 1987). Until very recently, however, when a small amount of money was set aside for a pilot project on pay flexibility, such advice was unheeded. This was not necessarily out of stubbornness or inertia, but owing to beliefs about the supply side (see below) and, more recently, in line with a general expectation that the take-off of the Self Governing Trust movement would diminish the importance of central pay bargaining.

Consider, for example, the attitude of the NHS to labour 'market forces', as revealed in the annual reports of the pay review body for nurses and professions allied to medicine (PAMs). This body was set up in 1983, following an industrial dispute, to provide the government with independent advice. It has produced eight pairs of reports to date (Review Body, annual 1984 to 1991). These reveal that the two 'sides' took classic positions in their submissions. The workers based their cases for large increases on arguments of fairness and comparability, pointing out that the NHS, as an employer, dominates the market for nursing and PAM labour and that staff were not, therefore, free to move jobs - the ultimate market sanction against niggardly employers. In technical terms the NHS is what economists would term a monopsonist - the sole buyer in the market.

For the first three years, the management's case for small increases was firmly based on the conventional argument of self interest that they were not at that time experiencing any difficulty in recruiting and retaining staff at the then current pay levels.

They were unable to back this argument with any hard data (perhaps an indication of how much this was then a buyer's market) but the Review Body did the best it could to provide itself with some independent and objective evidence on the state of the market and, with a few qualifications, confirmed the management's view.

But this of course still begs the question of whether the NHS may be exploiting its position as a monopsonist - it does not address the employees' claims that *fairness* should be the basis of wage rates in a market where existing trained staff have very few alternative employers.

The 4th and 5th Reports (Review Body, 1987a, 1987b, 1988a and 1988b) revealed a growing awareness of a change in the state of the market, but also exhibited a tendency for management to regard the problem as confined to particular skill groups (e.g. occupational therapists) and particular locations (London). By the sixth report, this line of argument was no longer tenable and the management side appeared to adopt a rather ambivalent attitude towards the power of market forces. With respect to nurses:

> Demographic trends meant that the NHS would find increasing difficulty in meeting demand from the traditional source of suitably qualified school leavers. In the Department's view, however, pay related solutions based on successive real terms increases were likely to prove both costly and ineffective and would lead to leap-frogging levels of settlements between competing employers. They would prefer a more accurately directed response to particular skill and geographical shortages. (Review Body, 1989a, p.4)

But with respect to PAMs, against a background of unfilled vacancies:

> The Department said that, because the results of our survey of vacancies related to the position at 31 March 1988, they would not give any indication of the effect of the 1988 pay award on recruitment and retention. They would, however, expect the position to improve as the impact of the subsequent pay increase was felt. (Review Body, 1989b, p.4)

There are three possible interpretations of this evidence. The first is that this is simply an example of a common tendency amongst those involved in pay negotiations to use the 'market forces' argument when convenient and ignore it when not. The second is that the NHS continues

105

to believe that market forces operate rather less effectively where female labour is concerned. Under this interpretation the management's dismissal of the comparability argument used by the other side can be made intelligible. It is argued that women are not pay/career minded and female dominated jobs have always been less well paid than male dominated ones. The shortage of labour within the NHS therefore cannot be blamed on comparatively low wage rates and there is no point in reacting to a shortage by paying them more - they wouldn't respond. The evidence for and against this view is examined in more detail in Chapter 8.

A third interpretation is that the NHS management is taking an anti-market forces' line, not because it doubts the effectiveness of such forces on supply, but because it genuinely believes it cannot afford to pay its workforce market-determined wage rates. Virtually all official publications comment on the high percentage of NHS expenditure devoted to the purchase of labour (e.g. see the CPA reports discussed in Chapter 1. The nursing wage bill alone accounts for over a third of the annual cost of the NHS, the bill for the other associate professions is a little under 10 per cent. So real increases in wage rates, especially for nurses, have large repercussions. Thus management could well feel that, constrained by the budget, it really cannot afford to respond to economic advice to pay higher wages. Of course, it is not surprising to find an employer saying such things, and economists should indeed be sceptical of such claims. But on the other hand the NHS does work under a rather unusual budget constraint.

In 1989 the Department of Health (DoH) asked the Review body to set aside £5m to finance a pilot flexible pay scheme for nurses. This they did, and the matter is discussed in subsequent reports (Review Body, 1990a and 1990b). Essentially the scheme is predicated on the argument that there is no general shortage of labour, rather staff shortages are seen as occurring only in particular locations and for particular types of skills. Thus, so the argument goes, large across-the-board pay rises would be a costly means of tackling the problem. A cheaper solution is the use of selective supplements to general pay levels, applied only in identified shortage areas. The particular scheme piloted was for discretionary supplements, up to a maximum value of £1,000 over the year, on posts judged appropriate by local management. The DoH subsequently asked the Review Body both to extend and develop the scheme for nurses and to introduce a similar one for PAMs. The Review body declined. Its ground for doing so was the failure of the DoH to monitor the scheme. It indicated that it was not prepared to see the scheme spread until it had evidence of its cost effectiveness, and it 'expected' the DoH to provide a full evaluation of the existing pilot for the next year's review. The Department of Health duly submitted the results of a monitoring exercise which was reported in the 1991 volume for nurses. A questionnaire was sent to participating managers and a small number of non-participating ones. This aimed to elicit basic factual data on management opinions on how the schemes were going. The Department concluded that a general scheme could contribute at a comparatively modest level to tackling recruitment and retention problems but noted that it is not guaranteed to work and not always appropriate. Thus it recognised that a general scheme would have to be introduced with care if the NHS is to avoid industrial relations problems and difficulties over differentials. There was little or no explicit discussion of economic issues however. The opinion of RHA chairmen was also sought, and they appeared to be strongly in favour of such developments. The staff side was more critical of the monitoring exercise on grounds that it was nothing more than the opinion of managers. The Review Body (1991) was not impressed with the quality of the monitoring exercise undertaken. Criticising the Health Departments for their failure to meet in full the conditions in the case of the pilot scheme, the Report commented that no firm conclusions can be drawn from the exercise:

- the monitoring exercise produced 'variable quality data'

- the lack of adequate controls make it impossible for managers to judge whether flexible pay, as opposed to other things, were affecting recruitment and retention.

It concluded: 'Given the need for care in applying flexible pay if effective results are to be secured, we hope that our concerns will be kept in mind in the forthcoming discussions on a more extensive scheme for flexible pay'. (Review Body, 1991, paragraphs 56 and 58.)

The DOH did not press its proposal to extend the existing pilot scheme. Instead it proposed negotiations with the staff side on the introduction of a general scheme apparently intending to do nothing more till those negotiations are over. The Review Body stated that it 'awaits with interest the outcome of the negotiations'.

Non-pay measures for aiding recruitment could also be important (see the discussion in Chapters 6 and 13 for a detailed case). This has not figured too heavily in the Review Body's deliberations. Child care vouchers were discussed in the 1990 PAM report but are not mentioned in the 1991 volumes. There are just a few comments in both reports about there appearing to be much interest in non-pay measures for aiding recruitment and retention, but little action as yet. Given the conclusions in Chapters 6 and 13 this may require further attention if and when labour markets do tighten again.

And there, for the moment, the matter rests. The DoH, however, is clearly interested in exploring the idea of flexible pay. The literature surveyed here is, with the exception of the Review Body reports, remarkable only for its silence on this topic. Yet the Review Body is quite right, there are issues which ought to be examined before such schemes become widespread and entrenched:

(i) It is not immediately obvious that local pay flexibility will work as a solution to a problem of 'patchy' labour shortage under any and all scenarios. For example, the effect of the wage supplements may be to induce some increase in total supply, but is also likely to cause some relocation of existing supply. Therefore, the cost effectiveness of the policy is likely to depend on how those two effects compare and on the extent to which the original problem was one of a plentiful, but mislocated, supply of labour as opposed to one of a general labour shortage, mild enough to manifest itself only as an inability to fill the least attractive posts. Clearly, therefore, the NHS needs to know something about the conditions under which local pay flexibility might be expected to work and to be a cost effective solution to a 'patchy' labour shortage problem.

(ii) It is plausible to assume that labour supply responds to wage signals with a time lag. Now most parties seem to be agreed that, although it has yet to manifest itself in any very serious way, a potential general shortage of nursing and PAM staff is imminent. This raises the question of the extent to which the existing pay structure should be designed to anticipate the future rather than current state of the labour market. To answer such questions the NHS needs to know something about those time lags.

(iii) It is not obvious how well such schemes will sit with the internal market. If the objective with respect to the geographical location of health care facilities is that of equal access (i.e. there should be one hospital per so many head of population) and if wages in general vary across the country, then there might be a case for a centrally funded scheme permitting local flexibility in wages such that RHAs in high labour cost areas are able to hire enough staff to permit them to provide the same level of service as those in low labour cost areas. However, the objective behind the internal market is supposed to be that of efficiency. Hospitals able to offer cheaper contracts are supposed to expand at the expense of others. Among other things this should mean that, *ceteris paribus*, hospitals in low labour cost areas expand relative to those in other areas. If the government uses central funds to allow hospitals in high labour cost areas to compete, it will be queering its own pitch.

7.2 Workforce planning

Neoclassical economics predicts that as the relative costs of inputs (e.g. labour, materials and capital), change, so does the method of production, and hence the quantities of each type of input required. In other words there can be a *trade-off* between factors - if doctors become more expensive, then more of their marginal activities can be undertaken by paramedics and nurses. There is, of course, enormous resistance from the professions and trades to seeing jobs in this light - hospitals have replaced printing works as the theatre for demarcation as an art form. Two of the reasons why the 'internal market' has been introduced have been first, to attempt to de-institutionalize production methods thereby affording managers more flexibility, and secondly to introduce an accounting system to measure, for the first time, the actual costs of production.

But up to now there have been few studies of the NHS demand-for-labour function. Lindsay (1980) applies a (very American) bureaucratic model to the NHS and finds some evidence of 'vote buying' via investments in marginal constituencies. Cohen (1972) and Hurd (1973) investigate the effects of hospital monopsony power in the nursing market and conclude that it does hold down wages and thereby creates 'shortages'. These are American studies and thus their conclusions are not directly applicable. However, both consider the motivations of non-profit (in the American sense) hospitals and so provide food for thought on how to approach the issue in the British context.

There appears to be very little, if any, published work which gives a pure economic analysis of the NHS demand for labour in the sense of being constructed around a demand function, as normally understood by economists. There is, however, a literature on the determination of staffing requirements within the NHS, to which we now turn. This work is generally carried on under the umbrella of *workforce planning*, which also contains a supply side element which is examined in Chapters 8 and 10.

The contention resulting from a review of this literature is that the NHS has not done all that it could do to reduce its demand for labour in the face of its shortages. To some extent, this point cannot be separated from the previous one, namely that wage rates have been highly inflexible. If, at the highest level, management fails to respond to a worsening labour market by raising the wage rate, then management lower down in the hierarchy has no incentive to economise on that labour. This economic point should not be overplayed, however. The dominant theme to come across from this literature is that, at least until fairly recently, inefficiency in the use of labour resulted mostly from poor - and not uncommonly non-existent - information and inadequate managerial skill at all levels of the organization.

This conclusion is drawn, in particular, from a study of the series of reports by CPA and NAO already referred to in Chapter 1. These two bodies are, of course, concerned with financial control over public expenditure. Their comments on staff planning within the NHS arose from concern over the rapid growth in employment of nurses and P&T staffing throughout the 1970s and early 1980s. As mentioned in Chapter 1, there were reasons to expect some growth in employment, but at least part of the increase was thought to have been a rather uncontrolled, budget-led expansion of questionable efficiency. Thus in the first of these reports (Committee of Public Accounts, 1981) the CPA, after considering possible explanations for the growth in NHS staff between 1971 and 1979, was highly critical of the DHSS for lack of central control. It highlighted: (a) very poor information on staffing at the centre; and (b) the failure of the centre to investigate, or even comment upon, differences between HAs in their employment levels. Two subsequent reports continued to nag away at the same point (CPA, 1982 and 1984).

What the CPA revealed was that staffing requirements were being determined low down within the hierarchy of the NHS with little guidance and no control from above. The centre knew little about how individual HAs were determining their staffing requirements and had no means of assessing their efficiency. Amongst other things, this exposure sparked the DHSS into investigating the methods used by HAs to determine their nursing requirements (DHSS Operational Research Service, 1980). This revealed a variety of methods at varying levels of sophistication - but, with few exceptions, very little emphasis was placed on economic constraints.

'Top down' approaches

These approaches predict workforce requirements on the basis of a chosen relationship between a measure of workforce and one or more measures of demand for care and/or activity. That relationship may be one which has been observed to hold in the past or elsewhere within the system, or it may be a policy choice as to what constitutes a best/adequate/minimum acceptable level of staffing. Thus, for example, a simple nurse/bed ratio may be used to predict future requirements for ward nurses from forecasts of future hospital bed provision and occupation. Three levels of sophistication were identified as shown in Table 7.1.

Only the third of these methods makes any reference to the relative cost and availability of manpower. Factor substitution is simply not recognised as an issue. Most approaches therefore parallel the classic employment functions used in labour economics in the 1960s and early seventies which emphasise the link between employment and some measure of activity (typically output). Since the 1970s there has been a radical reassessment of the appropriate method of modelling labour demand. This puts much greater emphasis on the role of factor prices. For a review of this literature see Briscoe and Wilson (1992).

'Bottom up' approaches

Staffing requirements for individual wards are predicted from the number and characteristics of patients cared for, on the basis of work study appraisals which seek to determine the workload generated by different categories of patients. Compared to 'top down' methods, they are likely to produce more accurate measures of current workload but they are really

110

low level decision making aids rather than strategic planning/control ones.

Table 7.1
Methods of prediction of future nursing requirements

a) Norms or simple ratios (e.g. the nurse/bed ratio)	Where the centre offered guidance, it tended to be in this form. These are therefore fairly common. Because workload is being indicated by one very simple surrogate (e.g. occupied beds) they are crude (e.g. will not reflect factors such as possible variations in the degree of nursing dependency of whoever occupies the beds). They are also capable of being misused through a failure to appreciate how the norm or ratio was chosen (simple continuation of past practice, policy variable plucked out of the air, policy variable based on some sort of scientific appraisal, etc.).
b) Multiple linear regression	Rare. Two models are quoted: the Trent model (Trent RHA/ Trent Regional Nursing Officers Dept., 1978; and West Midlands RHA, 1980); and the ORS model (DHSS/Operational Research Service, 1980; and DHSS/ORS, 1982). The way the Trent model was used is particularly interesting in view of the subsequent development of 'performance indicators'. In it, the determining variables are a number of measures of activity. The regression coefficients are re-estimated annually from data from all hospitals in the Region. They are then used to estimate, for each hospital individually, its staffing needs if it had applied 'regional average practice' to its particular activities. Hospitals which show a significant divergence between actual employment and estimated staffing needs are then highlighted for further investigation.
c) Models including financial constraints	Rare. Only one quoted: the Wessex model (Cree, 1978; and DHSS/Maplin, 1981). This is not actually a formal model, but it is of interest since it is the only one to give explicit consideration to the possible constraint imposed on staffing requirements by the budget. Strategies are identified by first identifying areas of care where there is a gap between desirable standards and actual practice and then by determining priorities between them according to the budget constraint.

111

They are in relatively common use. Mention should be made of the Aberdeen formula (Scottish Home and Health Dept., 1969; and Gault, 1982) since it was, for a time, adopted by the whole of Scotland. The most widely copied example of this type of approach is, however, that due to Barr (Barr, 1964; Oxford RHB, 1967; and Mulligan, 1973). Within their own terms, these approaches suffer from two weaknesses. They are vague on the question of variability in workload - should the staffing establishment be that necessary to cover the maximum workload or the average one? They are also vague on the question of quality of care - the work studies to determine 'necessary' time required for any given type of patient care activity leave unclear whether that is the time necessary to provide top quality care, adequate care, or the minimum care acceptable. In economic terms, they ignore the budget constraint and the relative cost and availability of labour.

Three further studies comment on the extent to which any form of systematic method of staffing determination is used. NAO, asked to investigate the control of nursing manpower by CPA, observes that a number of HAs fail to use any 'formula' for determining their nursing requirements and, of the rest, some are merely historically set ratios (National Audit Office, 1985a and 1985b). Not surprisingly, given the variety of methods and non-methods in use, staffing ratios are found to vary across HAs. A similar story is revealed in its report on the control of P&T staffing, again for CPA (NAO, 1987): no common method for determining staffing needs; a tendency to rely on historically determined staffing establishments; little evidence of fundamental review of requirements and wide variation in staff/workload ratios across HAs.

A survey of HAs conducted in 1984 and reported in Long and Mercer (1987, ch.7) confirms the picture. They report a general movement towards the adoption of some kind of workload based (i.e. 'bottom up') approach, but this is still far from universal and is only used as a supplement to professional judgement. Corroboration for this finding is provided by the All Wales Nurse Manpower Planning Committee (1985) This committee explicitly restricted its search for a method to adopt in its area to 'bottom up' ones, on the grounds of their acceptability to nurse managers. Further, it emphasises that, whatever method they finally decide to adopt, the role of 'professional judgement' will continue to be recognised as an important one.

The Long and Mercer survey is also of interest in that it found staffing requirements to be determined at a low level within HAs; usually that of the departmental head. It is tempting to draw inferences about the degree of importance therefore accorded to workforce planning and control. The implication pursued by the authors is that requirements are therefore determined on a staff group by staff group basis (see Table 7.2). Inevitably, they find that professional interests tend to dominate: 'One is left with the impression that staffing is planned more to support professional interests than to provide staffing teams with skills and experiences appropriate to meet patient needs' (*ibid.* p.141).

Table 7.2
Manpower planning as a multi-disciplinary approach

% all groups

	Totally	To some extent	Unacc-eptable	Don't know
Estimated staffing requirements on a staff group basis	74	21	4	1
Planned staffing requirements across staff groups: a multi-disciplinary approach	8[a]	80[b]	4	8
Pursuit of the WHO objective of manpower planning, specifying teams and their composition	0	46	51	3

Source: Long and Mercer (1987).
(a) Currently in use.
(b) Either seen as a useful approach and beginning to be adopted, or seen as a useful approach and pursuing it in the future.

It might be added that it is also likely to imply a failure to consider efficiency questions of skill mix and factor substitution. This is indeed an area rarely referred to in the internal literature. However, an econometric analysis of Scottish hospital cost data over the period 1951-81 does suggest that the NHS manages at least sometimes to substitute factors in response to changes in relative costs (Gray *et al.*, 1989). Whether it does so with efficiency is another matter and one not capable of being answered by the approach adopted in that study.

Wagstaff (1989a), in his survey of British econometric studies on health economics, mentions three other studies as giving some (though not central) consideration to the issue of factor substitution: Feldstein (1967); Lavers and Whynes (1978); and McGuire and Westoby (1983). He is, however, rather dismissive and suggests that little reliance should be placed on their conclusions. Part of the problem arises because the NHS is not a profit-motivated, market-orientated organization. As Wagstaff says, in criticising the approach adopted by McGuire and Westoby and

Gray and McGuire, one cannot assume cost minimising behaviour. It might be added that one also cannot assume factor costs are market clearing prices (We have argued above that wages may be far from what their equilibrium levels would be in a more competitive environment). Very little of the traditional economic approach to the estimation of production and cost functions is self evidently applicable to the NHS, and much work therefore remains to be done in order to develop more appropriate models.

Grade mix within the nursing profession, and among PAMs is now, of course, a live issue. Regrading exercises have taken place throughout the NHS in order to make workforce planning more systematic. Middle managers (ward sisters and the tier just above, laboratory managers, speech therapy service managers etc.) have been obliged to define their staffing requirements in terms of job descriptions and responsibilities, rather than professional qualifications.

The NAO report on the nursing workforce (National Audit Office, 1985a and 1985b) suggested that there is likely to be scope for efficiency gains from its consideration, and the All Wales Nurse Manpower Planning Committee (1985) identified skill mix as a priority area for study. HSRU received the research commission. Much impetus is likely to come from the reform of nurse training. The reform itself is discussed in more depth in a later section but, in brief, its relevance here is that proposals to upgrade the training (and therefore the cost) of qualified nurses are succeeding in concentrating minds on the question of the qualified/unqualified nurse mix. Maynard (1987), thinks there is scope for substituting unqualified for qualified labour, and this was demonstrated simply by Robinson et al. (1989). The Audit Commission (Audit Commission for England and Wales, 1991) has recently reiterated some of the conclusions of the NAO, in a report which also offers hostages to fortune in its commendation of the professional system of primary nursing.

The DHSS has published one study on grade mix (Wright-Warren, 1986) but, as the author emphasises, it is a strictly limited reconnaissance of uncharted territory. It contains an instructive literature review. Their literature search revealed only one study which looked explicitly at the effect of varying grade mix and that was American and 20 years old (Miller and Bryant, 1965). Otherwise, the literature refers only to recommended or target qualified/unqualified ratios chosen largely on the basis of opinion (and professional interest) rather than systematic study. Wright-Warren concludes:

> However, the study found little evidence of specific studies having been undertaken at district or ward level to evaluate historical staffing patterns or justify the target ratios of qualified to unqualified staff which were sometimes quoted. The more systematic evaluation and analysis that could be undertaken for the sample of geriatric wards studied confirmed the influence of historical district and hospital

patterns in determining ward staffing levels. (Wright-Warren, 1986, p.vii)

and continues:

We were concerned, but not surprised, to find that staffing and skill mix levels were set on the basis of past staffing patterns rather than from a systematic assessment of patients' needs. It would be easy to recommend further national research to develop, for example, acceptable methodologies for setting staffing levels and grade mix. We have not done so. In our view, the overriding problem is not one of further research but that a higher priority should be given by management to achieving the best value for money by adoption of methods of allocating staffing resources more closely related to the needs of patients and ward objectives. (*ibid.* p.viii)

7.3 Some recent developments

Some more recent studies have been undertaken, or recently started, which acknowledge that in certain circumstances one type of labour may be substituted for another. These are in contrast to most previous studies which have been concerned, as we have shown, with norms for particular professional groups without considering the possibility of trade off between different types of staff. These studies are: the publication of a description of a multi-disciplinary project to determine the desired nursing staff level and grade mix for wards in a new hospital (Ball *et al.*, 1989); the publication of the findings of a study by two US economists into the effect of nurse staffing levels on patient health and cost of care (Flood and Diers, 1988); a study at the University of Warwick financed by the Welsh Office, of skill mix within the context of ward decision making; and the initiation, at the Centre for Health Economics (CHE) University of York, of two DoH-funded studies in this area. The Warwick study, with complex objectives, has not yet reported, but should provide some evidence concerning the degree to which explicit nursing models, including grade mix, are adhered to, and implicitly therefore, the 'room for manoeuvre' in determining a cost effective mix of staff. An outline of what is intended for the two new studies at the CHE is given in the CHE Newsletter, issue No. 7 (Aug. 1990). The first is entitled skill mix and effectiveness of nursing care. The only output thus far is a literature survey (Gibbs, McCaughan and Griffiths, 1990). The second study is quoted as aiming to investigate the ability of the American DRG (Diagnosis Related Group) patient classification system to map the patient-related variability in nursing workload. It is entitled DRGs and Nursing Workload. Again it has yet to be published.

Ball *et al.* (1989) reports a project funded by Mersey RHA which involved applying an existing human resource planning methodology called *Criteria for Care*, to determine both the level and, with some adaptation, mix of staffing for the wards of a new hospital. The general approach estimates only the overall staffing level and requires the collection of three pieces of information for a sample of wards: (i) ward workload, as indicated by patient dependency; (ii) staff activity, as indicated by an analysis of time spent on different categories of activity, by grade; and (iii) quality of care provided, as indicated by number of items checked as done on a list of quality objectives. A staffing formula for each speciality is developed from a cross-analysis of the workload and activity pattern of those wards within that speciality which were scored as achieving 70 per cent or more of the quality objectives. Essentially, this approach is in the tradition of the non-economic methodologies described above. In introducing a quality of care dimension, this approach explicitly attempts to identify a normative standard of staffing - i.e. the amount of staffing necessary to provide a pre-determined minimum standard of care. There is, however, no explicit reference to evidence that high scores on the quality of care check list correlate with better patient outcomes and, of course, there is no formal appreciation of the possibility of trade-off between standard of care and staffing costs.

For the purposes of the Mersey RHA project, this general approach had to be adapted to produce a recommended grade mix, in addition to the recommended overall staffing establishment. How this was done is of some interest. First, the project team note that activity analysis reveals that a significant percentage of trained nursing time is spent on 'work which could more suitably be done by support staff', *op.cit.* (p.ii). That is '... between 18-28 per cent of nursing time is spent on activities listed under the heading "associated work", most of which are regarded as non-nursing, i.e. cleaning, housekeeping ...', *op.cit.*, (p.12). To determine a normative grade mix, therefore, this study had to consider the question of the types of task that ought to be performed by each grade, rather than the range of tasks they actually undertake. It began to do this with the aid of a questionnaire sent to nursing staff asking their opinion on the competence of each grade to perform the activities included in the activity analysis. The responses suggested that, in the opinion of those asked, only trained staff, or at least untrained staff under the supervision of trained staff, were competent to carry out quite a number of the 'associated tasks'. Bluntly, the project team were unhappy with this result and simply rejected it in favour of their own opinions that these 'non-nursing' duties ought to be performed by care assistants, hotel workers and ward clerks. Thus they recommended that the grade mix should contain a lower proportion of trained to untrained staff than is currently the case. Note, this recommendation is again reached without any formal assessment of the effect of grade mix on patient outcome and without consideration of the relative cost effectiveness of different grade mixes.

To play devil's advocate, the currently relatively narrow differential between the pay rates of trained and untrained nursing staff suggests that the financial saving from substituting one for the other is relatively small and compared to the differential between, say, trained nurses and medics one might conclude that studies about the intra-nursing grade mix are barking up the wrong tree. Essentially, this is one of the points made by Robinson *et al.* (1989). The predicted forthcoming shortage of young trained nurses, together with moves towards 'professionalisation', does of course mean that this is only the argument of the devil's advocate. Moreover, the decision to grade most auxiliaries at A means that the gap between them and D graded staff nurses is greater than if more use had been made of the intermediate B and C grades. Nonetheless, it serves to emphasis another point made by Robinson *et al.*, that there is a confusion of objectives behind many grade mix arguments. There are three rather different 'performance indicators' for policy actions on grade mix; cost containment/reducing demand for labour skills in shortage; improving the attractiveness of the trained nurse's job and therefore reducing the outflow of skilled labour; and improving the quality of patient care. Because they may have different objectives, therefore, it would not be surprising to find nurse managers and NHS general managers disagreeing over the desired direction of change in grade mix. This issue has to be resolved before properly conducted and monitored experiments with different staff levels/grade mixes can begin. There is a clear need for those types of experiments.

The contrast between the study described by Ball *et al.* (1989) and the American one (Flood and Diers, 1988) is quite stark, and shows that the American literature in this area is at a higher level of economic sophistication. Flood and Diers report a small study using a simple methodology and its conclusions are by no means the last word on the topic. Nonetheless, the study makes a genuine attempt at an economic analysis. It compares patient outcomes in a ward staffed at its establishment level against those achieved in a similar ward which, compared to its establishment, was short-staffed. The evidence is that patients experience a higher incidence of complications and remain in higher dependency categories for longer in the ward which is understaffed. This evidence is then used as the basis for a case that the cost of care can actually rise due to inadequate staffing levels.

7.4   Performance indicators

It is apparent from this literature that the NHS demand for nursing and P&T staffing is determined at an extremely low level within the organization and by a variety of methods which, by and large, lack sophistication. The attitude of the Government that inefficiencies must be endemic in an organization which has in the past paid scant regard to market forces is reflected in the terms *efficiency savings* and *cost improvements* which are cost reductions which spending departments of the NHS are expected to achieve. There is certainly some evidence (e.g. a study done in Brighton) that sisters underestimate their needs for adequate staffing. Also there are suggestions in the literature (e.g. Hart, 1989) that nurses routinely work overtime and therefore contribute to cost savings. However, the introduction of cost containment strategies increased and systems of financial control may lead to a loss of goodwill of this kind and increase costs.

Since different methods must produce different estimates of staffing needs, variability across Health Authorities in staffing levels and skill mixes is hardly surprising. This indeed is what is observed (Audit Commission, 1991). An obvious implication of that variability is that staffing requirements in total could be reduced if all HAs achieved the standards of the cheapest - we hesitate to use the words 'most efficient' but this is clearly what the NAO has in mind when it talks about there being 'scope for efficiency savings' (National Audit Office, 1985a, 1985b and 1987). Those savings could be reaped, it suggests, through comparative exercises between HAs using recently developed 'performance indicators'.

Performance indicators (PIs) have been introduced across the whole of the public sector. However, their origin within the NHS owes much to the CPA reports discussed at the beginning of this chapter, which were critical of the DHSS for its lack of information and lack of control over the HAs - with regard to staffing and other issues. Another of the ways in which the DHSS responded was with the introduction, in 1982, of a system of 'annual reviews' between successive hierarchical levels within the NHS.

Thus each DHA had to report to its RHA, and each RHA to the DHSS on its performance in the past year. Clearly, for this to be something more than an informal exercise, objective measures of performance were required. Hence the development of performance indicators. Given the previous lack of interest in collecting such information, they had to start from scratch, and the first set of indicators were decidedly crude (e.g. they are often equivalent to the 'norms' in Table 1.1). They are improving and based on better data, but it is still early days. They should, therefore be used with great care. Useful general references on PIs are Long and Harrison (1985, ch.6); Birch and Maynard in Maxwell (1988); and Smith (1987).

Within the economics literature, the profession has responded to the political climate of the times with a renewed interest in various cost minimizing or efficiency maximising techniques which take into account both inputs and outputs. These have been applied to a number of public sector activities, two of which seem particularly relevant: Wagstaff (1989b) (Spanish hospital sector) and Hughs (1988) (English residential child care). These techniques are being applied to the NHS in some areas, such as the maternity sector (Boussofiane, Thonassoulis and Dyson, unpublished).

Such techniques would seem to present a more rigorous way of investigating cost inefficiency in general and variations across HAs in particular. There will remain the difficulty of accurately measuring the quality and quantity of both inputs and output - when output is measured in terms such as 'number of cases treated' it is impossible to distinguish, by any method, whether a hospital with a particularly low 'cost per case' is really more efficient than the rest or providing cheap but ineffective care in the interest of 'economy' - but the methodology is probably less crude than that of simple performance indicators.

8 Demand and supply within the NHS: Supply issues

Labour supply models

In contrast to Chapter 2, which focused upon the background demographic elements which underly the overall supply of labour, and Chapter 6, which concentrated on the general factors influencing labour supply, the present chapter turns to a discussion of the evidence concerning the factors which affect the share of the labour force which can be captured by the NHS. Unfortunately, a study of the literature in this area reveals it to be restricted in three senses: most studies concentrate on nursing, very few even mentioning the PAMs; most also concentrate on quit rates, there having been very little investigation of life cycle participation patterns, return to work decisions and hours of work decisions; and finally, most of the empirical work lacks sophistication.

8.1 Labour supply and the wage rate

The critical question is how the supply of labour responds to changes in the wage rate.   Both the tone of some of the submissions from the management side to the Pay Review Body, discussed in Chapter 7, and the conclusions of some of the attitude surveys, discussed in this chapter, suggest that the supply of nurses (and PAM staff) is rather unresponsive to this economic variable.   However, this view may reflect perceptions of how people think this group of employees ought to behave rather than what actually governs key supply decisions.

It is crucial that managers should learn the lesson of Chapter 6 that the econometric evidence on female labour supply is that it does respond to economic variables in general, and own wage in particular. Why should nurses and PAM staff be any different? Although this issue is at the very heart of the worry over forthcoming shortages, it has until recently attracted little investigation. One exception is the work of Hoskins on the supply of nurses (Hoskins, 1982a and b) who finds that relative pay is a key factor for full-time staff, though less so for part-timers. More recently, Phillips (1990) has confirmed these general results.

By contrast, American writers on nurse supply and nursing shortages (the USA tends to have periodic shortages too) are much more likely to use straightforward economic analysis. For example, Link and Settle (1979 and 1981) are centrally placed in the neoclassical tradition. The older of these two studies estimates a typical neoclassical labour supply function for nurses - and finds that their responsiveness to own wage, husband's income, children's age, etc. is much as expected. One might use this as evidence that nurses have more in common with the rest of the female labour force than they do with the angelic host. Link and Settle (1981), however, find evidence of a backward bending supply function. (This means that there is a level of wages above which an increase in the wage rate brings about a reduction in hours offered, usually because as people become relatively rich they may choose to reduce their hours of paid work.) As they say, the implication of these studies is that increasing the wage rate may not necessarily be an effective way of coping with a shortage. The question of whether or not the supply function is backward bending in the UK clearly requires further research. What seems beyond doubt is that economic factors do influence nursing supply.

Dusansky et al. (1986), building on the earlier work of Benham (1971), developed a three equation model of the nursing market in order to investigate alternative policies for increasing supply. In addition to a normal participation equation, there is also a 'stock' equation, which essentially determines the geographical distribution of people with nursing qualifications, and a demand equation, which allows for substitution between grades of nurses according to relative wage rates. They find that participation is responsive to earnings, though geographical location is not (the most important variable in the determination of the latter is lagged number of graduations from training courses - something which accords with the British experience of a tendency to remain in the hospital in which training was given).

The model could not be applied to the British context without some adaptation and, because wage rates are (at present, with very few exceptions) determined nationally, could not be applied to cross section data. Nonetheless, it stimulates ideas on developing a rigorous model for the UK situation.

There is one recent and substantial econometric study using British data, Phillips (1990). This estimates labour supply functions (in terms of both participation in the market and hours of work supplied) for a sample of female nurses and members of PAMs. The evidence from this study is that nurses are very like other female workers. Their responsiveness to increases in their wage rate is strongly positive, both in their willingness to undertake employment (participation) and in the number of hours they choose to work. On this evidence then, rises in relative rates of pay *are* likely to prove effective in attracting and keeping staff, and so in combating any impending shortage. Furthermore, and again as for other women, childcare responsibilities have a strong adverse effect on willingness to work. There is even evidence of a sizeable 'fixed cost' to the nurse from working - something that might be explained in terms of high childminding costs, etc. Thus, the suggestion, discussed in the next section, of a childcare voucher scheme made by the staff side in the 1990/91 pay review round could be a sensible one.

8.2 Labour supply and non-pay-measures

It was pointed out in Chapter 2 that although the number of school leavers is set to decline, the total female labour force will actually increase. This will occur largely through growth in the number of working women in the 35-44 age cohort. A potential shortage in nursing and P&T staff can be averted, therefore, if the NHS can change its employment practices so as to be more attractive to women in the older age cohort, and since this is such an important issue we devote Chapter 13 of this book to it. The latest literature to appear from within the NHS suggests that this point has been appreciated, if not acted on. There is wide discussion of the necessity to introduce equal opportunity and non-pay-related measures to attract qualified female staff back to work.

The topic of non-pay-related measures for attracting and keeping staff crops up in both nursing and PAM staff pay review reports (Review Body, 1990a and 1990b). In the PAM report, the staff side suggests a specific policy; a nationwide child care voucher scheme whereby staff working 18 or more hours a week would be eligible for a voucher worth £1,000 p.a. and those working less than this would be eligible for one worth £500 p.a. The management rejects this suggestion in favour of a flexible pay scheme. However, the Review Body recommends that the idea be discussed further. The staff side in the nurses' report argues that significant increases in basic pay should be reinforced by equal opportunity measures such as better maternity leave arrangements, child care provisions and more part-time jobs and job sharing. The Review Body is again supportive and, consistent with its comments in the PAM report, suggests that the management side might consider a pilot scheme to investigate the effectiveness of child care provision policies. The general impression gained from reading these reports is of a growing awareness of the need for equal opportunity measures but, as yet, little action. Given the conclusions of Chapter 6 and 13 of the present volume this could be a particularly important area if and when labour markets do tighten once again as the economy recovers from recession.

The impression of little action being taken so far is reinforced by the literature emanating from the RHAs. For example, in explicit response to Conroy and Stidston (1988), West Midlands has initiated a series of reports under the general heading of *Staying Power*. The first two of these (West Midlands RHA, Manpower Planning Section, 1989 and 1990) give a rehearsal of the above argument before turning to consider a range of possible policy options; job sharing; flexible employment contracts; improved promotion prospects; career break management; crèches; etc. These policies are being discussed, but still in a rather general way. There is no reference to any pilot scheme to assess them and none to their immediate implementation. In short, they are aware of the issues and possible solutions, but still at an early stage in implementation. Chapter 9 of the Welsh commentary on its districts' manpower resource plans reveals a similar situation (WHCSA Manpower Planning Division, 1990). A study by Mersey RHA makes a similar point (Mersey RHA, 1988).

Further confirmation is gained from two reports by the Institute of Manpower Studies (Meager, Buchan and Rees, 1989; and Bevan, Buchan and Hayday, 1989). The first reports a survey of HAs to elicit their practices and experiences with regard to job sharing schemes. This reveals job sharing to be a relatively new and still infrequently used measure, usually adopted as a reaction to a specific staff request or a specific difficulty in filling a post, rather than as a proactive human resource strategy. The second of these two concerns a study commissioned by the MPAG. The remit was to provide evidence from which to construct policies on utilisation and retention of female hospital pharmacists. The fact that the study was commissioned at all is further evidence of the awareness of the problem. What it reveals, however, is a familiar story. Within NHS hospitals, 62 per cent of pharmacists are female (mostly young females). However, only 28 per cent of pharmacy managers are female. Amongst these managers, the females are more likely than the males to be single and/or childless. Very few female managers work part-time. The conclusion, of course, is that the NHS has not yet adjusted to the needs and aspirations of female employees. It is recommended that equal opportunity measures are considered.

Although awareness of the issues seems prevalent, it has to be said that the literature does not reveal any strong analysis of the costs and benefits of alternative schemes. Compared to the advances being made in the modelling of supply, for example, there is no reference to attempts at formal quantification of the likely cost and yield (in terms of whole-time equivalent years of service) from any of these measures (the results of Worthington, 1988 and 1990 are relevant here too) and little indication that monitored pilot schemes are underway.

8.3 Supply-side workforce planning

The workforce planning techniques which are discussed below are different from the economic models reviewed in Chapter 7 in that they do not attempt to get beneath the observed labour market behaviour and explain it; they are satisfied with what logicians term naive induction - the sun has always risen in the East. But, so called, manpower planning is a ubiquitous and influential discipline, so much so that Chapter 10 is devoted to a general summary of its development and use in the UK

Some HAs, for example Trent, Wessex and the Welsh NHS, are using nurse workforce supply models to assist them in the development of their human resource planning strategies (Welsh Health Common Services Authority, Health Intelligence Unit, 1989 and 1990; Resource Analysis Team, Wessex RHA, 1987; and, for Trent, Beaumont, 1988; Jones 1989; and Wren 1990. Trent is in the early stages of developing a similar model for other qualified staff (Trent Manpower Studies Section, personal communication). These are workforce planning models similar to that developed by the Institute of Manpower Studies for the RCN (Royal College of Nursing, 1985) and surveyed below. Worthington (1988 and 1990) and Manpower Planning Advisory Group (1991) discuss this general approach to supply modelling from the perspective of operations researchers.

The traditional 'stocks and flows' model forecasts the future workforce on the basis of the current one adjusted for expected recruitment and wastage (IMS; Welsh NHS and one version of Trent). The newer 'participation' approach estimates the future age-related population of trained nurses and then forecasts the future workforce on the basis of expected age-related participation rates (Wessex and the other version of Trent). As Worthington says, the two approaches are formally consistent, but may produce different predictions because they make use of recruitment, wastage and participation rates which are empirical estimates derived from different sources of data. Nevertheless, Jones (1989) compares the predictions to 1993/4 for the Trent region arising out of their two-version model and finds them very similar.

Worthington provides an interesting assessment of this type of supply modelling. Four of his points are selected as being of general interest, and noted here:

(i) Good quality data is very important. With reference to the 'stocks and flows' model the particular problem in this respect is in identifying a true wastage rate; most estimates used to be of the turnover rate, and therefore include movement within the NHS. (In theory, this should cease to be a problem as the statistics generated by the Körner reforms start to appear.) With respect to the 'participation' model, the problem is in inferring the size of the population of trained nurses from extrapolations of census data; the information on qualifications is insufficiently detailed to permit really accurate estimation. It is hoped that the development of a 'live' UKCC register will eventually lead to more useful estimates of the potential workforce for this purpose. The LFS provides another source for this type of information as outlined in Chapter 11, although once disaggregated by region problems of sampling error become significant.

(ii) Because there is a strong life-cycle pattern to female labour supply, and because the age structure of both the workforce and the population changes, accurate predictions require the use of age-specific estimates of both the wastage and the participation rate, (and possibly also the return-to-work-rate), as opposed to the broad averages used in a number of early versions of the 'stocks and flows' model.

(iii) The models have a limited capacity to assist management in investigating the effects of their possible actions on the future size of the labour force. For example, they cannot calculate directly the effect on labour supply of equal opportunities policies like opening creches. Management has to estimate the effect of those policies on, for example, the wastage rate and then feed the expected change in that rate into the model. Furthermore, of course, some degree of interaction within the model must be anticipated. If, for example, a management action has the effect of permanently reducing the wastage rate, then it must also have an eventual effect on the return to work rate (if fewer people leave, then there are fewer to come back).

(iv) Because the models use critical rates (wastage rates, etc.) which are estimated from past data (however good) they are capable of error, should the future turn out to be different from the past. Wastage rates, in particular, are known to be rather unstable.

The first point that must be made in commenting on the new literature is that it reveals an active area where progress is clearly being made and where, potentially at least, the results are of great interest. That said, the absence of any economic incentives within the models has to be noted. Particularly with reference to point (iv) above, but also to some extent to point (iii), the effect is to make the variability in the critical rates unpredictable and problematic. That variability might be somewhat less unpredictable if it was explicitly recognised that recruitment, wastage and participation rates are functions of relative wage rates and other economic factors, as well as of age. In particular, it is a little worrying that both Worthington and the Trent Manpower Studies Section seem to be working under the assumption that the participation rate is stable compared to the wastage rate. Economic analysis of female labour supply suggests, of course, that the participation rate is responsive to economic variables (See Chapter 6).

8.4   Training

This section focuses on the supply of newly trained nurses, since the changes now taking place in nurse training are by far the most important labour market development in the NHS.

Reform of nurse training

The training of nurses is undergoing a dramatic change, universally known as 'Project 2000', (United Kingdom Central Council for Nursing, Midwifery and Health Visiting (UKCC),1986). The context of these changes is a move within the nursing profession to increase the standing of nurses by upgrading the nature of their professional qualification. The original proposals emanated from a committee commissioned by the nurses' professional body, the RCN (Royal College of Nursing, 1985a). This committee commissioned the Institute of Manpower Services, Sussex, and the Centre for Health Economics, York, to investigate respectively the staffing and cost implications of their proposals. These studies appear in RCN (1985b) and the latter also appears as Bosanquet and Goodwin (1986). Almost simultaneously, the body in charge of training and registration, the UKCC, also investigated the issue: they produced a very similar set of proposals (UKCC, 1986) . This time the staffing and cost implications were investigated by Price Waterhouse (Price Waterhouse, 1987), though this study drew heavily on the earlier work of the IMS and the CHE. After discussion, a modified set of proposals were submitted to the Departments in February 1987. By 1991 most DHA's were implementing, or had plans to implement, Project 2000 training.

Prior to Project 2000 there were two levels of qualified nurse, the state registered nurse (SRN) and the state enrolled nurse (SEN); and an untrained grade, the nursing auxiliary (for obvious reasons the professional literature does not refer to the latter as 'nurses', but NAs are often included as such in official statistics). The register kept by UKCC also covers midwives and health visitors - theoretically these are freestanding qualifications but in practice most midwives and all health visitors first qualify as SRNs. Further, although most nurses have pursued a general training (RGN), some have taken narrower specialist courses in nursing those with mental illnesses (RMN); sick children (RSCN), etc. Due to the resulting variety of different syllabi, there were acknowledged problems to do with standards and of post-registration courses, transferability, etc. Hence, part of the reforms were about simplifying this situation, a matter largely outside the remit of the present report. However, there is the possibility that a better and more general basic training, followed by a more rational development of post-registration courses, could reduce the tendency of unpromoted SRNs (staff nurses) to be highly mobile. Evidence reviewed later shows that staff nurses are in any given job for a very short space of time and frequently take breaks from work to attend a variety of courses, i.e. they seem to feel the need to broaden their experience. Though it should be noted that, decisions to go on courses usually involve employer as well as employee. Attendance (e.g. on midwifery post registration) is usually via secondment and has a service element (so may not entail 'a break from work' albeit involving a job change). The trainee is almost certainly not supernumerary, and the number of available places on courses is not infinitely flexible - courses may only run within set numbers of places and, at least to some extent, these are determined by the service scene.

The entrance requirements for SEN training were below the 5 GCSE minimum requirement for SRN training and the training period was only 18 months to two years, compared to three for the latter. Both spent the majority of their training period in clinical locations, making a 'service contribution' within an apprenticeship model of training. By contrast, those studying for degrees in nursing receive a more classroom-orientated education over a 3 year period. The latter used to qualify as SRN. Project 2000 schemes, which are three year non-degree schemes, will replace the old SRN with the new registered general nurse (RGN) qualification. These are to be taught in new colleges of nursing, replacing the old nursing schools. Their service contribution will be much lower than the traditional SEN and SRN schemes, particularly at the start of the course. This has led to concern that this will exacerbate any future labour shortages (Jones 1989; and Welsh Health Common Services Authority, Manpower Planning Division, 1990).

Position of the SEN

The SEN was known officially as a 'second level' nurse and that is indicative - the qualification was seen as inferior to the SRN and had limited opportunities for personal advancement (although 'conversion' courses to RGN level did exist). A related criticism concerned the lack of distinction in practice between the job of the SEN and the staff nurse - something confirmed by the regrading exercise which resulted in many examples of SENs and SRNs being graded D. This is partly a status issue, but there is also the argument that less well qualified SENs were often (especially in the continuing care setting) given inappropriate levels of responsibility.

In reviewing the research evidence, the UKCC (1986, p.39) suggested that SENs were misused by being treated as one level at one moment, another at the next. They were often abused, by being treated as inferior to the first level nurses and lacking in knowledge and judgement. They were also frequently denied opportunities for advancement and development. Many professional conduct hearings show SENs used interchangeably with colleagues with a three year training, and the distinction between these in practice being ignored. With the introduction of Project 2000 a decision was taken to phase out enrolled nurse training, and recruitment to courses has now ceased. Conversion courses are available to enable enrolled nurses to upgrade their training to registered nurse status. But there is evidence from the nursing press that demand for such places is not being met, adding to enrolled nurses' fears that they will be further marginalised.

The relative unattractiveness of the SEN grade is evidence that pay, promotion, status, etc., do matter to female school leavers. This is hard evidence based upon observable behaviour rather than the more questionable evidence from questionnaires such as that used in the IMS study (RCN, 1985b).

The service contribution of learners

Whilst pre Project 2000 learners were on the wards they were counted as part of its staff establishment and therefore formally seen as working, not learning. The criticisms were that they are therefore exploited as 'pairs of hands' and often given responsibilities for patient care beyond their competence. In addition, this system implied a relatively low proportion of qualified staff in the ward's establishment, and thus a reduced chance for the learner to receive instruction whilst working. As the RCN (1985a, p8-9) noted,

> ..it is precisely the present structures which subordinate educational to service requirement functions. Only 58 per cent of all nursing staff employed by the NHS in England in 1982 were formally qualified (38.4 per cent Registered, plus 17.8 per cent Enrolled). Almost a quarter were unqualified, and 20 per cent were trainees. The trainees are therefore regarded as an integral part of the workforce. That arrangement is, in the long run, good for nobody and certainly not the patient.

Quality of training schools

DHA training schools have been criticised for being too small, lacking a full range of expertise, and planning intakes with a view to providing hospitals with a constant flow of 'service contributions'. Because training schools provide both a flow of cheap labour in the form of the trainee's service contribution and a locally controlled flow of newly qualified labour, every DHA wanted one. The result was a large number of often very small schools. Because they were small, the clinical teaching establishment was small and so nurse tutors had to be generalists rather than specialists. Because the wards were dependent on a constant flow of non-supernumerary trainees to do the work, a number of small intakes per annum were required - so there was much repetition of teaching. In short, the training was poor:

> the weight of research evidence and the growing body of opinion suggests that the system must be seen as fundamentally flawed. The constant grind of up to six intakes per annum and of repeated

teaching with no time for research or professional development; the frequent need to make compromises in terms of learning experiences to ensure that wards are staffed; the daily need for pairs of hands to get things done, are some of the factors which erect immense barriers to educational improvement. (UKCC, 1986 p.10)

In the event the staged introduction of Project 2000 led to students on these courses being accorded full student status and receiving a non-means tested tax-free bursary. Project 2000 courses are being established in colleges of nursing and midwifery, many of which have been formed from the amalgamation of smaller schools. Linked with institutions of higher education they can award a professional qualification as a first level nurse as well as an academic qualification at diploma level. Legislative change has been initiated to transfer responsibility for financing nursing, midwifery and health visiting education and training to the NHS. This means the Regional Health Authorities in England and health boards in Scotland. In Wales the Manpower Resources Group is to be the responsible body but in Northern Ireland management of colleges will remain in the hands of the National Board.

In summary, the current and near future position appears to be as follows:

- there will be larger, more independent colleges of nursing
- they will award diplomas which allow registration (RGN)
- they will have closer links with higher education institutions but will continue to be under control of the RHA's etc.
- students on such courses will be paid a bursary (less than the current training allowance).

The decision on whose budget the bursaries will come out of has yet been taken. The current arrangements are pilots/temporary ones whereby DHA's bid for funds to introduce Project 2000 courses. However, the new Project 2000 courses currently being introduced are pilot schemes being run alongside the traditional ones. Presumably the former will eventually replace the latter. But many of the critical decisions - like how much control DHA's will eventually keep, have yet to be made (or at least, have yet to be made public).

Staffing implications of Project 2000

There will be, therefore, two major labour supply implications arising from the implementation of Project 2000. The first will occur because of the loss of the SEN grade. This used to be known as the 'second level' nursing grade - second to the SRN and used to offer a route into nursing for the less academically qualified applicant. Under the reformed system, there will be one and only one qualification permitting entry into the nursing profession; all nurses will, in the first instance, train to be RGNs. This qualification is intended to be on an academic par with the old SRN qualification and therefore above that of the SEN. Thus people with fewer than 5 GCSEs may, in future, find themselves unable to gain places on nurse training courses and the NHS may, in consequence, find that it experiences a contraction in the flow of newly qualified nurses into NHS hospitals. This danger has been recognised and there are plans to develop pre-registration nursing courses which will offer a second entry gate into RGN training for the less academically qualified. Whether this will be effective remains to be seen.

The second implication will be a reduction in the amount of labour supplied by student nurses. Under the old system, trainees spend the vast majority of their time on the wards rather than in the classroom. Though in theory they were receiving on-the-job training, they counted as part of the ward's staff establishment and most of their time was spent working rather than learning. In effect, trainees were a cheap source of labour to their training hospitals. That being so, every DHA counted its own training school and the result was a large number of often very small schools. Many were too small to offer the full range of clinical expertise within their nurse tutor establishment. In addition, in order to maintain the flow of trainee labour onto the wards, the schools tended to take in up to six small intakes per annum. Thus there was much repetition of teaching. In school, the training was poor. The Project 2000 reforms will replace this system with one in which training is carried out in larger Colleges of Nursing, linked to institutions of higher education and with some independence from DHA control. During training, the trainees will be treated as students rather than workers and though practical experience on the wards is still regarded as vital, the time spent on the wards will be reduced and more carefully directed at ensuring the student gains a proper training. On paper, at least, these reforms should improve the quality of nurse training. However, they also imply that the NHS will have to substitute for much of the labour which the trainees once supplied. Thus there is likely to be an increase in the demand for qualified and unqualified nurses. Again, the problem has been recognised and there are plans to develop a lowly trained grade - the care assistant - as a cheap and appropriate replacement for student labour.

Taking these two implications together, the Project 2000 reforms seem likely to exacerbate the potential shortage created by the demographic time bomb. The first could restrict the stock from which the NHS has traditionally drawn its nursing labour, the second could increase the demand for that labour. There could be countervailing effects, however. The improved training could increase the attractiveness of nursing as a career to academically well qualified and ambitious school leavers, leading to an increase in the proportion of school leavers with five or more GCSEs who opt to apply for nurse training, which in turn could improve both the quantity and quality of entrants into training. Improved training would also result in an improvement in the productivity of nurses, once qualified, and in a reduction in the need for so many to take post-registration courses. These two things could provide off-setting reductions in the demand for qualified labour. Finally, improved training could result in a reduction in the training wastage rate and, if it creates qualified nurses who are more able to cope and therefore happier in their jobs, a lowering of the qualified wastage rate. Much of this, however, is speculation. RCN (1985b) and Price Waterhouse (1987) attempted some degree of qualification of the likely effect of Project 2000, but were hampered by lack of information.

The main advantages of the Project 2000 reforms were argued to be:

(a)   To make the profession more attractive to high quality applicants.
(b)   To reduce the level of training wastage.
(c)   To improve the quality of qualified nursing care.
(d)   To reduce the level of wastage of qualified staff.
(e)   To adapt training such that it reflects the growing importance of community, as opposed to hospital, care.
(f)   To permit the integration of part-time training courses for mature applicants and refresher courses for returnees.

From the point of view of the NHS, there are obvious disadvantages as well. The loss of DHA control reduces their ability to plan staffing - this is clearly implied, but the literature is careful to avoid the topic. There is evidence from the study being carried out by HSRU on decision making and staffing in Wales (funded by the Welsh Office) that, owing to the various requirements of nurse tutors, the nursing service deliverers have on some sites effectively lost control of learners' deployment. The real problems, however, are the workforce and cost implications of the reduced service contribution of students and to a lesser extent the loss of the cheaper SEN. The purpose of commissioning the research studies was to see if the possible benefits listed above could be made to outweigh these costs. Clearly, a number of those benefits are difficult to estimate. Attention has centred, therefore, around those where there is at least a fighting chance of objective measurement - the wastage rates.

The cost of Project 2000

The Centre for Health Economics (CHE) report for the RCN (incorporated into RCN, 1985b, and reprinted as Bosanquet and Goodwin, 1986) also concentrates on the effect of the supernumerary status proposal, rather than that of one grade of qualified nurse. They estimate and compare the recurrent costs of three nurse training courses: traditional training in DHA schools; degrees; and diplomas, as proposed by the RCN Commission. Their cost model recognises three classes of cost:

131

(i) formal costs
   (a) direct tuition costs
   (b) training allowance/bursary/grant,

(ii) informal training costs
   (resource costs of informal tuition received on wards from nurses other than nurse tutors, etc.),

(iii) replacement costs
   (service contribution valued at replacement cost - i.e. a negative cost).

The net cost per trainee is then the sum of formal plus informal minus replacement costs.

The cost per qualifier is calculated by allowing for training wastage. The wastage rate in DHA training schools is taken from the IMS study. Thus it is assumed to be 10 per cent dropout during the course (for costing purposes, assumed evenly spread over the three years) and 10 per cent exam failure. The third source of training wastage on the IMS definition, failure to take up a post immediately following qualification, was ignored here - this was estimated at 10 per cent and so produces the total figure of 30 per cent quoted earlier when discussing the IMS study. The wastage rate for the degree course is assumed to be 10 per cent, all occurring at the end of the first year of study - this comes from the information collected by the Commission, discussed above. In line with the Commission, the CHE study assumes that diploma courses would achieve a wastage rate comparable to that of degree courses.

Applying these assumptions, as relevant, net costs per qualifier are then estimated to be (1982/3 prices):

DHA schools £8,750,
degrees £17,350,
diplomas £10,250.

The CHE study estimates that tuition costs are larger and replacement costs smaller for degree and diploma courses than for DHA schools. There are counteracting influences: training grant and the wastage rate are smaller than for DHA schools and would thus act to reduce costs. But the net effect is for the degree and diploma courses to be more expensive per qualifier.

The CHE study concentrates on estimating cost per qualifier - not cost of a target qualified workforce. The possibility that the reforms might reduce qualified wastage and the 'excessive' desire to take time off work to attend post registration courses, and increase the productivity of qualified staff is thus not accounted for. (The authors of the CHE study mention that these possibilities are argued by the Commission, but do not include estimates in the main body of their formal analysis. It is of course possible to extend their analysis by incorporating the 'guesstimates' made in the Price Waterhouse (1987 or 1988) reports on these matters. It is thus possible that although the reforms might raise the cost per qualifier, they could still lower the cost of achieving a target qualified workforce.

In economic terms, a further criticism relates to their cost model. What is being estimated is the financial cost to the public sector, narrowly defined, not the true opportunity cost. The latter, properly defined, would consist of the opportunity cost of training resources, direct and informal, and the value of the forgone output of the trainee, net of the value of their service contribution. It would not include the value of the payment made to the trainee. This is a transfer payment/reward for the service contribution. Its value affects the distribution of the cost, - i.e. how much is borne by the student as opposed to the state - rather than its size. The inclusion of the grant in the estimates of formal costs will tend to imply that the size of the increase in cost per qualifier resulting from the reforms is being underestimated - because the reforms also propose switching from a training allowance to a smaller bursary-cum-grant.

Thus it is more accurate to say that the reforms would have a larger increase in the opportunity cost of training than estimated, and also a redistribution of that cost away from the public purse and towards the trainee. (It does not, of course, follow that the trainee's welfare is necessarily reduced, merely that their command over marketed resources is - the trainee might be quite happy to take a smaller payment in return for a better education and less 'exploitation' as a pair of hands.)

A second implication of the choice of cost model is that a benefit to other employers is ignored. The value of the forgone output of the trainee in alternative sources of employment is ignored. This means that the lower wastage which is assumed to result from the reforms is regarded as of benefit only to the extent that it reduces the cost, to the NHS, of training - but lower wastage reduces NHS demand for trainees and so releases labour for alternative employment.

Rough calculations suggest that this additional source of cost savings is unlikely to change the sign of a properly estimated 'change-in-cost' estimate of the reforms - but in a situation where demographic factors will cause a contraction in supply and therefore increase the scarcity value of fairly well educated school leavers, there is the possibility that evidence on the past wages of this category of labour significantly underestimates the near-future value of its output to other employers. It is perhaps worth adding that this may become more of an issue in the future with the move to trust status of many units and the increase in private sector provision serving to increase competition for this sort of labour.

9 Labour turnover within the NHS

Three critical factors determine the supply of trained staff to the National Health Service, in addition to the flow from training which has been discussed in Chapter 8. These are: the rate at which staff leave the NHS; the rate at which they return; and the number of hours' work per week which they offer. A fourth factor might also be regarded as relevant: the propensity to change posts within the NHS - though strictly speaking this factor is a potential influence upon the productivity, rather than the number, of hours supplied. The literature in this area concentrates on the first of these (though data limitations usually mean that the fourth interferes with the drawing of conclusions). Further, it rarely extends beyond an interest in the leaving rates of the nursing profession.

9.1 Estimating turnover

The estimation of turnover within the NHS is hampered by the fact that the effective employer is usually the DHA. Thus, where records can be made to yield any kind of data at all, it tends to be data about joining and leaving a DHA, not the NHS as a whole. Therefore, for example, estimated 'quit rates' tend to be an amalgam of quit rates proper and internal movement. Most references on this topic make the point that there is no single adequate measure of turnover and therefore that a number of such measures need to be used in combination. However, data limitations usually severely restrict the choice of measure when it comes to actual estimation. There are three commonly used measures:

(i) Turnover rate   =   no. leavers during   x   100/no. in post over
    (often called   any given period time   that period
    wastage rate)

This statistic is affected by the choice of: (a) basic unit - i.e. bodies
or WTE; and (b) method of measuring the divisor i.e. the number at
beginning of period, end, middle, average, etc.   It is potentially
misleading; it cannot distinguish between a general turnover of all
posts at any given rate and a situation of variability between the
turnover of subsets of posts which produce the same average rate.

A variant is :

Cohort   =   no. in cohort who   x   100/total no. in cohort
turnover rate   leave during period

Cohort may be age, date of recruitment, etc.

(ii) Stability rate   =   no. staff in post x   100/no. staff in post
                          who have been
                          there for N years

Used in conjunction with the turnover rate, this will indicate internal
variability in turnover.   Care is still required in interpretation
however - a short time in post need not imply a short time in the
work setting since internal promotion may have occurred.

(iii) Vacancy rate   =   no. posts vacant x   100/total no. posts

This statistic is affected by:

(a) whether total number of posts is measured as establishment,
    number actually in post, or WTE actually in post,

(b) whether a vacant post is defined literally or as one which has lain
    vacant for some minimum period of time or as one where
    attempts to fill it have been unsuccessful.

This third indicator is more properly interpreted as a measure of the
state of the market rather than of supply.

Mercer (1979) is a study of turnover among qualified nurses below
administrative grades, based on data from 14 District General Hospitals in
9 Yorkshire DHAs collected in 1975/6.   Arguably this is a small,
unrepresentative sample, however many of Mercer's basic findings are

replicated in later studies. The crude turnover rate across all qualified grades (numbers not WTE) is estimated to be approximately 25 per cent - though this figure is not, on its own, very informative because 'leaving' simply means leaving a DGH. More interestingly, the rate is found to vary across grades: staff nurses having the highest rates of turnover, sisters the lowest, and SENs lying in between. For one of the hospitals, Mercer was able to calculate the turnover rate back to 1971. He found that it varied, possibly in relation to the local unemployment rate. However, the calculated correlation coefficient turned out to be low.

The stability rates are perhaps the most interesting statistics. Across all grades: 37 per cent of respondents had been in post for under 1 year; 80 per cent under 5 years; and only 6 per cent more than 10 years. The average length of time in post, in years, was 3.1 (mean), 1.7 (median) and 1.5 (mode). Thus the distribution of the sample across years in post was found to be positively skewed. Because of the way the data was collected, little can be concluded about the quantity of labour supplied - but predominance of very short length of service in any given post might well have implications for productivity.

The differences in stability rates between grades are consistent with the observations on turnover. Staff nurses were the least stable group with 60 per cent having been in post for under 1 year, 94 per cent under 5 years and none over 10 years. Ward sisters were much more stable, and SENs, once again, in the middle. Responses to questions on work history reveal that the instability is a function of the grade, not the individual i.e. SRNs are highly mobile when staff nurses but settle down when they are promoted to sisters. The general pattern revealed is that, on qualifying, most took a job in the hospital in which they trained. There is an early peak in the number of leavers after 3-6 months then a larger resurgence after 1 year. Very few of the leavers go to jobs outside the NHS. The largest group are leaving the labour market for the usual reasons of pregnancy, etc. Many, however, are simply transferring within the NHS - for promotion, to undertake further training, or even just for a change. This pattern evidently concurs with the informal experience of internal commentators, and is widely quoted. It is difficult to interpret however. For example, given that SENs cannot get promotion to sisters, it is hardly surprising to find that their rates of stability and turnover lie in between those for unpromoted and promoted SRNs. It is therefore dangerous to use these figures as data in arguments about the merits of the SEN grade. Further, given the institutional arrangements for training it is hardly surprising to find that newly qualified nurses are mobile - for their first post, they take what amounts to the easy option of a job in the place in which they trained, but they move on fairly quickly. It is also risky to jump too quickly to conclusions about, for example, job stress causing instability.

Young et al. (1983) report a study, again on nursing, carried out by a team of mathematicians and sociologists. The study area is the whole of

Northern Ireland and the data is drawn from the period 1978-81. Movement between NHS posts within Northern Ireland is traced, thus 'leavers' exclude those who transfer between jobs within the Northern Ireland section of the NHS. Making allowance for this difference, Mercer's basic picture is supported in Tables 9.1 and 9.2:

Table 9.1
Turnover rates for Northern Ireland as a whole

%

Year	Trained staff	Nursing auxiliary
1978	18.0	16.3
1979	16.0	14.2
1980	14.8	13.4
1981	13.0	8.2

Source: Young *et al.* (1983).

Table 9.2
Trained nurses: length of service in present post, 1981

months

NI area	Lower quartile	Median	Upper quartile
Eastern	11	24	42
Northern	13	30	78
Southern	12	30	79
Western	10	29	73

Source: Young *et al.* (1983).

Amongst trained staff, the turnover rate for staff nurses is again measured as higher than that for SENs. This study also reports that there is some evidence of a correlation between hospitals with high trainee densities and high turnover/low stability of trained staff. (The Eastern area in Table 9.2 includes Belfast, which has an unduly large percentage of Northern Ireland's training schools.) Again, there is some evidence of correlation between turnover and unemployment: this study found, not

137

only that turnover had declined over the period 1978-81, but also that those districts within Northern Ireland with the highest unemployment rates had the lowest turnover rates. The authors do not extend their analysis beyond those observations.

An attempt was also made to examine return to work behaviour, though the conclusions must be regarded as compromised by data limitations. The data consists of observations on those who had left after 1977 and had since returned - i.e. it covered a short period and did not distinguish between alternative destinations of leavers.

The basic assumption of the model seems to be that the probability of returning will decrease as the time lapse since leaving increases. Whilst that seems to be a reasonable assumption for many situations, it is not appropriate where the reason for leaving is child birth. The conclusions drawn were that, for trained nurses, half will never return and, of those who do, most return within a year. For nursing auxiliaries, very few leavers ever return.

Gray *et al.* (1989) reports the results of a pilot study, by economists, of turnover amongst all non-medical staff. Data was collected from English Health Authorities for 1987/88; the sample size varied depending on how many authorities were able to supply any given piece of information. Only turnover rates are reported. Some of their results are summarised in Tables 9.3-9.5.

With respect to Table 9.3, the turnover rates for (qualified) nurses are broadly consistent with those estimated in earlier studies. Two new pieces of evidence emerge. First, turnover rates for Professional and Technical (P&T) staff are calculated and, in this table, would seem to be of roughly the same order of magnitude as those for nursing. Second, turnover rates show considerable variation across DHAs.

Tables 9.4 and 9.5 show the influence of age and length of service (which is undefined - it could be in total or in last post) in one RHA. The pattern for nursing is again broadly consistent with the earlier studies - people are more mobile in the early years of their career, when they are young. An interesting feature of these tables is that turnover rates are calculated separately for full and part-time staff. For nurses, there would seem to be little difference. The situation is not so for P&T staff however.

Part-time P&T staff under the age of 30 would, on this evidence, appear to have very much higher turnover rates than the full timers or both groups of nurses. By contrast it is full-time PSMs who are out of line in Table 9.5, where the peak in their rate of turnover is revealed to occur after a greater number of years service than is the case for the other groups.

Table 9.3
Annual turnover by major staff groups in ten district health authorities

%

District	Turnover rate for:				
	Domestic & ancillary staff	Administrative & clerical staff	Nursing & midwifery staff	Professional & technical staff	All non-medical staff
Bath	43.3	21.2	17.3	17.8	20.9
Bradford	50.4	21.1	18.6	20.9	25.2
Dewsbury	36.2	29.2	11.3	17.2	17.4
East Yorkshire	143.3	22.6	22.3	37.2	41.7
Leeds West	77.4	23.0	20.9	20.2	30.4
Milton Keynes	110.8	41.9	33.0	33.1	42.1
Northampton	59.1	27.6	19.5	25.2	27.8
Portsmouth	31.0	20.6	14.4	17.3	18.6
Southampton	28.8	18.6	19.8	21.8	21.4
West Berks	64.8	55.0	28.1	30.3	35.6

Source: Gray, Normand and Currie (1989).

Table 9.4
Turnover by staff group and age, Yorkshire RHA, 1987-88

Staff group	Age			
	25-29	35-39	45-49	55-59
Full-time				
Ancillary	27	17	17	15
Admin. and clerical	21	11	5	9
Nursing & midwifery (qualified)	23	10	6	13
Prof. and Tech. (PSMs)	24	15	7	8
Prof. and Tech. (technician)	16	11	4	5
Part-time				
Ancillary	39	35	27	24
Admin. and clerical	40	18	13	13
Nursing & midwifery (qualified)	19	12	8	13
Prof. and Tech. (PSMs)	33	19	11	11
Prof. and Tech. (technician)	19	16	12	5

Source: Gray, Normand and Currie (1989).

Table 9.5
Turnover by staff group and length of service, Yorkshire RHA, 1987-88

Staff group	Years of service						
	1	2	3	4	5	5+	Total
Full-time							
Ancillary	42	37	23	23	21	18	24
Admin. and clerical	15	28	21	22	16	11	16
Nursing & midwifery (qualified)	10	28	25	20	21	12	16
Prof. and Tech. (PSMs)	13	17	24	45	19	12	19
Prof. & Tech. (technician)	16	23	15	13	15	9	13
Part-time							
Ancillary	37	46	38	34	31	27	34
Admin. and clerical	41	32	15	17	14	10	21
Nursing & midwifery (qualified)	15	27	20	13	15	11	14
Prof. and Tech. (PSMs)	29	45	25	23	3	12	21
Prof. & Tech. (technician)	27	28	19	19	21	8	17

Source: Gray, Normand and Currie (1989).

Gray *et al.* provide some evidence on the proportion of leavers who are really transferring jobs within the NHS. Only 5 Authorities were able to provide data, each for only one year. Furthermore, the way the data are presented raised doubts about whether a consistent definition of leaver was being used. Finally, two of the observations cover all non-medical staff (including unskilled groups) and, whilst the other three include only nurse leavers, only one of them is explicit in stating qualified nurses (i.e. the other two could include NAs). Bearing in mind their limitations, the data reveal that between 8 and 15 per cent of leavers are actually moving within the NHS - a lower proportion than assumed in the IMS study discussed in Chapter 8. The authors give this conclusion some prominence in their summary (this is a report for the DoH), maybe more than the data limitations warrant.

Finally, mention should be made of Thomas *et al.* (1988). This study (again by non-economists) is specifically interested in the effect the expanding private sector has had on the availability of nurses to the NHS. A small but well designed random sample of DHAs and of private hospitals/nursing homes were asked to provide information on all qualified nurses joining their institutions in the year 1985 - previous post; qualifications; and personal characteristics. The results suggest that there was, in 1985, a net outflow of qualified nurses from the NHS to the private sector, but that the outflow was small - calculated to be something of the order of 5.5 nurses per DHA. Of those moving from the NHS to the private sector, some had only recently completed their training but, on average, they had provided 5 years' service to the NHS prior to their move. In other words, the NHS was getting some return for its investment in their training. However, there was also some evidence that the flow into private hospitals, unlike that into private nursing homes, came from a fairly narrow and perhaps critical section of the NHS nursing workforce: under 30 and with specialist skills, particularly theatre nursing. To summarise, this study suggested no general cause for concern but a possible worry over loss of specific skills.

With respect to the issue of whether the NHS is losing an excessive amount of trained staff, these studies are less helpful than might have been hoped. They concentrate on the propensity to leave whilst saying very little on the probability of return or expected length of time away and absolutely nothing on the expected hours supplied whilst working for the NHS. Furthermore, they tend to conflate two different issues: the problem of instability due to excessive mobility within and across NHS boundaries; and that of loss of trained staff.

Finally it is far from clear what constitutes 'excessive' mobility or loss of staff. Mercer does refer briefly to NES data in an attempt to say something about the relative instability of the nursing profession. Young *et al.* claim that the rate of turnover among nurses is above what might be expected for their skill level, a conclusion they seem to reach by using primary school teachers as a comparison group.

The recent implementation of the Körner reforms is beginning to raise the standards of work in this area. For example, West Midlands RHA, Manpower Planning Section (1990) gives a statistical report of its nursing staff which is much more detailed than anything published previously. Age-, grade- and contract-specific wastage and stability rates are estimated. A similar level of detail is provided on the joiners data. The picture revealed is the now familiar one of a highly mobile workforce, as shown in Tables 9.6 and 9.7. Strictly speaking these are turnover rates rather than wastage rates, i.e. they show the percentage of staff leaving the RHA, rather than that leaving the NHS. As Table 9.8 shows, many are moving within the NHS and therefore, this cannot really be described as 'wasted'.

It was hoped that the Körner returns would, by providing information on the destination of leavers, permit a deeper interpretation of turnover figures derived from payroll data. As can be seen from Table 9.8, the returns provide a rather esoteric list of possible destinations and, for the West Midlands in 1989/90 at least, the 'not known' category is by far the most popular. This is disappointing and it is to be hoped that the list can be reformed to include a more helpful set of mutually exclusive categories. A further incidental point worth emphasising is that the variability in the wastage rate across age groups, shown in Table 9.7, confirms Worthington's argument that nurse supply models should use age-specific wastage rates rather than broad average ones. Observed differences in wastage rates, for example across regions, could turn out to be due to nothing more than differences in the age structure of the workforce.

Another source of information is arising out of the MPAG's 'National Lead Region Initiative'. Under this initiative, particular regions are selected to become centres of information on particular staff groups. Thus Trent, for example, is the lead region for physiotherapy. Beaumont, Thornton and Sleaney (1989) is its first report in the role. Its analysis of workforce flows is based on a survey carried out by the Chartered Society of Physiotherapists in 1987/8. Here it is possible to separate turnover from wastage - revealing that over half of those leaving were moving within the NHS, a much higher figure than that mentioned in Gray, Normand and Currie (1989), reviewed above. (See Tables 9.9 - 9.11.) Buchan and Pike (1989) quote information from similar surveys, carried out by the professions themselves, which suggest that much the same pattern of leavers' destinations applies across all PAM groups (Table 9.13).

The data with regard to the PAM staff groups does not permit analysis of the effect of age on wastage rates. However, the Beaumont et al. study does give a breakdown of wastage by regions for physiotherapists. As Table 9.12 reveals, there is a high degree of variability across the country.

Whilst the production of this type of information is indisputably improving, it has to be said that the statistical analysis is still relatively naive and therefore capable of misleading. For example, simple bivariate

Table 9.6
Nursing wastage rates in West Midlands, 1989: by length of service

per cent

Length of service (Years)	Full-time		Part-time	
	Male	Female	Male	Female
<1	73	80	121	92
1 -2	6	8	12	10
2 -3	8	8	22	9
3 -5	9	10	5	8
5 -10	4	5	11	6
10-15	3	4	3	5

Source: West Midlands RHA (1990).

Table 9.7
Nursing wastage rates in West Midlands, 1989: qualified and unqualified nurses

per cent

Age	Qualified		Unqualified	
	Full-time	Part-time	Full-time	Part-time
21-25	34	34	11	51
26-30	23	23	15	25
31-35	15	19	8	19
36-40	10	14	7	14
41-45	7	15	8	13
46-50	6	10	6	10
51-55	7	9	7	9
56-60	17	21	9	15
61-65	40	28	21	10

Source: West Midlands RHA (1990).

Table 9.8
Destination of nurses leaving West Midlands, 1984

percentage of total leavers

	Full-time	Part-time
Other RHA	16	3
Death	1	1
Maternity	5	7
Retirement	8	9
Redundancy	1	4
Dismissal	1	1
End of contract	7	8
Private sector	5	4
Public agency	1	1
Other	5	3
Different employment	6	7
Not working	8	15
Abroad	1	0
Not known	32	38

Source: West Midlands RHA (1990).

Table 9.9
Trends in numbers of physiotherapy leavers and joiners in England, 1984-1988

per cent of in post

Period	Leavers	Joiners
1984-85	18.7	20.1
1985-86	19.3	20.4
1986-87	20.7	20.8
1987-88	22.0	21.5

Source: Beaumont, Thornton and Sleany (1989).

Table 9.10
Physiotherapist leaver destinations: England, 1988

Destinations of the 1,818 WTE leavers recorded by the 1988 CSP Staffing Survey for England

-    56 % of leavers remain within the NHS

     Of these 30% move on promotion
             68% leave to a job of a similar grade
             2% move to a lower grade

-    14% of leavers move abroad

     Of these 64% continue to work in physiotherapy
             29% go for holiday/travel reasons
             7% are returning to their home country

-    6% of leavers move to physiotherapy work outside the NHS. The majority of these are in private practice, the remainder in clinics or in industry

-    2% of leavers move to non-physiotherapy work.

-    4.5% of leavers reach retirement

-    13.5% of leavers move for maternity and domestic reasons

-    4% of leavers move for other reasons, including ill health 1%, further study 1%

-    0.3% are unemployed and currently seeking employment

Source: Beaumont, Thornton and Sleany (1989).

comparisons can fail to identify the true reasons for variations in wastage rates (the above point about regional variations possibly being due to no more than differences in age structure is an illustration). Multivariate analysis using either econometric techniques or statistical modelling, as described in Barry, Soothill and Francis (1989), are much to be preferred. Similarly, the current method of calculating wastage rates (i.e. non-cohort) makes them prone to variation due to the past rate of growth in the total workforce. For example, a constant length of service will produce a constant wastage rate if the workforce size is also constant but a declining

Table 9.11
Sources of physiotherapist joiners: England, 1988

In 1987/1988, of the 1,780.4 WTE joiners recorded by the CSP Staffing Survey in England:

- 51% of joiners came from another NHS post

- 37% of joiners were newly qualified staff

- 5% of joiners were returning after a career break

- 3% of joiners returned from non NHS posts

- 4% of joiners were returning from abroad

Source: Beaumont, Thornton and Sleany (1989).

Table 9.12
Physiotherapist wastage rate from English NHS by region, 1988

per cent

	Wastage
Northern	10.8
Yorkshire	8.3
Trent	8.2
East Anglian	8.5
North West Thames	12.9
North East Thames	13.3
South East Thames	11.0
South West Thames	12.0
Wessex	8.3
Oxford	10.6
South Western	9.8
West Midlands	8.8
Mersey	7.2
North Western	7.1
ENGLAND	9.9

Source: Beaumont, Thornton and Sleany (1989).

Table 9.13
PAM staff leaving health authorities in Great Britain from
1/4/87 to 31/3/88

| | Total known staff leaving | % as of total WTE | % to other employment | | | % no longer working because of: | | |
| | | | Within NHS | Non-NHS Employment | | Maternity | Retirement/ ill health | Other [b] |
				In UK	Abroad			
Chiropody	227.5[a]	13.4	46.7	18.7	7.0	7.6	9.4	9.7
Dietetics	256.2[a]	19.3	58.4	9.8	5.1	7.8	2.4	13.9
Occ. Therapy	1,107.5	18.2	59.9[d]	17.9[e]	5.7	6.6	1.7	8.2
Orthoptics	67.8[a]	12.0	51.6	5.9	7.4	13.3	6.2	15.6
Physiotherapy	2,112.4[a]	19.5	55.5	7.9	13.9	9.0	5.5	7.4
Radiography	877.2[a]	10.6	48.5	9.0	12.3	10.7	6.8	12.7
TOTAL	4,648.6[d]		54.9	11.1	10.7	8.7	4.8	9.2

Source: Buchan and Pike (1989)

Notes: (a) Unspecified leavers included.
(b) Others include leavers who left for further study, for other domestic commitments, are unemployed or looking for another job.
(c) Figures exclude Special Health Authorities.
(d) Includes staff moving within health authorities.
(e) Includes 95.4 WTE moving to Local Authorities.
(f) Totals may not equal the sum of components because of rounding.

Percentages have generally been calculated on rounded figures.

rate if the workforce is expanding. Of course, it is still early days and no doubt the level of sophistication will improve as familiarity with the issues grows. The paper by Barry *et al.* mentioned above is a useful attempt by statisticians to talk to nursing managers about the tricks of their trade in this respect, and hopefully it is only the first of many.

9.2   Explaining turnover - attitude surveys

Factors which are conventionally regarded as affecting turnover can be grouped into three categories:

  (i)   personal
             - e.g. age and sex
  (ii) institutional
             - level of skill and responsibility
             - degree of job satisfaction/job related stress
  (iii) market
             - unemployment, relative pay, etc.

Attempts to explain turnover within the NHS have tended to concentrate on the first and second categories.   Young *et al.* (1983) seek the explanation for what they seem to regard as a higher level of turnover and instability among nurses than might be expected, given their levels of skill and responsibility, in an attitude survey.   That is, they adopt a sociological framework and assume that the explanation is institutional.   The survey revealed a large measure of job satisfaction and a strong sense of corporate identity.   It also suggested that, whilst nurses saw themselves as underpaid, this caused little resentment.   The 'problem' seemed to lie in the 'stress' of the job.   Respondents tended to be critical of the quality of the training they had received and complained of a lack of supervision and support in the period immediately following qualification - i.e. they felt inadequately prepared to cope on their own.   There was also evidence of concern over the instability of ward staff, particularly with regard to support for trainees, and inexperience of ward sisters (many felt that their promotion had come too quickly simply because of rapid turnover).   They also tended to feel that they were working too many hours and were too busy, though the authors suggest this is probably not true - i.e. the feeling is the result of stress, not the cause of it.

Three other studies of nursing are based on questionnaires designed to elicit attitudes and opinions.   Waite and Hutt (1987) is another of the studies commissioned by the RCN from the IMS.   Since only RCN members were surveyed, the sample is biased.   As Waite and Hutt say, individuals who decide to withdraw from the profession are unlikely to maintain their membership of the RCN.   It might also be added that, whilst the RCN is the largest of the nursing unions, it is not the only one - and one would not expect the choice between the 'establishment' RCN and the more 'militant' COHSE, NUPE, etc. to be random.   It is difficult, therefore, to know to what extent their findings can be generalised. When asked for their opinions on possible reasons for leaving NHS employment, respondents (most of whom were of course still in the organization) tended to mention factors such as stress, bad atmosphere, excessive workloads - but also the desire to broaden their experience. Questioned about their opinion on which factors might influence the retention and return of staff to the NHS, respondents seemed to attach greater significance to better pay, but continued to mention 'more realistic' staffing levels.

The responses to other questions are consistent. When asked directly, respondents revealed a fairly low level of satisfaction with their pay, but when questioned about what they regarded as most important, they tended to regard pay as a 'second most important' factor - second to things such as job security, good atmosphere and doing a worthwhile job. When asked about their perceptions of changes in the NHS environment over recent years, increased workload and responsibility, increased frustration in trying to 'get things done' and decreased morale were the most common types of response. Consistent with one of the findings of Young *et al.* 'good support and counselling' were usually rated as fairly important, and were commonly felt to be lacking.

A methodological drawback of such studies is the common failure to provide the factual, as opposed to perceived, background. The device of claiming that 'perceptions become their own reality' is, of course, counter-scientific mystification. In this study there is, for example, no attempt to determine whether staffing levels really have worsened and workloads really increased, so causing stress, or whether the 'feeling' that this is the case is an expression of stress, rather than a cause.

Similarly, one wonders about the wisdom of asking members of a profession strongly imbued with an ethos of caring and dedication whether they are 'in it for the money' in quite such an open and straight forward manner - is the wage really of only secondary importance, or is that what the respondent believes ought to be the case?

An interesting contrast is provided by Mackay (1988). This reports the findings of a smaller, but well balanced, survey in one DHA in the north of England - the questionnaire was administered to a random sample of 1 in 3 nurses in post and all who had left the DHA in the previous 15 months. The respondents were asked to rate the importance of 11 possible ways of encouraging the retention of trained nurses. Pay was revealed to be the most prominent factor - 94 per cent of both samples rated it as important or very important. Other high scorers were regular training opportunities, better promotion prospects and crèche and nursery facilities. It is not necessarily the case that this finding is any nearer the truth than those of Waite and Hutt but it does offer an important counter to the quite widely held view that 'pay doesn't matter'.

The third study is Price Waterhouse (1988). It, also, merely asked nurses for their opinions and intentions and came to no very surprising conclusions: evidence of dissatisfaction with pay and stress from pressure of work was found.

Francis, Peelo and Soothill (1988), from the same research team as Mackay, report work which makes novel use of attitudinal data. The motivation for the analysis is that it should not be presumed that nurses are a homogeneous group. Thus latent class analysis was used and 4 groups, categorised according to attitudes towards the job, were identified. Interestingly, the group into which the largest percentage of respondents capable of being classified were placed (28 per cent) was the non-career-minded one, dubbed 'nursing, just a job'. The other three groups ('nursing come what may'; 'nursing but for how much longer'; and 'nursing, battling it out') attracted a little under 20 per cent each. The conclusion drawn is that it would be futile to pursue a one-solution strategy towards human resource management for nurses.

Beardshaw and Robinson (1990) describes an otherwise unpublished report for Trent RHA by Hart (1989). This is again an attitude survey, but an interesting point is made about the clash between the NHS management's desire to see turnover rates reduced and a nursing culture which regards variety of experience as important and therefore positively encourages job mobility. It is suggested that some nurse managers might therefore have mixed feelings about implementing policies which treat staff retention as the sole aim.

9.3 Explaining turnover - observing behaviour

Mercer (1979) uses multiple linear regression to investigate the influence of socio-psychological variables on turnover. His dependent variable is a dichotomous stay/leave one. His determining variables are age, education, length of service and a prior expression of 'intention to move'. The results are weak and not very informative: the explanatory power of the 'intention to move' variable dominates all others. Further, the econometrics is flawed; as Missiakoulis et al. (1980) and Knapp et al. (1981 and 1982) point out, MLR is inappropriate with a dichotomous dependent variable.

Pfeffer and O'Reilly (1987) is an American study of nursing turnover and is worthy of mention, not because it is a seminal piece of work (for reasons given below, it is considered seriously flawed) nor because it is an example of the economic approach, seriously lacking in the British literature (the background of the authors is in business studies), but because its viewpoint is different.

The general hypothesis considered is that organizations with more heterogeneous employees will experience greater turnover. The particular version of that hypothesis tested in the Pfeffer and O'Reilly paper defines heterogeneity in terms of variation in size of entering cohorts. The argument used to back that hypothesis is that variations in cohort size will cause unequal and fluctuating probabilities of promotion and unequal and fluctuating burdens upon experienced staff.

If the idea is interesting, the test is not. The authors look for statistical relationships between turnover and two 'indices of inequality', whilst allowing for the influence of other factors known to affect turnover: unemployment; relative wages; presence or absence of collective bargaining; and hospital type (private or government funded). The statistical tests are correlation coefficients and simple multiple linear regression. The problem arises in the way the variables are measured. The turnover rate is the crude overall one rather than a cohort specific measure. More critically, the 'indices of inequality' are measures of the distribution of staff across 4 categories based on length of service. In other words, they are based on the alternative measure of turnover discussed above - stability rates. Thus the finding of a highly significant relationship between the turnover rate and these measures of inequality comes as no great surprise. It is difficult to see any link between the original concept of cohort heterogeneity and these empirical measures - perhaps the choice of measure for cohort heterogeneity was constrained by the data. Whatever the reason, one can only conclude that the empirics are not a fair test of the hypothesis, but the hypothesis might be worth developing and testing properly.

Gray *et al.* (1989) take a different viewpoint again. As noted above, the authors are economists and the hypothesis tested reflects this. It is that differences in turnover between DHAs can be explained by differences in their local labour markets. The test used is again based upon simple multiple linear regression. Once again the idea is interesting but its development is limited. Eight measures of factors prevailing in the local economy are tried: the unemployment rate; the change in that rate over the past three years; the percentage of the working age population who are economically active; the percentage of the economically active population who are employed in producer service and high tech. industries; the number of private nursing home beds; average manual female earnings; average non-manual female earnings; and average house prices. The choice of variables is *ad hoc,* justified on the basis of no more than a sentence of *a priori* reasoning and without any reference either to existing theories on quit rates or to possible statistical worries over multicollinearity, etc. A follow-up project, funded by the DoH, entitled *Recruitment and Retention of NHS Staff: A local labour market approach,* has yet to be made public.

Finally, one point to emerge from Moores *et al.* (1983) is of interest. The responses of married nurses to questions about their husband's occupation and earnings suggest that the probability of their working, and working full-time, decreases against their social class and alternative sources of household income - i.e. financial necessity is a prime reason for working. Again one must not put too much reliance on this finding, for the sample was non-random and the statistical analysis very simple. Nevertheless, it is reassuring to report that a study asked a sensible question and could then interpret the answers in a sensible manner.

151

10 Manpower planning in the NHS: A critical review

10.1 Introduction and summary

Objectives

The objective of this chapter is to provide a brief but critical review of the literature on what has traditionally been termed manpower planning, with special reference to the health service. Although this terminology appears increasingly out-dated, given pressures towards equal opportunity and the use of non-sexist language, the term is still in regular use, even in the health services where the majority of the workforce are female. The present review, has not attempted to use alternative terminology. However, the term manpower planning should be understood to refer to the management of all human resources. Given the focus of the present volume the emphasis is on nurses rather than doctors, although some brief reference is made to the latter.

National manpower planning

Section 2 summarizes the literature on general manpower planning, both at a national and company level. This discussion includes a review of the methodologies adopted as well as a summary of the main criticisms of the approach and the manpower planner's response to such criticism.

Manpower planning first became prominent during the early 1960s when economists were concerned about problems of both structural unemployment and manpower shortages. Initially it was hoped that governments would be able to intervene, especially on the supply side of the labour market, in order to ensure a balance between the demand for and the supply of skills.

The initial optimism of the planners was soon dented, both by technical and practical problems in producing accurate forecasts, as well as a barrage of theoretical criticism which questioned the whole rationale for manpower forecasts. Although these criticisms have been rejected to some extent, the nature of the manpower forecasting undertaken in the 1990s is now very different from that attempted in the 1960s. Forecasts of both the demand for (and in a few cases the supply of) skills at the national level are regularly undertaken in most of the major OECD economies. However, these assessments are very different from the indicative type planning exercises attempted by the pioneers of the 1960s. In particular, the attempt to link the changing pattern of demand for skills to regulation of the intake into education and training courses has now been recognised as impractical.

Current assessments emphasise the implications of past patterns of change for the future demand for skills, often using quite sophisticated econometric models. The aim is to present policy makers with information on the labour market environment that they may face if such trends continue. They may also attempt to assess the effect of different courses of action. The information provided by such assessments is only one of the necessary inputs into decisions about the scale and content of different education and training programmes which government officials, educationalists, companies and trade unions will need to use in developing their strategic thoughts. Current thinking is that the scale of education and training programmes needs to reflect the demand from individuals, the latter making choices based upon a vast range of micro as well as macroeconomic information, which a bureaucrat would not be able to take into account.

Company manpower planning

In parallel with the development of national manpower models there was a growing interest in personnel planning at a microeconomic level. Company manpower planning also began in earnest during the 1960s although some institutions had undertaken this kind of exercise for many years. Much intellectual effort has been put into understanding the problems of wastage and recruitment in order to ensure that companies have the skills they require. Most major companies and other large employing institutions are now well aware of the importance of human resource planning. Many now have personnel officers in quite senior positions whose main responsibilities are to deal with such problems.

As at the macroeconomic level, the nature of such planning has changed over the years, with much less emphasis on mechanistic manpower models. Nevertheless, there is a considerable amount of effort devoted to forecasting wastage and assessing future recruitment needs.

Section 3 of this chapter moves on to consider manpower planning within Health Services. This provides examples of both 'macroeconomic' type manpower planning and the more company level type of exercise. In the case of the former these may cover whole countries or somewhat smaller geographical areas (such as the Regional Health Authorities in the UK). In the case of the latter, manpower planning is conducted from the individual ward level up to whole hospitals. In the context of nursing manpower planning the most relevant work is probably that undertaken by certain UK Regional Health Authorities although the studies at other levels are also of some relevance. Considerable attention has also been placed on planning the labour market for doctors. Although this is not a key concern here, it would be remiss to ignore this body of work completely. A very brief overview is therefore included in Section 3.

As a general rule, the methodology adopted in the manpower models developed within the health services is not technically very sophisticated. On the demand side a simple fixed coefficient approach is the general rule, with the provision of particular types of service being linked directly to the requirement of specialised nursing and other skills. Rarely, if ever, has an attempt been made to assess the scope for substitution of skills, although the whole subject of 'skill-mix' has become increasingly topical in recent years. The latter reflects a growing interest in changing the skill-mix used to provide health services in response to financial considerations (e.g. greater use of auxiliaries in place of nurses). This is of course a classic example of substitution in economic terms but such considerations have not figured in the manpower planning forecasts in terms of linking changes in parameters to wage changes.

Considerable attention has also been placed on the analysis of wastage, especially amongst nurses. Much of this analysis has focused on what might better be termed turnover rather than wastage, much of the loss representing people moving from one employer to another, rather than the complete loss of such skills to the health service as a whole.

Other aspects of supply have also received some attention but, as with wastage and the demand side generally, there is little or no emphasis on economic considerations in attempting to model these phenomena. Fixed coefficients or constant rates of inflow or outflow are generally assumed. While this may be a reasonable starting point for analysing future manpower developments, it begs a number of questions, especially if the forecast horizon extends more than a year or so.

Much of the methodology that has been used seems to reflect the availability of existing data (often collected for administrative purposes) rather than theoretical considerations of what is important. For example, there is very little emphasis on the total supply of health service personnel and the economic activity rate decision. Rather the focus is on the stock of those currently employed, the age structure of this stock, wastage rates etc.

Main conclusions

The first conclusion from this brief review is that manpower planning can provide a useful aid to policy makers in making decisions about training, recruitment and personnel issues. The second conclusion however, is that there are strong limitations to what such exercises can do. They do not offer a crystal ball from which the future can be gleaned. Rather they spell out the implications of a series of assumptions about future developments based on certain relationships with past patterns of behaviour.

The value of such exercises will depend crucially on the quality of the data upon which they are based, as well as the validity of the various assumptions built into the forecasts. To some extent the latter will depend upon the degree of sophistication of the models adopted. Naive, mechanistic models are, unless used very carefully, likely to mislead rather than inform. On the other hand, increasing complexity and sophistication of such models can rapidly run into decreasing returns, unless backed up by data and analysis of equivalent quality.

With regard to manpower planning in Health Services, the review suggests that, while a considerable amount of work is going on in this area, it is generally not very sophisticated from a technical viewpoint. Often this reflects the fact that manpower planning has been conducted using data readily available from administrative records rather than information specifically collected for the purpose.

On the demand side two main methods have been used. The first is the manpower requirements approach, based on fixed coefficient links between the demands for service (i.e. patient care) and skill requirements. The second method is based on surveys of employers. The former has been adopted most frequently in the health services. Generally speaking, the 'bottom up' variant, in which the coefficients are based on micro level analysis of skill requirements at the ward level has been most popular. However, this has been criticised as more relevant to low level decision making than strategic policy on human resource planning.

On the supply side two main methods have been adopted. The stock-flow approach projects future stocks from current levels by predicting inflows and outflows. This is usually done on the basis of assuming fixed rates of flow based on past data. However, there is much evidence accumulating that such flows are dependent on economic and other variables. The focus of such models tends to be on the existing workforce and wastage rates. An alternative method has been proposed which focuses on the participation rate of all those qualified. While in principle this is consistent with the stock-flow model, this method tends to use different data sources, but the results from the two methods seem broadly equivalent. As with the stock-flow models such methods ignore the fact

155

that participation rates change in response to changing labour market conditions. Their use therefore requires considerable care when projections are being made beyond the short-term if misleading inferences about future demand-supply imbalances are not to be made.

10.2 A general review of manpower planning

Manpower planning: A brief history

Manpower forecasting has been undertaken in one form or another for many years and there is now an enormous literature covering work at both a macro and micro level. A number of useful reviews have been conducted to which the interested reader is referred for more detailed discussion (see, for example, Hughes, 1991a and 1991b; Colclough, 1990; Smith and Bartholomew, 1988; and Youdi and Hinchliffe, 1985). The present section attempts to provide a summary of the main features of this literature.

During the 1960s manpower forecasting became prominent at a national level as economists attempted to advise governments on how to avoid imbalances between the supply and demand for skills (whether appearing as structural unemployment or skill shortages impeding economic growth). At that time it was hoped that manpower plans could be developed which could be used to guide policy decisions relating to the provision of educational and training programmes at a very detailed level (i.e. for particular levels of qualifications or specialisms).

In practice the methods adopted tend to be rather naive and mechanistic. As a result, these early forecasts were usually very inaccurate, especially on the supply side. The typical methods adopted involved linking the demand for particular skills to output projections for different industries, often via some form of input-output model (see for example Parnes, 1962; and Hollister, 1967). The links were generally a series of fixed coefficients. This assumption was heavily criticised as failing to recognise the possibility of substitution of one factor of production (or skill) for another, (see for example, Ahamad and Blaug, 1970).

Criticisms of manpower planning

Three main criticisms of the general manpower requirements approach have been offered (see Colclough, 1990):

(i) that national level manpower planning is irrelevant because markets will respond of their own accord to ensure that the correct skills are produced;

(ii) that the fixed coefficient approach is invalid since it ignores the possibilities of economic substitution;

(iii) that inaccuracies in the assumptions will be compounded making the projections of little value.

These criticisms have all been rejected by manpower planners. With regard to the first criticism, they point to evidence of market failure (reflected in persistent skill shortages) and to the long-lags in training (which can lead to temporary but long-lasting imbalances in occupational labour markets). With regard to the second point they highlight empirical evidence that the elasticity of substitution for skills is low and argue that wage structures tend to exhibit stability over the long-term. The third criticism is rejected on the grounds that the problem of forecasting inaccuracy is not unique to manpower forecasting but applies to any economic projections. Evidence does not suggest that manpower forecasts are significantly more inaccurate than any others and it appears that policy makers have found them useful, (see Corcoran and Hughes, 1991).

Manpower planning in the 1990s

As a consequence manpower planning has continued to be practised, albeit in a less mechanistic and indicative fashion. Most developed countries now undertake regular labour market projections although these are used as general aids to policy makers to illustrate the implications of a continuation of past economic and labour market trends for the future, rather than as an indicative input into educational planning. It is emphasised by most practitioners that such assessments should be regarded as broad-brush guides to the sort of environment that policy makers may face rather than a crystal ball.

Manpower forecasts can be subject to wide margins of error but this does not invalidate them, any more than it does other economic forecasts. One of the key problems in all social science forecasting is of course that the forecast itself may alter behaviour and indeed this is often a key objective. In any event, as Cairncross (1969) notes, forecasts should not be taken too literally or as telling policy makers what to do. A manpower forecast should be treated as one among many pieces of information which planners need to assess before taking decisions. As such, they can be used to help evaluate the risks which exist in the present situation. Manpower forecasts can contribute to the decisions which have to be taken with regard to education, training, and choice of occupation by providing, as Colclough (1990, p.20) argues, 'a detailed, consistent and plausible picture (if properly done) of how the future might look.'

Methodological approaches: demand

Manpower forecasting has adopted a variety of different methods. The fixed coefficient **manpower requirements approach** is the most common method of dealing with the demand side. As noted above, this has usually involved making a series of links from Gross National Production (GNP),

157

to individual industry output, to employment, to the demand for particular skills. In most of the early manpower models these links were all in the form of fixed coefficients. More recently the models used have been more sophisticated, allowing for changing coefficients and responses to economic variables such as prices and relative wages.

Surveys of employers, asking them what their future demand will be has been another popular approach. The latter was the subject of especially strong criticism. This centred upon the lack of any firm theoretical foundation as well as the practical problems of ensuring that all respondents are adopting common assumptions about the future scenario and that their responses are mutually consistent (for example, all the firms in an industry cannot increase their market share). Such methods have been used more recently by Rajan and Pearson (1986) and can, if deployed with care, produce useful results. Their main value is where the available data are inadequate to build more sophisticated time series econometric models (and as such they are still widely used in developing countries).

Methodological approaches: supply

On the supply side, the typical approach has been to develop simple **stock-flow models** relating the total stock of manpower in period t to that in period t+1 using an accounting identity linking the main inflows and outflows to the stock. Supplementary models to determine the proportion of the stock that are economically active (and if it is a particular occupation that is of interest, the proportion actively engaged in that particular job) are also used. The main outflows considered are those due to death, retirement and other exits from the workforce and emigration. The main inflows relate to the flow of new entrants (qualified as appropriate), re-entrants to the workforce and migration. If the focus is on particular occupational categories then inter-occupational mobility also needs to be considered.

Quite sophisticated systems of demographic accounts were developed in the 1960s to parallel the national economic accounts. However, lack of government interest has meant that these have not been developed in line with the financial accounts. As a result manpower models have not flourished to the same degree as the macroeconomic models based upon the economic accounts. Nevertheless, manpower forecasters have made attempts to fill the information gaps from various *ad hoc* surveys and to build models which allow for some response in flow and activity rates to economic and other factors.

In the more sophisticated models, detailed econometric analysis of time series data has been undertaken to explain historical trends in rates of flow and economic activity rates and to project them into the future. Where data are more limited these rates are assumed fixed or extrapolated from a few observations. Data limitations have meant that the more sophisticated models are restricted to particular occupational categories, where good information on the various stocks flows are available, (see for example Wilson *et al.*, 1990).

Company level manpower planning

Companies and other employing institutions also have an obvious interest in monitoring their workforces and assessing the implications for recruitment of such factors as the age structure of the workforce, wastage rates, and changing patterns of demand. Company level manpower planning (or personnel planning to use a less sexist term) is now a well established management function. Larger companies and employing institutions often have a specialist personnel manager in quite a senior position to undertake this function.

At the company level, the range of models and methods is, of course, even broader ranging from very simple rules of thumb to quite complex models paralleling the national level ones described above. These tend to focus more on the short-term than the national models, reflecting the different interests of governments and individual companies. The former are generally more concerned with the longer term development of the economy and the provision of education programmes which involve long lags between entry and qualification. They are therefore much more interested in projections 5-10 years ahead. Companies on the other hand tend to be more concerned with immediate problems connected with recruitment and wastage.

Manpower planning in Health Services may cover both these two extremes depending upon whether it is being conducted at micro or macro level. Where the focus is more upon the short-term, the assumptions of fixed coefficients is more sustainable. However, the longer-term the forecast being undertaken, the more important it is to recognise that such coefficients may be changing because of long-term trend influences as behaviour responds to changing economic circumstances.

10.3 Health services manpower planning

Manpower planning at the national level

Manpower planning within health services has also been conducted for many years. It is possible to distinguish the more general macro level approaches adopted to plan human resource allocation at a national or regional level, from the more micro level studies that are concerned with meeting needs at the level of individual wards or hospitals. A further distinction is between planning for nursing and planning for doctors. A key criticism of much human resource planning within the health service, is that these two elements have been kept quite separate, despite the possibilities of substitution of doctors for nurses or other health staff (and *vice versa*).

At the national level, as for manpower planning in general, there has been a gradual change in emphasis from formal, mechanistic, quantitative manpower forecasts to more qualitative types of analysis, as the limitations of the former methods were realised. In the UK, for example, there has been considerable discussion in recent years about the future of the National Health Service (NHS) and the labour market, in the context of demographic changes. However, although various studies have been undertaken to examine possible future scenarios, (see for example, Beardshaw and Robinson, 1990; Reid, 1986; Royal College of Nurses, 1985a and 1985b; Conroy and Stidston, 1988; Committee of Public Accounts, 1987; and Price-Waterhouse, 1987) these have not been based upon a formal national manpower forecasting model. Certain elements have of course been quantified, but indicative planning, which assumes a series of fixed links between the demand for health services and the requirements for particular skills, has not been attempted. Indeed, the Committee of Public Accounts (CPA) in the UK has taken the Department of Health and Social Security (DHSS) to task for its lack of control on staffing in the NHS. Its 1981 report (CPA, 1981) highlighted the lack of information at the centre and the failure of the centre to recognise or investigate very large differences in staffing levels in different Health Authorities. This resulted in the DHSS undertaking an investigation of methods used (DHSS, 1983) which revealed a variety of methods of varying degrees of sophistication. However, generally speaking, they all failed to take account of any economic constraints or the responsiveness of supply to economic incentives. Subsequent CPA reports suggest that matters have not greatly improved. Dawson et al. (1990) represents a notable exception which does explicitly consider financial aspects.

With regard to doctors there is a long history of manpower planning which has been the responsibility of a whole series of official committees since the 1940s. Their work has been reviewed and criticised by Birch et al. (1986). The latter, while recognising that improvements have been made, argue that the current methodology is still inadequate and in particular suffers from the lack of recognition of the need to consider the allocation of labour resources generally throughout the NHS.

A considerable amount of research has been undertaken in the UK in the context of proposals within the nursing profession to increase their standing by upgrading the nature of their professional qualification. The original proposals emanate from a committee commissioned by the nurses' professional body, the RCN (Royal College of Nursing, 1985a). This committee commissioned the Institute of Manpower Services, Sussex, and the Centre for Health Economics, York, to investigate respectively the staffing and cost implications of their proposals. These studies appear in RCN (1985b), and Bosanquet and Goodwin (1986). Almost simultaneously, the body in charge of training and registration, the UKCC, also investigated the issue: they produced a very similar set of proposals (United Kingdom Central Council for Nursing, Midwifery and Health Visiting, 1986). This time the staffing and cost implications were

160

investigated by Price Waterhouse (Price Waterhouse, 1987), although this study draws heavily on the earlier work of the IMS and the CHE. The IMS report for the RCN (RCN, 1985b) is interesting because it developed a simple workforce planning model which could in principle be adapted to provide a useful framework to investigate general staffing issues. However, although the IMS study developed a potentially useful model it did very little with it. For an example of how such a model can be used to guide policy it is necessary to turn to the introductory Commentary to RCN (1985b) in which the Commission used the model to argue their case for the reforms they proposed.

There has in recent years been some recognition that health service personnel, although driven by a strong sense of vocation, are subject to the same economic and social incentives and disincentives as other groups of workers (see the discussion in both Chapter 6 and Chapter 8). Rising real incomes in other parts of the economy and pressures towards equal opportunities for women are both impinging on the supply side of the equation, while the financial constraints imposed on the total scale of public expenditure have provided a budget limit on the scale of labour demand in many countries. Health services the world over are therefore facing the problem of skill shortages. Nevertheless, in formal modelling terms there are still very few examples of manpower planning models which explicitly take financial considerations into account.

Manpower planning at a sub-national level

There has been much more work on nursing workforce planning undertaken at the sub-national level in the UK although this still stretches across a broad spectrum from Regional Health Authorities down to individual wards. Some of the most relevant work has been conducted by certain Regional Health Authorities, such as Trent, and Wales. The Comptroller and Auditor General has also published a review of procedures in Northern Ireland. Most are using nursing manpower supply models to assist in development of human resource planning strategies (Welsh Common Services Authority, Health Intelligence Unit, 1989 and 1990; and for Trent, Beaumont, 1988 and Beaumont *et al.* 1989). These are workforce planning models similar to that developed by IMS for the RCN. Trent is also developing models for other occupational categories. Many other Health Authorities have also developed less sophisticated models. Much of the emphasis has been on assessing staffing requirements, often at the ward level.

Demand: two main approaches

As noted in Chapter 7, it is possible to distinguish two main approaches to the 'demand' side of the picture. The **'top-down'** method attempts to relate labour requirements to various measures of the demand for care or the level of a particular clinical activity. This may be based on past

161

observed relationships (including, in more sophisticated variants, some measure of trend change) or a policy choice of what constitutes a best/acceptable/adequate level of staffing. Neither of these alternatives can be regarded as properly measuring demand for skills in the true economic sense, since relative costs and the possibilities of substitution of one skill for another are simply not recognised. In this sense they still parallel the national manpower planning of 20-30 years ago with its emphasis on fixed coefficients.

This type of approach characterises much of the medical manpower planning undertaken for doctors. It has also been adopted in a number of Regional Health Authorities in the UK such as Trent, and Wales for planning nursing requirements. It has also been used in the United States (see Leenders, 1985). It has tended to be adopted as a strategic planning and management tool, aimed at providing an early warning of impending shortages or surplus (in conjunction with models of supply).

The second approach is termed **'bottom-up'**. This is typically undertaken at the more microeconomic level of individual district Health Authorities starting at ward level. Staffing requirements are based on work study appraisals of the workload generated by patients with particular medical problems or are based on 'professional judgement'. These methods tend, from a clinical point of view, to provide more accurate work-load measures than the top-down method. However, they are essentially low-level decision making aids rather than strategic planning control ones. As with the top down approach they entirely ignore financial and economic considerations. Even in their own terms they are often vague on the question of variability in workloads (for example, do they represent minimum or average requirements?) and the question of the quality of care provided to the patient. Nevertheless, they are in widespread use, often based on now well established 'formulae' or rules of thumb.

Whichever approach is adopted the methods used include adjustments to allow for part-time working, everything being expressed in whole-time equivalents. The contribution by trainee sources also needs to be taken into account when comparing supply and demand.

With the recent interest in 'grade-mix' within the context of reform in the NHS a live issue, the whole question of the possibility of substitution of unqualified for qualified staff has been raised once again within the UK. It is also a subject of much interest in the United States. However, there appears to be little literature on just what the scope for substitution may be and on the implications for patient care per pound spent. The DHSS has published a study on grade mix (Wright-Warren, 1986) which contains a useful literature review. The author finds little evidence of systematic evaluation or analysis.

More recently Ball et al. (1989) have published a description of a multi-disciplinary project to determine the desired nursing staff level and grade mix for wards in a new hospital. This project, funded by Mersey

RHA, is reviewed in detail in Chapter 7. Essentially, it is in the tradition of the non-economic methodologies. In introducing a quality of care dimension, this approach explicitly attempts to identify a normative standard of staffing - i.e. the amount of staffing necessary to provide a pre-determined minimum standard of care. There is, however, no explicit reference to evidence that high scores on the quality of care check list correlate with better patient outcomes and there is no formal appreciation of the possibility of trade-off between standard of care and staffing costs. As noted in Chapter 7, there is a marked contrast between this study and American ones such as Flood and Diers (1988). Flood and Diers' report using a simple methodology makes a genuine attempt at an economic analysis. It compares patient outcomes in a ward staffed at its establishment level against those achieved in a similar ward which was short-staffed. The evidence that patients suffer as a consequence of a ward which is understaffed is then used as the basis for a case that the cost of care can actually rise due to inadequate staffing levels.

The general situation in the UK within the NHS, however, seems to be that nursing and related staffing levels are determined at a relatively low decision making level by methods which lack sophistication. Different Health Authorities adopt different rules of thumb and subsequently have often quite different staffing levels for similar clinical needs. However, there is increasing pressure on the NHS to achieve efficiency savings by ensuring that all Health Authorities produce various 'performance indicators' and attempt to achieve the 'best' or 'most efficient' standards.

Supply

On the supply side, there are few examples of attempts to build national level supply models for nurses or other groups apart from doctors. In the case of the latter, increasingly sophisticated models have been developed, culminating in that used by the Advisory Committee for Medical Manpower Planning, (1989). Detailed data are available from administrative records and concerns about the need to get an adequate balance between supply and demand for doctors have resulted in considerable resources being devoted to developing a computerised model. Such a comprehensive approach has not, by and large, been attempted for nurses or other health staff. For those other groups there are, however, many examples of quite detailed studies focusing on particular issues such as wastage, labour supply decisions etc. As with the demand side, the literature is not characterised by a great deal of economic sophistication. Key factors such as wastage rates, recruitment into training and economic participation rates are assumed fixed and immune from changes in economic or other influences.

Manpower planning models for nursing have been developed by the IMS, and by some RHAs, for example, Wales, Wessex and Trent. These adopt a traditional stock flow approach to modelling the future workforce. Current stocks are combined with information on expected recruitment

163

and wastage in order to develop projections of the future stock. But there is little behavioural content, rates of flow generally being exogenously fixed. In an alternative approach Trent and Wessex focus on the participation rate of trained nurses. Forecasts of the active population are then based on projections of age-specific participation rates. As Worthington (1988 and 1990) notes, this method is in principle not inconsistent with the stock-flow method, but the two approaches are likely, in practice, to produce different results because they rely on different data sources, (see also Manpower Planning Advisory Group, 1991). Jones (1989) compared the two alternative projections and found them broadly similar.

Worthington's review of this literature stresses a number of key points (see Chapter 8 for a more detailed discussion). First, good data is very important. With stock-flow models a key issue is identifying a true wastage as opposed to total turnover rate. In the case of the participation approach the difficulty is in obtaining regular censuses of the total qualified population. His second point is that the strong life-cycle pattern to female labour supply means that age specific data on wastage or participation rates are crucial if misleading inferences are not to be made (as was the case in early versions of the stock flow models which used broad averages for wastage rates). The third point is that the models lack much behavioural content. Responses to changes in wage rates or other variables such as provision of crèche facilities are not generally incorporated. The related final point is that all such models assume that wastage or participation rates are fixed or based on trends extrapolated from past data. Evidence suggests that these rates can and do change, often quite dramatically (especially wastage rates). Without a proper understanding of why these rates alter, forecasting will tend to be a hazardous business.

Both Worthington and the Trent researchers implicitly assume that participation rates are less unstable than wastage rates. While this may be true, it is clear from the more general labour supply literature that female participation rates do respond to changing real wage rates, so this assumption may be unnecessarily complacent.

Much attention has been focused on the question of wastage, (see for example, Mercer (1979), Young et al. (1983), Thomas et al. (1988), Gray et al. (1989), Beaumont et al. (1989), Buchan and Pike (1989) and West Midlands RHA, Manpower Planning Section (1990). This literature is reviewed in detail in Chapter 9. Various different measures of turnover have been examined although these tend to reflect data available from existing records rather than any attempt to measure the rates of flows which a manpower model would ideally require. For this reason much of the data is inadequate, reflecting total turnover between district Health Authorities rather than true wastage of personnel from the health service. In the Irish context the issue of international migration might also be a more important factor.

Much of this literature is descriptive rather than analytical. However, some attempts at analysing turnover/wastage have also been made, (see for example, Young *et al.*, 1983; Mackay, 1988 and 1989; Price Waterhouse, 1988; Francis *et al.*, 1988; Barry *et al.*, 1989; and Beardshaw and Robinson, 1990). Many studies involve simple attitudinal surveys and cross-tabular analysis. Often these studies fail to recognise the methodological limitations of the use of perceptions rather than factual background as explanatory variables. A few studies have been based on observed behaviour (Mercer, 1979; Moores *et al.*, 1983; Pfeffer and O'Reilly, 1987; Gray *et al.*, 1989) but even these are somewhat basic both from an economic theory and econometric viewpoint. Nevertheless, they suggest that there is considerable scope for modelling such behaviour using conventional econometric models.

The flow of newly qualified entrants into the workforce has not been the subject of much research within the UK. Firby (1990) contains a useful review. Existing models use simple rules of thumb rather than behavioural approaches to explain such flows. Again this contrasts with more general economic analysis of labour supply division which has highlighted responsiveness to wages and other socio-economic variables.

On the issue of economic participation (i.e. whether persons qualified as nurses actually work as such) the literature is much less well served. Chapter 6 provides a general review but Phillips (1989c and 1990) presents a more detailed analysis. Both the general literature on female labour supply and more specific studies on nurses suggest that health service workers behave in a manner consistent with economic theory and that their decisions to work in their chosen profession will depend positively on the wage offered (as well as on many other factors).

The review of the literature in Chapter 8, confirms that these conclusions are supported by various American studies. For example, Link and Settle (1979 and 1981) and Dusansky *et al.* (1986) build quite sophisticated supply models, incorporating economic incentives in order to analyse alternative policies for increasing the supply of nurses. This kind of evidence suggests that nurses and other medical staff respond as much to economic incentives as any other group. This suggests that models of supply based on fixed parameters must be used with great care if misleading inferences are not to be drawn about future labour market imbalances. It also highlights the fact that there is considerable scope for improving the analysis of such issues in the UK and suggests that this area should be a priority one for further research.

11 The supply of nursing skills: Evidence from the LFS

11.1 Introduction

Managers in Regional Health Authorities need to have information about the labour market environment they face. Only very limited data are available in published statistics although there is considerable potential for exploiting various underutilized data sources, given time and resources.

This chapter presents evidence on the supply of nursing skills extracted from the Labour Force Survey (LFS). The LFS represents the most important source of information on the supply of labour skills apart from the Census of Population. The LFS contains a wealth of data on the numbers and characteristics of people in the labour force. The present chapter focuses on those questions which have some bearing on the labour market facing the health services for the UK as a whole. It deals with those who have nursing qualifications or those who are employed as nurses. The chapter concentrates primarily on numbers of people rather than their characteristics although some analysis of hours worked etc. is provided. The initial objective was to provide a time series database covering the period from 1979. In practice problems of changing definitions, changing coding practices etc. have meant that, in order to maintain continuity, attention is currently restricted to 1983-1989. Chapter 12 provides corresponding analyses for two Regional Health Authorities. These have been selected fairly arbitrarily. Similar tables could be produced for all RHAs.

Section 11.2 describes the method of extraction of data from the annual component of the Labour Force Survey (LFS) in order to provide information on the distribution of persons in the UK with and without a nursing qualification, by occupation, age group, usual weekly hours worked, economic status and industry, for the years 1983 to 1989 inclusive. It thus extends the research undertaken by Elias (1987) who was concerned with examining data for 1984 alone.

Section 11.2 also describes the methods used to code, edit and reclassify the responses to various questions that are relevant to this enquiry. A fuller description of the LFS, in terms of sampling procedure, the relevant questions for this enquiry and the interviewing methodology is contained in Appendix A whilst Appendix B gives an indication of the changes in mnemonics and technical characteristics of the LFS across different years. Section 11.3 contains the tables and a short commentary. The results in this chapter provide some indication of the wealth of information available from the LFS. There remain, however, many areas for extending this analysis which could give policy makers further insight into the labour market environment they face. Section 11.4 contains conclusions together with suggestions for such additional work.

11.2 The Labour Force Survey

This section is concerned with describing the methodology used to code, edit and reclassify the responses to the relevant questions for the annual boosts to the LFS for the years 1983 to 1989 inclusive. It briefly describes the differences in questionnaire design and possible responses that are of relevance to this enquiry. As mentioned in the introduction, a fuller description of the LFS and the methodology underlying the questionnaire design is contained in Appendix A. Any one not familiar with the LFS may find it informative to read Appendix A before continuing with the rest of this report.

The data from which the tables presented in Section 3.3 are drawn relate to the annual boost to the Labour Force Survey conducted in the spring of each year since 1984. Previous to that date the survey was conducted in the spring at two-year intervals ending in 1983. The topic of interest, the distribution of persons with nursing qualifications by age group, sex, occupation, economic status, hours usually worked and industry, is derived from replies to a range of questions that form an integral part of all Labour Force Surveys. Several of these questions are repeated in different guises throughout the survey to enable checks to be made on the replies given.

The main difference in questionnaire design, and more importantly interviewee response, concerns the questions used to elicit the economic status of the respondent. As an illustration of these differences we can observe that the 1983 LFS allows 26 possible responses, the 1984 LFS also allows 26 categories of response, albeit in part different to the 1983 responses, whilst the 1985 LFS, through greater disaggregation, increases the number of potential responses to 52. The number of responses was reduced to 28 for 1986, 1987 and 1988 and further reduced to 26 in 1989.

It is possible to disaggregate the responses to all of the LFS questionnaires to a much wider degree by utilising the response to other questions. For example, the 1985 LFS disaggregates most economically active individuals by self-defined part-time and full-time status, whilst for 1987 this same disaggregation is not directly recorded in answers to the question concerning economic status. However, it can be obtained by utilising the response to an alternative question that asks whether the respondent was working full-time or part-time. Thus by utilising the answers to a range of questions in the LFS, the respondents can be reclassified into 10 categories of economic status of which two, full-time and part-time employees may be disaggregated further into three occupation categories; nursing, midwifery and other. Several economic status codes have been merged to give a less disaggregated and hence more easily interpreted table. For example, in the previous research by Elias (1987) those individuals who stated that they were unemployed were subdivided into six distinct categories. Here we present the data under two categories, those actively seeking employment and those who are not seeking employment. These changes reduce the number of rows in the tables from 21 to 14 - thereby making interpretation easier. This gives a consistent and matched set of responses across time. The results of the reclassification are given in Tables 11.3-11.10, which are discussed in detail in the following section.

Occupational descriptions are coded after the interview by the interviewer to one of 350 occupation 'operational' codes. Two of these categories have been selected for detailed analysis here. However, the disaggregation of economic status to include midwifery, occupation 'operational' code 351, is only possible prior to 1985. For the years since 1985, the occupational descriptions do not allow this element of detail and midwives are included within the occupation 'operational' code (043) which also comprises 'Nurses and nurse administrators', including 'nurse auxiliaries'. Amongst others, this latter category includes hospital sisters and matrons together with school matrons.

Prior to 1984 data on occupations were coded by the central office rather than by the interviewer. According to OPCS this should not make any significant difference. However, results of an exercise conducted by IER as part of the development of the new Standard Occupational Classification leave us less sanguine about the impact of this change. In addition to occupation, employed respondents are coded by the interviewer to one of 315 industry codes. This information has been used to recode individuals from five activity groups defined in terms of the 1980 Standard Industrial Classification activity headings as shown in Table 11.1.

These five headings constitute what might be termed a 'health services' group. All other industry codes have been combined in an 'other sectors' group.

Hours usually worked per week have been recoded into five groups (less than 10, 10-19, 20-29, 30-39, 40 and over) whilst the age of the respondent has been recoded into six categories (under 20 years, 20-29, 30-39, 40-49, 50-59 and 60 years and over). In the case of the latter variable it should be noted that data for the '60 years and over' category is only available for female employees from the 1983 LFS.

Finally, it is possible to obtain information on the qualifications of the respondents who give details of their three 'highest' qualifications. The rank order of these qualifications is given in Table 11.2.

Table 11.1
Main activity heading

Activity heading	Description
9510	Hospitals, nursing homes, etc.
9520	Other medical care institutions
9530	Medical practices
9540	Dental practices
9550 etc.	Agency and private midwives, nurses,

Table 11.2
Qualification categories

Higher degree
First degree
Other degree level
BTEC, BEC, TEC, Higher
Teaching qualification secondary
Teaching qualification primary
Nursing qualification
BTEC, BEC, TEC, General
City and Guilds
'A' level etc.
'O' level etc.
CSE
Other professional qualification
None
Don't know

Thus a respondent may reply that their highest qualification is a degree, followed by a nursing qualification and then 'A' levels. In the 1987 LFS, of those people giving a nursing qualification as one of their three

169

qualifications, 95 per cent stated that it was their main (highest) qualification.

There have been a number of changes to the classification of individuals who make no reply or who reply none/don't know when asked about their qualifications. In the more recent Labour Force Surveys some of these individuals have been classified as 'missing' observations'. In addition, since 1985, women aged 65 and over and men aged 70 and over, have been classified as missing observations in response to the question about qualifications. Thus, the data on the retired persons and those in these older age categories need to be interpreted with considerable caution. The extracted data have therefore been altered to specifically exclude all persons aged under 16, men aged 65 and over and women aged 60 and over. The LFS has used a number of alternative approaches to coding individuals who are aged over the standard age of retirement and were still in employment. In the early LFS these data were included for disaggregation by economic status whereas in more recent years they were coded as missing data. Thus by omitting the data a more consistent data set is obtained. Fortunately, the omission of these groups of individuals is of little consequence for the present analysis.

In order to avoid problems caused by reclassification of 'missing' data, and those individuals who responded as having no qualification or 'don't know', the following conventions have been adopted. The qualifications data have been recoded such that the disaggregation of data by qualification refers to the following three categories:

(i)   those who have a nursing qualifications as one of their three 'highest' qualifications;

(ii)   those who do not have a nursing qualification but have an alternative qualification which can be considered as very broadly equivalent to or higher than a nursing qualification. (These include degrees, BTEC, BEC, and TEC qualifications, teaching qualifications and 'A' levels);

(iii) those who do not have a qualification equivalent to nursing or who are recorded as not giving an answer to the question about occupation (i.e. 'missing' data) but do answer the other labour force questions e.g. those about age, occupation, hours worked etc.

Responses have been weighted to yield population estimates. Further information about sample structure, coding, editing and the weighting procedures are given in, for example, the published report of the 1983 and 1984 Labour Force Surveys (OPCS, 1986).

11.3 Results for the UK

Health warning

As noted above, despite efforts to ensure comparability over time some anomalies may still remain. These may reflect changes in the questionnaire, changes in coding practices, changes in coding frames or changes in editing procedures used to extract the data. Another important point to note is that there are significant sampling errors associated with some of the smaller numbers in the tables. This should be borne in mind when making comparisons between years.

It should also be remembered that the data in the LFS are based on an individual's response and hence self classification. In addition prior to 1984 data on occupations were coded by the central office rather than by the interviewer. These and other changes in coding practices make comparison across the year fraught with difficulties. For example, as noted in the introduction, the 1984 LFS allowed 26 categories of potential response to questions on the economic status of the respondent whilst in 1985 this increased to 52 potential responses and in 1986 it was reduced to 28 and further to 26 in 1989 (although not the same 26 potential responses as 1984). In the present analysis data have been reclassified into 10 categories of which two are further sub-divided by three occupation categories; nursing, midwifery (only available for 1983-4) and other.

Economic status

Tables 11.3 to 11.10 show the distribution of the estimated population of the United Kingdom aged 16 and over, excluding men aged 65 and over and women aged 60 and over, by 10 categories of economic status in the reference week of the survey. Full-time and part-time employees are further disaggregated into the occupations, nursing, midwifery and other, where possible and the individual tables are also separated according to qualification and by gender.

Tables 11.3 and 11.7 refer to individuals who have a nursing qualification as one of their top three qualifications, whilst Tables 11.4 and 11.8 cover other individuals with a qualification which can be considered broadly equivalent to or higher than a nursing qualification. Tables 11.5 and 11.9 contain information about those with no qualifications, this includes three categories of individual: those with no qualifications, those with qualifications that are not considered equivalent (i.e. inferior) to a nursing qualification and those recorded as missing values. Finally, Tables 11.6 and 11.10 provide information on the total UK population regardless of qualification (i.e. they present the sums of the entries in the earlier tables).

From Table 11.6 and 11.10 it can be seen that, for the UK, the number of full-time female employees classified in the occupational groups 'nursing and nurse administrators, including nursing assistants and

171

auxiliaries' and 'midwifery' has shown a small increase from 329 thousand in 1983 to 344 thousand in 1989, a rise of 4½ per cent over the entire period. However, the comparative increase for males has been more significant moving from 53 thousand in 1983 to 60 thousand in 1989, an increase of 14 per cent over the period as a whole.

For the same two occupational groups the number of part-time employees has increased from 214 thousand to 273 thousand (or by 27½ per cent) for females and from 1 thousand to 2 thousand for males over the same period (although this latter figure should be treated with caution as it may suffer from small sampling error bias). Whilst males make up a significant proportion of full-time employees engaged in 'nursing' or 'midwifery' (14-15 per cent throughout the period) they only accounted for between ½ per cent (in 1983) and ¾ per cent (in 1989) of all part-time 'nursing' employees.

In comparison, the full-time data for other occupations show male dominance with a fairly constant 68 per cent of full-time employees in other occupations being male (compared to 14-15 per cent for nursing). In 1983 4½ per cent of UK males in categories other than nursing were classified as part-time employees whilst by 1989 this figure had risen to 10 per cent (compared to less than 1 per cent for nursing).

Turning attention to those individuals who state that one of their top three qualifications is a nursing qualification (see Table 11.3 and 11.7) some clear trends can be easily identified. There has been an increase in the number of individuals with a stated nursing qualification over the period. For females this reached a peak of 713 thousand in 1986 but the 1989 figure of 680 thousand, although lower, represents an increase of 7½ per cent on the 1983 figure of 633 thousand. What is more significant is the increase in the numbers with a nursing qualification who are currently employed in a nursing occupation. In 1989 a total of 57 per cent of females with a nursing qualification were currently employed (either full- or part-time) in a nursing occupation compared to 51½ per cent in 1983. Females in full-time nursing having increased by 7½ per cent over the six year period from 1983 to 1989 whilst females in part-time nursing saw a huge 38 per cent increase over the same period.

The main source of the increase in females with a nursing qualification working as nurses appears to be increased female participation in the labour market, as there has been a large fall in the numbers with a nursing qualification who either state that they are looking after the home or family or are unemployed but seeking employment. Thus in large part the changes can be explained by increases in the numbers of female returners. Some possible reasons for their return to employment may be gleaned from the analysis in Chapter 6.

The data for males do not show the same pattern. Over the period as a whole there has been a decline from 66 thousand to 55 thousand in the number of males who are recorded as stating that they have a nursing qualification as one of their top three qualifications, although this figure did increase to a peak of 73 thousand in 1988. In 1989, over 60 per cent of these males with a nursing qualification were employed as full-time nurses (compared to 32½ per cent of females) with a further 3 per cent in part-time nursing (compared to 24½ per cent for females). The numbers of males with a nursing qualification working full-time in other occupations has halved from 19½ thousand to 10 thousand over this same six year period. A partial explanation for this may lie in the way in which males answer the questionnaire. They may only report a nursing qualification if they are working as nurses.

Finally, referring to Tables 11.4 and 11.8 we can see that, although the numbers of individuals with other approximately equivalent or higher qualifications than nursing has increased, those who are employed either full- or part-time in a nursing occupation has remained more or less the same. Tables 11.5 and 11.9 refer to those individuals who either have a qualification that cannot be considered broadly equivalent to nursing, have no qualification at all or whose answer to the question about qualification has been coded as missing. These tables show that females in these qualification categories who are working part-time in a 'nursing' occupation have increased by 13½ per cent. The numbers of females in full-time nursing showed a decline during the middle of the period but have more recently increased to roughly the 1983 number by 1989.

Hours worked

Tables 11.11, 11.12 and 11.13 focus upon female employees who have a nursing qualification and are working either full-time or part-time. These women are reclassified into two broad occupational groups: those working in the two occupations 'nursing and midwifery' (henceforth referred to as nursing) and those working in other occupational groups (henceforth referred to as other or non-nursing occupations).

Table 11.11 and 11.12 show the distribution of usual weekly hours for both of these groups. They also allow a comparison between part-time and full-time employees. Throughout the period approximately half the part-timers in nursing occupations work between 20 and 29 hours per week with between 25-30 per cent working fewer than 20 hours. The comparative figures for non-nursing occupations show a different pattern with over half the part-timers working fewer than 20 hours throughout the period and one-third working between 20 and 29 hours. The tables also show fairly dramatic changes in the self-designated part-time employment, particularly in the 30-39 hours category for nursing. However, one problem with all of these data is that they are by self-designation. Thus some so-called part-timers are apparently working more than 40 hours per week!

It appears that part-timers in nursing occupations choose to work (or are expected to work) longer hours than in other occupations. The reasons may be due to differences in work practices with part-time work in nursing being organized on say half-time contracts whilst the greater range of occupational activities allow those in non-nursing occupations more flexibility in the choice of hours that they can work. Alternatively the difference in hours worked may be a reflection of the age structure of those in nursing with certain age categories preferring to work longer hours and nursing occupations attracting those age categories. Another possible explanation is that the presence of part-timers leads managers to use them, rather than full-timers to make up staffing shortfalls and nurses working part-time on a bank or agency basis may clock up very many hours.

Table 11.11 indicates that a very high percentage of those employed in nursing occupations work in excess of 40 hours per week. This figure rises from 42 per cent in 1983 to 50 per cent in 1988 although these figures are sensitive to relatively minor changes in numbers employed as nurses. The data for non-nursing occupations show approximately 46-47 per cent working more than 40 hours with only slight variation throughout the period.

In conclusion, it is clear that there have been increases in both dimensions of labour activity for the nursing occupational category i.e. an increase in both average hours worked and the number of nurses employed. Thus there has been a significant overall increase in the total number of available 'nursing hours'. This is probably a major part of the explanation of why the demographic timebomb has, thus far at least, failed to explode as far as the NHS is concerned. (The other major factor is probably the depth of the current recession with consequent effects on demand for labour from other employers.)

Age structure

Tables 11.14-11.16 show the age structure for the same group of individuals; i.e. females with a nursing qualification. In the main there has been relatively little change in the age structure of part-time employment. As noted above, the total numbers of part-timers in nursing occupations has grown by 37 per cent over the six year period (or 5½ per cent per year) whilst for non-nursing occupations the growth rate has been lower; 21 per cent over the entire period (or 3¼ per cent per year).

For those working part-time and in non-nursing occupations, over half are aged over 40 with a further third aged 30-39. In contrast, a smaller and slightly decreasing proportion of part-timers in nursing occupations are aged over 40 (approximately 40 per cent) with the 20-29 age range showing a relatively large share at around 18-20 per cent (compared to a more variable figure, ranging from 6 to 15 per cent, for non-nursing).

The data further show that there have been very large increases (in both absolute and percentage terms) in part-time employment for nursing occupations for those in the under 40 age categories. For example, the 30-39 age group shows a 50 per cent increase from 46 thousand in 1983 to 69 thousand in 1989 (the same percentage increase is experienced in the 20-

29 age group). Thus, much of the increase in female participation has been for younger age groups moving into part-time employment.

The age structure of full-time employment shows more marked changes across time. The total numbers of full-timers in nursing occupations shows a modest 7½ per cent (about 1 per cent p.a.) increase over the period with that of non-nursing growing by 43 per cent (6 per cent p.a.), the reverse situation to the trends in part-time employment where the largest growth rate was experienced by part-time employment. In addition most age groups show an increase in numbers employed but this has been uneven across age groups resulting in changes to the age structure of the full-time workforce.

In 1983, 65 per cent of full-time employees in nursing occupations were aged 20-39 but this had fallen to 57 per cent by 1989, the main increases in proportions being in the 30-39 range. In contrast, non-nursing occupations show a decline from 48 per cent to 39 per cent in the proportion of those aged over 40.

It seems that of those females who have a nursing qualification and are working full-time, there has been a clearly indentifiable shift in the age structure, with younger women preferring to work in non-nursing occupations and older women returning to full-time nursing, as there are large increases in the numbers of older women employed in nursing occupations. For example, for the age group 40-49, there has been an increase from 40 thousand to 57 thousand full-time employees in nursing occupations (the equivalent increase for non-nursing is 15 thousand to 19 thousand) whilst those aged 20-29 have seen a fall in numbers from 83 thousand to 78 thousand (compared to an increase from 17 thousand to 26 thousand for non-nursing occupations). This contrasts with the changes reported above for part-time employment.

Sectoral breakdown

Finally, Tables 11.16-11.19 give the sectoral breakdown for those female employees who have a nursing qualification. As can be seen the vast majority of full-time and part-time employees working in nursing occupations are employed in the health service sector (about 85 per cent in 1989). For those working in 'other' occupations an increasing percentage of those full-time women employees with a nursing qualification are employed in the health service sector. This has more than doubled from 10 per cent in 1983 to 22 per cent in 1989. This is in contrast to part-time employment where 17 per cent of women with nursing qualifications are employed in the health service sector in both 1983 and 1989 with slight variations in the intervening years.

Not surprisingly, of those employed in the health service sector the majority find employment in hospitals and nursing homes etc. with a sizeable proportion of the remainder being employed in other medical institutions.

175

11.4 The potential of the Labour Force Survey

This chapter has reported the first attempt to extract a time series of information from various Labour Force Surveys concerning those with nursing qualifications. This exercise has highlighted the difficulties of such a task arising from changes in questionnaire design, coding etc. Nevertheless, some useful information on trends in nursing labour supply has been assembled which throws new light on the way in which supply trends have impinged on the nursing labour market.

Amongst the important points highlighted are: the large and significant numbers of those with nursing qualifications with jobs outside nursing; significant but declining numbers looking after the family/home (a figure that may increase in the future); and the significant numbers of persons working in nursing type jobs who are not qualified as such.

The analysis presented in this chapter can be extended in a number of ways. Clearly the time coverage can be extended to include further years as data become available. Another extension is to consider the regional breakdown. This is explored in Chapter 12.

There is also a host of other potential developments which might form the subject of further work. One example might be to extend the 'characteristics' dimension of nurses or those with nursing qualifications. There are many ways in which this can be done. For example, it is possible to disaggregate the data by marital status, ethnic origin and region. It is also possible to find information on the number of children in the family and their characteristics together with the spouse's occupation and other work characteristics. It is also possible to discover what percentage of people have a nursing qualification as their main, second or third qualification. On a wider scenario it is possible to find out if respondents have a second job and it may be possible to discover if they are looking for a part-time job whilst being fully employed, i.e. that they are dissatisfied with their working hours.

Another exercise which might be of interest would be concerned with comparing nurses to a similar occupational group. An obvious group would be teachers (occ code 033) or librarians (occ code 026). Alternatively, a similar review to the current analysis could be undertaken for different occupations in the health sevice e.g. medical practitioners, physiotherapists, chiropodists, pharmacists, radiographers, opticians, therapists etc. or other related medical occupations. However, the small numbers involved could pose problems here.

Table 11.3
The distribution of females, with nursing qualifications, by occupation and economic status, United Kingdom

(thousands)

Economic status	Occupation	1983	1984	1985	1986	1987	1988	1989
Full-time employee	Nursing	189.4	187.7	210.8	225.0	232.6	231.3	220.3
	Midwifery	15.4	12.6	0.0	0.0	0.0	0.0	0.0
	Other	56.2	60.0	71.7	79.4	78.7	80.9	80.6
Part-time employee	Nursing	111.6	129.5	140.6	142.8	157.7	156.1	167.7
	Midwifery	9.9	8.7	0.0	0.0	0.0	0.0	0.0
	Other	42.6	52.2	51.4	66.0	60.3	64.4	51.9
Self employed		19.2	22.5	23.5	21.7	23.2	24.0	21.1
Employment status/time not stated		8.5	0.3	0.0	0.0	0.4	0.0	0.0
Government scheme		3.0	1.1	1.6	3.4	0.3	2.9	0.8
Unemployed actively seeking work		24.4	27.2	27.1	28.2	19.5	18.6	18.0
Unemployed - not seeking		19.1	22.5	27.1	29.6	24.5	24.3	20.8
Sick/holiday/disabled/retired		16.2	16.9	16.5	15.9	21.6	20.6	30.0
Student		5.5	2.2	5.2	2.4	4.0	5.0	4.8
Looking after home/family		112.2	98.6	100.0	98.7	83.1	79.1	64.5
TOTAL		633.2	642.0	675.5	713.1	705.9	707.2	680.5

Source: Own calculations based on Labour Force Survey tapes.
Note: The figures refer to persons of working age. Those under 16, men 65+ and women 60+ are excluded.

Table 11.4
The distribution of females, with other qualifications, by occupation and economic status, United Kingdom

(thousands)

Economic status	Occupation	1983	1984	1985	1986	1987	1988	1989
Full-time employee	Nursing	22.5	16.8	25.4	21.6	19.3	17.9	20.0
	Midwifery	0.3	0.1	0.0	0.0	0.0	0.0	0.0
	Other	1025.3	1043.4	1128.1	1143.4	1209.8	1277.8	1465.6
Part-time employee	Nursing	5.4	2.9	4.0	6.8	8.0	5.6	6.1
	Midwifery	0.0	0.3	0.0	0.0	0.0	0.0	0.0
	Other	243.2	317.4	328.2	375.9	379.8	415.6	461.4
Self employed		98.6	121.4	132.5	137.6	148.6	150.3	186.3
Employment status/time not stated		14.7	2.7	0.0	1.9	1.3	0.0	0.4
Government scheme		22.5	0.9	9.7	12.8	14.9	17.3	12.2
Unemployed actively seeking work		96.9	138.4	112.5	122.5	112.7	101.4	95.3
Unemployed - not seeking		59.2	83.5	85.3	89.7	89.8	72.1	72.7
Sick/holiday/disabled/retired		22.7	29.6	28.9	41.2	38.3	42.7	47.0
Student		237.0	166.2	212.6	159.1	178.0	166.8	185.7
Looking after home/family		386.4	345.3	360.8	316.7	298.8	303.2	278.6
TOTAL		2234.7	2268.9	2428.0	2429.2	2499.3	2570.7	2831.3

Source: Own calculations based on Labour Force Survey tapes.
Note: The figures refer to persons of working age. Those under 16, men 65+ and women 60+ are excluded.

Table 11.5
The distribution of females, with no qualifications, by occupation and economic status, United Kingdom

(thousands)

Economic status	Occupation	1983	1984	1985	1986	1987	1988	1989
Full-time employee	Nursing	100.4	102.7	82.5	82.5	82.9	94.1	103.7
	Midwifery	1.2	0.4	0.0	0.0	0.0	0.0	0.0
	Other	3516.9	3649.9	3540.3	3575.0	3573.7	3724.7	3895.2
Part-time employee	Nursing	87.2	91.7	91.4	92.4	97.6	93.9	99.1
	Midwifery	0.0	0.5	0.0	0.0	0.0	0.0	0.0
	Other	2711.1	3133.0	3064.2	3259.0	3307.6	3400.0	3420.0
Self employed		382.3	438.8	480.4	470.8	530.5	554.4	554.1
Employment status/time not stated		139.0	11.2	2.2	4.8	7.6	4.6	3.7
Government scheme		129.6	25.0	142.6	118.7	169.1	182.0	171.1
Unemployed actively seeking work		836.7	973.0	865.3	891.3	898.3	750.7	660.7
Unemployed - not seeking		534.9	748.0	897.8	836.2	820.0	777.6	612.7
Sick/holiday/disabled/retired		394.8	531.5	671.5	555.8	573.3	609.9	650.0
Student		664.3	427.5	641.7	385.6	378.8	358.3	355.0
Looking after home/family		3741.0	3170.4	3059.0	2969.3	2865.1	2756.3	2601.9
TOTAL		13239.4	13303.6	13538.9	13241.4	13304.5	13306.5	13127.2

Source: Own calculations based on Labour Force Survey tapes.
Note: The figures refer to persons of working age. Those under 16, men 65+ and women 60+ are excluded.

Table 11.6
The distribution of females, with all qualifications, by occupation and economic status, United Kingdom

(thousands)

Economic status	Occupation	1983	1984	1985	1986	1987	1988	1989
Full-time employee	Nursing	312.3	307.2	318.7	329.1	334.8	343.3	344.0
	Midwifery	16.9	13.1	0.0	0.0	0.0	0.0	0.0
	Other	4598.4	4753.3	4740.1	4797.8	4862.2	5083.4	5441.4
Part-time employee	Nursing	204.2	224.1	236.0	242.0	263.3	255.6	272.9
	Midwifery	9.9	9.5	0.0	0.0	0.0	0.0	0.0
	Other	2996.9	3502.6	3443.8	3700.9	3747.7	3880.0	3933.3
Self employed		500.1	582.7	636.4	630.1	702.3	728.7	761.5
Employment status/time not stated		162.2	14.2	2.2	6.7	9.3	4.6	4.1
Government scheme		155.1	27.0	153.9	134.9	184.3	202.2	184.1
Unemployed actively seeking work		958.0	1138.6	1004.9	1042.0	1030.5	870.7	774.0
Unemployed - not seeking		613.2	854.0	1010.2	955.5	934.3	874.0	706.2
Sick/holiday/disabled/retired		433.7	578.0	716.9	612.9	633.2	673.2	727.0
Student		906.8	595.9	859.5	547.1	560.8	530.1	545.5
Looking after home/family		4239.6	3614.3	3519.8	3384.7	3247.0	3138.6	2945.0
TOTAL		16107.3	16214.5	16642.4	16383.7	16509.7	16584.4	16639.0

Source: Own calculations based on Labour Force Survey tapes.
Note: The figures refer to persons of working age. Those under 16, men 65+ and women 60+ are excluded.

Table 11.7
The distribution of males, with nursing qualifications, by occupation and economic status, United Kingdom

(thousands)

Economic status	Occupation	1983	1984	1985	1986	1987	1988	1989
Full-time employee	Nursing	35.1	31.9	33.7	41.0	34.4	34.4	33.1
	Midwifery	0.0	0.0	0.0	0.0	0.0	0.0	0.0
	Other	19.5	12.8	20.0	17.6	14.8	21.7	10.0
Part-time employee	Nursing	1.0	0.6	1.6	0.7	0.8	0.7	1.6
	Midwifery	0.0	0.0	0.0	0.0	0.0	0.0	0.0
	Other	0.0	1.6	0.8	0.7	1.7	0.5	0.7
Self employed		2.4	2.3	3.5	2.8	3.8	3.7	0.5
Employment status/time not stated		0.2	0.0	0.0	0.0	0.0	0.0	0.0
Government scheme		0.0	0.0	0.0	0.0	0.0	0.0	0.2
Unemployed actively seeking work		2.5	2.4	2.5	4.4	2.6	3.2	2.3
Unemployed - not seeking		0.6	0.4	0.0	0.3	0.9	1.0	1.1
Sick/holiday/disabled/retired		2.8	3.7	6.2	2.7	5.3	5.6	4.7
Student		1.1	0.4	1.9	0.3	0.0	0.4	0.4
Looking after home/family		0.4	0.4	0.0	0.0	0.0	1.5	0.0
TOTAL		65.6	56.5	70.2	70.5	64.3	72.7	54.6

Source: Own calculations based on Labour Force Survey tapes.
Note: The figures refer to persons of working age. Those under 16, men 65+ and women 60+ are excluded.

181

Table 11.8
The distribution of males, with other qualifications, by occupation and economic status, United Kingdom

(thousands)

Economic status	Occupation	1983	1984	1985	1986	1987	1988	1989
Full-time employee	Nursing	5.2	3.8	4.5	3.7	3.9	5.7	6.6
	Midwifery	0.0	0.0	0.0	0.0	0.0	0.0	0.0
	Other	2680.4	2710.4	2847.0	2828.5	2861.1	2970.8	3032.4
Part-time employee	Nursing	0.0	0.0	0.5	0.0	0.0	0.0	0.0
	Midwifery	0.0	0.0	0.0	0.0	0.0	0.0	0.0
	Other	35.4	58.7	34.7	59.1	76.6	82.4	88.9
Self employed		334.4	366.4	407.5	424.0	438.1	465.5	503.4
Employment status/time not stated		13.1	2.3	0.3	1.6	2.0	0.3	0.4
Government scheme		35.1	2.9	13.2	17.1	26.1	24.5	18.1
Unemployed actively seeking work		163.5	171.2	159.4	171.3	167.6	129.1	126.5
Unemployed - not seeking		38.1	43.1	50.1	45.2	36.8	34.0	26.4
Sick/holiday/disabled/retired		83.9	84.1	94.3	104.0	117.4	104.6	101.3
Student		293.3	239.3	283.1	241.1	252.1	232.5	234.1
Looking after home/family		4.0	2.8	2.1	3.4	4.1	4.0	3.5
TOTAL		3686.4	3685.0	3896.7	3899.0	3985.8	4053.4	4141.6

Source: Own calculations based on Labour Force Survey tapes.
Note: The figures refer to persons of working age. Those under 16, men 65+ and women 60+ are excluded.

Table 11.9
The distribution of males, with no qualifications, by occupation and economic status, United Kingdom

(thousands)

Economic status	Occupation	1983	1984	1985	1986	1987	1988	1989
Full-time employee	Nursing	12.3	11.0	8.0	12.1	8.7	12.0	20.4
	Midwifery	0.0	0.0	0.0	0.0	0.0	0.0	0.0
	Other	8584.5	8668.9	8393.9	8340.0	8165.4	8317.6	8423.3
Part-time employee	Nursing	0.0	0.4	0.0	0.4	0.7	1.4	0.3
	Midwifery	0.0	0.0	0.0	0.0	0.0	0.0	0.0
	Other	106.6	277.5	154.6	286.7	321.4	363.9	333.2
Self employed		1392.6	1587.1	1586.5	1593.7	1747.7	1863.5	2058.4
Employment status/time not stated		41.7	22.6	2.4	6.6	9.9	1.9	4.8
Government scheme		199.1	45.9	255.4	264.7	303.2	317.6	298.1
Unemployed actively seeking work		1604.6	1669.4	1494.2	1512.7	1483.4	1235.9	1004.8
Unemployed - not seeking		396.2	378.2	448.6	488.5	394.2	331.5	267.2
Sick/holiday/disabled/retired		876.3	944.7	1185.9	966.1	1033.8	1019.7	1070.7
Student		619.5	441.2	627.7	432.5	431.5	400.5	381.3
Looking after home/family		47.1	54.3	61.4	69.9	69.2	86.3	75.1
TOTAL		13880.5	14101.2	14218.6	13973.9	13969.1	13951.8	13937.6

Source: Own calculations based on Labour Force Survey tapes.
Note: The figures refer to persons of working age. Those under 16, men 65+ and women 60+ are excluded.

Table 11.10
The distribution of males, with all qualifications, by occupation and economic status, United Kingdom

(thousands)

Economic status	Occupation	1983	1984	1985	1986	1987	1988	1989
Full-time employee	Nursing	52.6	46.7	46.2	56.8	47.0	52.1	60.1
	Midwifery	0.0	0.0	0.0	0.0	0.0	0.0	0.0
	Other	11284.4	11392.1	11260.9	11186.1	11041.3	11310.1	11465.7
Part-time employee	Nursing	1.0	1.0	2.1	1.1	1.5	2.1	1.9
	Midwifery	0.0	0.0	0.0	0.0	0.0	0.0	0.0
	Other	142.0	337.8	190.1	346.5	399.7	446.8	422.8
Self employed		1729.4	1955.8	1997.5	2020.5	2189.6	2332.7	2562.3
Employment status/time not stated		55.0	24.9	2.7	8.2	11.9	2.2	5.2
Government scheme		234.2	48.8	268.6	281.8	329.3	342.1	316.4
Unemployed actively seeking work		1770.6	1843.0	1656.1	1688.4	1653.6	1368.2	1133.6
Unemployed - not seeking		434.9	421.7	498.7	534.0	431.9	366.5	294.7
Sick/holiday/disabled/retired		963.0	1032.5	1286.4	1072.8	1156.5	1129.9	1176.7
Student		913.9	680.9	912.7	673.9	683.6	633.4	615.8
Looking after home/family		51.5	57.5	63.5	73.3	73.3	91.8	78.6
TOTAL		17632.5	17842.7	18185.5	17943.4	18019.2	18077.9	18133.8

Source: Own calculations based on Labour Force Survey tapes.
Note: The figures refer to persons of working age. Those under 16, men 65+ and women 60+ are excluded.

Table 11.11
Distribution of hours worked: full-time women employees with a nursing qualification by occupation, United Kingdom

(thousands)

Occupation	Usual hours worked per week	1983	1984	1985	1986	1987	1988	1989
Nursing	Less than 10	0.3 (0.1)	0.0 (0.0)	0.0 (0.0)	0.7 (0.3)	0.3 (0.1)	0.0 (0.0)	0.0 (0.0)
	10 to 19	0.6 (0.3)	0.3 (0.1)	0.0 (0.0)	0.0 (0.0)	0.4 (0.2)	0.3 (0.1)	0.0 (0.0)
	20 to 29	2.1 (1.0)	0.4 (0.2)	1.1 (0.5)	1.9 (0.8)	0.7 (0.3)	1.2 (0.5)	0.8 (0.4)
	30 to 39	115.5 (56.4)	110.3 (55.1)	112.0 (53.1)	120.3 (53.5)	121.8 (52.4)	113.4 (49.0)	76.1 (34.5)
	40 to 49	76.2 (37.2)	76.8 (38.3)	89.5 (42.5)	92.2 (41.0)	102.6 (44.1)	106.5 (46.0)	14.2 (6.4)
	50 and over	10.1 (4.9)	12.5 (6.2)	8.2 (3.9)	9.9 (4.4)	6.5 (2.8)	9.9 (4.3)	1.1 (0.5)
	Not stated	0.0 (0.0)	0.0 (0.0)	0.0 (0.0)	0.0 (0.0)	0.3 (0.1)	0.0 (0.0)	128.2 (58.2)
	TOTAL	204.8 (100.0)	200.3 (100.0)	210.8 (100.0)	225.0 (100.0)	232.6 (100.0)	231.3 (100.0)	220.4 (100.0)
Other	Less than 10	0.0 (0.0)	0.0 (0.0)	0.0 (0.0)	1.3 (1.6)	0.0 (0.0)	0.0 (0.0)	0.0 (0.0)
	10 to 19	0.0 (0.0)	0.7 (1.2)	0.0 (0.0)	0.3 (0.4)	0.0 (0.0)	0.0 (0.0)	0.4 (0.5)
	20 to 29	3.8 (6.7)	3.5 (5.8)	3.4 (4.7)	1.8 (2.3)	1.8 (2.3)	1.7 (2.1)	1.7 (2.1)
	30 to 39	26.1 (46.4)	34.9 (58.2)	36.0 (50.2)	40.8 (51.4)	41.0 (52.1)	41.2 (50.9)	24.8 (30.7)
	40 to 49	20.3 (36.1)	17.6 (29.3)	25.2 (35.1)	26.9 (33.9)	25.3 (32.1)	29.7 (36.7)	5.7 (7.1)
	50 and over	6.1 (10.8)	3.3 (5.5)	6.8 (9.5)	8.3 (10.5)	10.2 (13.0)	7.9 (9.8)	2.5 (3.1)
	Not stated	0.0 (0.0)	0.0 (0.0)	0.3 (0.4)	0.0 (0.0)	0.4 (0.5)	0.4 (0.5)	45.6 (56.5)
	TOTAL	56.3 (100.0)	60.0 (100.0)	71.7 (100.0)	79.4 (100.0)	78.7 (100.0)	80.9 (100.0)	80.7 (100.0)

Source: Own calculations based on Labour Force Survey tapes.

Note: Percentage values are given in parentheses.

185

Table 11.12
Distribution of hours worked: part-time women employees with a nursing qualification by occupation, United Kingdom

(thousands)

Occupation	Usual hours worked per week	1983	1984	1985	1986	1987	1988	1989
Nursing	Less than 10	3.0 (2.5)	5.1 (3.7)	4.7 (3.3)	9.0 (6.3)	8.8 (5.6)	7.8 (5.0)	7.0 (4.2)
	10 to 19	26.9 (22.1)	30.1 (21.8)	29.2 (20.8)	28.5 (20.0)	34.1 (21.6)	32.7 (21.0)	21.9 (13.1)
	20 to 29	60.1 (49.4)	72.7 (52.6)	69.5 (49.4)	63.9 (44.8)	71.5 (45.3)	71.3 (45.7)	47.8 (28.5)
	30 to 39	29.0 (23.8)	28.6 (20.7)	35.4 (25.2)	37.7 (26.4)	39.7 (25.2)	40.5 (26.0)	20.0 (11.9)
	40 to 49	0.6 (0.5)	1.0 (0.7)	1.8 (1.3)	3.2 (2.2)	2.6 (1.6)	3.3 (2.1)	0.1 (0.1)
	50 and over	2.1 (1.7)	0.7 (0.5)	0.0 (0.0)	0.3 (0.2)	0.8 (0.5)	0.0 (0.0)	0.0 (0.0)
	Not stated	0.0 (0.0)	0.0 (0.0)	0.0 (0.0)	0.0 (0.0)	0.3 (0.2)	0.4 (0.3)	70.9 (42.3)
	TOTAL	121.7 (100.0)	138.2 (100.0)	140.6 (100.0)	142.6 (100.0)	157.8 (100.0)	156.0 (100.0)	167.7 (100.0)
Other	Less than 10	6.8 (16.0)	11.7 (22.5)	8.6 (16.7)	12.2 (18.5)	11.2 (18.6)	12.4 (19.3)	10.5 (20.3)
	10 to 19	13.7 (32.2)	17.6 (33.8)	19.9 (38.7)	20.6 (31.2)	23.2 (38.5)	22.1 (34.4)	13.1 (25.3)
	20 to 29	14.0 (32.9)	16.3 (31.3)	18.2 (35.4)	24.1 (36.5)	17.9 (29.7)	21.6 (33.6)	9.1 (17.6)
	30 to 39	6.6 (15.5)	5.7 (10.9)	4.3 (8.4)	8.1 (12.3)	7.6 (12.6)	7.7 (12.0)	2.0 (3.9)
	40 to 49	0.0 (0.0)	0.4 (0.8)	0.0 (0.0)	1.1 (1.7)	0.4 (0.7)	0.3 (0.5)	0.0 (0.0)
	50 and over	1.4 (3.3)	0.4 (0.8)	0.0 (0.0)	0.0 (0.0)	0.0 (0.0)	0.2 (0.3)	0.0 (0.0)
	Not stated	0.0 (0.0)	0.0 (0.0)	0.4 (0.8)	0.0 (0.0)	0.0 (0.0)	0.0 (0.0)	17.1 (33.0)
	TOTAL	42.5 (100.0)	52.1 (100.0)	51.4 (100.0)	66.1 (100.0)	60.3 (100.0)	64.3 (100.0)	51.8 (100.0)

Note: Percentage values are given in parentheses.

Source: Own calculations based on Labour Force Survey tapes.

Table 11.13
Distribution of hours worked: all women employees with a nursing qualification by occupation, United Kingdom

(thousands)

Occupation	Usual hours worked per week	1983	1984	1985	1986	1987	1988	1989
Nursing	Less than 10	3.6 (1.1)	5.1 (1.5)	4.7 (1.3)	9.7 (2.6)	9.1 (2.3)	7.8 (2.0)	7.0 (1.8)
	10 to 19	28.5 (8.6)	30.4 (9.0)	29.2 (8.3)	28.5 (7.8)	34.5 (8.8)	33.0 (8.5)	21.9 (5.6)
	20 to 29	64.0 (19.3)	73.1 (21.6)	70.6 (20.1)	65.8 (17.9)	72.2 (18.5)	72.5 (18.7)	48.6 (12.5)
	30 to 39	145.4 (43.8)	138.9 (41.0)	147.4 (41.9)	158.0 (43.0)	161.5 (41.4)	153.9 (39.7)	96.1 (24.8)
	40 to 49	77.7 (23.4)	77.8 (23.0)	91.3 (26.0)	95.4 (26.0)	105.2 (26.9)	109.8 (28.4)	14.3 (3.7)
	50 and over	12.5 (3.8)	13.2 (3.9)	8.2 (2.3)	10.2 (2.8)	7.3 (1.9)	9.9 (2.6)	1.1 (0.3)
	Not stated	0.0 (0.0)	0.0 (0.0)	0.0 (0.0)	0.0 (0.0)	0.6 (0.2)	0.4 (0.1)	199.1 (51.3)
	TOTAL	331.7 (100.0)	338.5 (100.0)	351.4 (100.0)	367.6 (100.0)	390.4 (100.0)	387.3 (100.0)	388.1 (100.0)
Other	Less than 10	6.8 (6.8)	11.7 (10.4)	8.6 (7.0)	13.5 (9.3)	11.2 (8.1)	12.4 (8.5)	10.5 (7.9)
	10 to 19	13.7 (13.8)	18.3 (16.3)	19.9 (16.2)	20.9 (14.4)	23.2 (16.7)	22.1 (15.2)	13.5 (10.2)
	20 to 29	18.5 (18.6)	19.8 (17.7)	21.6 (17.5)	25.9 (17.8)	19.7 (14.2)	23.3 (16.0)	10.8 (8.2)
	30 to 39	32.7 (32.9)	40.6 (36.2)	40.3 (32.7)	48.9 (33.6)	48.6 (35.0)	48.9 (33.7)	26.8 (20.2)
	40 to 49	20.3 (20.4)	18.0 (16.1)	25.2 (20.5)	28.0 (19.2)	25.7 (18.5)	30.0 (20.7)	5.7 (4.3)
	50 and over	7.5 (7.5)	3.7 (3.3)	6.8 (5.5)	8.3 (5.7)	10.2 (7.3)	8.1 (5.6)	2.5 (1.9)
	Not stated	0.0 (0.0)	0.0 (0.0)	0.7 (0.6)	0.0 (0.0)	0.4 (0.3)	0.4 (0.3)	62.7 (47.3)
	TOTAL	99.5 (100.0)	112.1 (100.0)	123.1 (100.0)	145.5 (100.0)	139.0 (100.0)	145.2 (100.0)	132.5 (100.0)

Source: Own calculations based on Labour Force Survey tapes.

Note: Percentage values are given in parentheses.

187

Table 11.14
Age distribution: full-time women employees with a nursing qualification by occupation, United Kingdom

(thousands)

Occupation	Age group	1983	1984	1985	1986	1987	1988	1989
Nursing	16 to 19	1.1 (0.5)	2.8 (1.4)	0.3 (0.1)	1.5 (0.7)	0.4 (0.2)	0.4 (0.2)	0.7 (0.3)
	20 to 29	83.5 (40.8)	77.3 (38.6)	79.6 (37.8)	95.3 (42.4)	107.5 (46.2)	96.1 (41.5)	77.9 (35.4)
	30 to 39	49.3 (24.1)	45.9 (22.9)	48.1 (22.8)	44.8 (19.9)	43.7 (18.8)	45.8 (19.8)	49.1 (22.3)
	40 to 49	39.7 (19.4)	46.5 (23.2)	48.4 (23.0)	50.8 (22.6)	50.8 (21.8)	50.5 (21.8)	57.3 (26.0)
	50 to 59	31.1 (15.2)	27.8 (13.9)	34.4 (16.3)	32.6 (14.5)	30.2 (13.0)	38.5 (16.6)	35.3 (16.0)
	TOTAL	204.7 (100.0)	200.3 (100.0)	210.8 (100.0)	225.0 (100.0)	232.6 (100.0)	231.3 (100.0)	220.3 (100.0)
Other	16 to 19	1.5 (2.7)	3.8 (6.3)	0.7 (1.0)	1.4 (1.8)	2.2 (2.8)	3.4 (4.2)	1.8 (2.2)
	20 to 29	17.0 (30.2)	14.1 (23.5)	26.7 (37.2)	28.1 (35.3)	27.8 (35.4)	24.5 (30.3)	26.2 (32.5)
	30 to 39	11.0 (19.5)	10.1 (16.9)	15.0 (20.9)	18.9 (23.8)	16.3 (20.7)	16.0 (19.8)	21.0 (26.1)
	40 to 49	15.1 (26.8)	18.1 (30.2)	17.9 (25.0)	15.6 (19.6)	20.1 (25.6)	22.0 (27.2)	18.9 (23.5)
	50 to 59	11.7 (20.8)	13.8 (23.0)	11.4 (15.9)	15.5 (19.5)	12.2 (15.5)	15.0 (18.5)	12.6 (15.7)
	TOTAL	56.3 (100.0)	59.9 (100.0)	71.7 (100.0)	79.5 (100.0)	78.6 (100.0)	80.9 (100.0)	80.5 (100.0)

Source: Own calculations based on Labour Force Survey tapes.
Note: Percentage values are given in parentheses.

Table 11.15
Age distribution: part-time women employees with a nursing qualification by occupation, United Kingdom

(thousands)

Occupation	Age group	1983	1984	1985	1986	1987	1988	1989
Nursing	16 to 19	0.3 (0.2)	0.0 (0.0)	0.0 (0.0)	0.0 (0.0)	0.0 (0.0)	0.0 (0.0)	0.0 (0.0)
	20 to 29	21.8 (17.9)	23.4 (16.9)	25.4 (18.1)	27.3 (19.1)	34.4 (21.8)	33.9 (21.7)	30.9 (18.4)
	30 to 39	46.1 (37.9)	54.7 (39.5)	50.7 (36.0)	51.0 (35.7)	63.8 (40.5)	61.9 (39.7)	69.4 (41.4)
	40 to 49	36.0 (29.6)	40.5 (29.3)	39.2 (27.9)	41.6 (29.1)	37.0 (23.5)	40.4 (25.9)	45.4 (27.1)
	50 to 59	17.4 (14.3)	19.8 (14.3)	25.4 (18.1)	22.9 (16.0)	22.5 (14.3)	19.9 (12.7)	22.0 (13.1)
	TOTAL	121.6 (100.0)	138.4 (100.0)	140.7 (100.0)	142.8 (100.0)	157.7 (100.0)	156.1 (100.0)	167.7 (100.0)
Other	16 to 19	0.3 (0.7)	0.5 (1.0)	0.0 (0.0)	0.3 (0.5)	0.7 (1.2)	0.8 (1.2)	0.3 (0.6)
	20 to 29	4.8 (11.3)	6.9 (13.2)	3.3 (6.4)	8.5 (12.9)	10.0 (16.6)	9.8 (15.2)	8.9 (17.1)
	30 to 39	14.8 (34.7)	19.5 (37.4)	18.5 (36.0)	22.4 (33.9)	19.7 (32.7)	21.6 (33.6)	17.1 (32.9)
	40 to 49	14.9 (35.0)	15.3 (29.4)	18.6 (36.2)	20.0 (30.3)	16.7 (27.7)	18.8 (29.2)	17.1 (32.9)
	50 to 59	7.8 (18.3)	9.9 (19.0)	11.0 (21.4)	14.8 (22.4)	13.2 (21.9)	13.3 (20.7)	8.5 (16.4)
	TOTAL	42.6 (100.0)	52.1 (100.0)	51.4 (100.0)	66.0 (100.0)	60.3 (100.0)	64.3 (100.0)	51.9 (100.0)

Source: Own calculations based on Labour Force Survey tapes.
Note: Percentage values are given in parentheses.

Table 11.16
Age distribution: all women employees with a nursing qualification by occupation, United Kingdom

(thousands)

Occupation	Age group	1983	1984	1985	1986	1987	1988	1989
Nursing	16 to 19	1.4 (0.4)	2.8 (0.8)	0.3 (0.1)	1.5 (0.4)	0.4 (0.1)	0.4 (0.1)	0.7 (0.2)
	20 to 29	106.1 (32.0)	100.7 (29.7)	105.0 (29.9)	122.6 (33.3)	141.9 (36.4)	130.0 (33.6)	108.8 (28.0)
	30 to 39	97.5 (29.4)	100.6 (29.7)	98.8 (28.1)	95.8 (26.0)	107.5 (27.5)	107.7 (27.8)	118.5 (30.5)
	40 to 49	76.9 (23.2)	87.0 (25.7)	87.6 (24.9)	92.4 (25.1)	87.8 (22.5)	90.9 (23.5)	102.7 (26.5)
	50 to 59	49.5 (14.9)	47.6 (14.1)	59.8 (17.0)	55.5 (15.1)	52.7 (13.5)	58.4 (15.1)	57.3 (14.8)
	TOTAL	331.4 (100.0)	338.7 (100.0)	351.5 (100.0)	367.8 (100.0)	390.3 (100.0)	387.4 (100.0)	388.0 (100.0)
Other	16 to 19	2.1 (2.1)	4.3 (3.8)	0.7 (0.6)	1.7 (1.2)	2.9 (2.1)	4.2 (2.9)	2.1 (1.6)
	20 to 29	22.0 (21.7)	21.0 (18.8)	30.0 (24.4)	36.6 (25.2)	37.8 (27.2)	34.3 (23.6)	35.1 (26.5)
	30 to 39	26.3 (26.0)	29.6 (26.4)	33.5 (27.2)	41.3 (28.4)	36.0 (25.9)	37.6 (25.9)	38.1 (28.8)
	40 to 49	30.3 (29.9)	33.4 (29.8)	36.5 (29.7)	35.6 (24.5)	36.8 (26.5)	40.8 (28.1)	36.0 (27.2)
	50 to 59	20.5 (20.3)	23.7 (21.2)	22.4 (18.2)	30.3 (20.8)	25.4 (18.3)	28.3 (19.5)	21.1 (15.9)
	TOTAL	101.2 (100.0)	112.0 (100.0)	123.1 (100.0)	145.5 (100.0)	138.9 (100.0)	145.2 (100.0)	132.4 (100.0)

Source: Own calculations based on Labour Force Survey tapes.
Note: Percentage values are given in parentheses.

Table 11.17
Sectoral distribution: full-time women employees with a nursing qualification by occupation, United Kingdom
(thousands)

Occupation	Sector	1983	1984	1985	1986	1987	1988	1989
Nursing	Hospitals, nursing homes etc.	154.9	147.0	158.5	167.1	161.6	174.3	161.8
	Other medical care institutions	34.5	32.3	38.9	38.9	31.5	25.4	25.7
	Medical practices	1.0	0.6	2.0	6.4	2.5	1.7	1.8
	Dental practices	1.6	0.9	1.2	1.1	1.4	0.5	0.8
	Agency and private midwives, nurses etc.	0.8	3.5	1.4	1.0	3.2	0.5	1.5
	TOTAL HEALTH SERVICE SECTOR	192.8	184.3	202.0	214.5	200.2	202.4	191.6
	Other sectors	15.5	17.2	12.1	13.3	35.0	32.6	30.3
	TOTAL ALL SECTORS	208.3	201.5	214.1	227.8	235.2	235.0	221.9
Other	Hospitals, nursing homes etc.	5.0	5.7	12.3	8.6	12.9	10.6	12.3
	Other medical care institutions	0.0	1.5	4.1	4.1	2.9	1.4	3.7
	Medical practices	0.0	0.7	1.7	1.1	1.5	1.0	0.9
	Dental practices	1.1	0.3	0.7	1.1	0.6	0.0	2.1
	Agency and private midwives, nurses etc.	0.7	0.4	0.7	1.4	1.4	0.4	1.0
	TOTAL HEALTH SERVICE SECTOR	6.8	8.6	19.5	16.3	19.3	13.4	20.0
	Other sectors	59.0	61.2	64.0	74.2	69.8	77.7	71.7
	TOTAL ALL SECTORS	65.8	69.8	83.5	90.5	89.1	91.1	91.7

Source: Own calculations based on Labour Force Survey tapes.

Table 11.18
Sectoral distribution: part-time women employees with a nursing qualification by occupation, United Kingdom

(thousands)

Occupation	Sector	1983	1984	1985	1986	1987	1988	1989
Nursing	Hospitals, nursing homes etc.	97.4	92.6	103.4	107.7	113.0	109.4	117.1
	Other medical care institutions	15.5	21.2	17.1	16.7	16.3	13.0	14.8
	Medical practices	1.9	7.6	7.4	7.6	3.8	5.5	8.6
	Dental practices	0.0	1.1	1.3	0.0	0.0	0.0	0.7
	Agency and private midwives, nurses etc.	3.1	3.9	3.3	5.3	7.2	2.7	1.9
	TOTAL HEALTH SERVICE SECTOR	117.9	126.4	132.5	137.3	140.3	130.6	143.1
	Other sectors	7.3	13.6	9.3	9.2	20.8	27.9	25.8
	TOTAL ALL SECTORS	125.2	140.0	141.8	146.5	161.1	158.5	168.9
Other	Hospitals, nursing homes etc.	5.6	5.6	5.4	7.0	5.9	6.6	7.7
	Other medical care institutions	0.4	1.1	1.1	4.0	1.1	1.2	0.2
	Medical practices	1.5	2.3	2.5	1.7	3.1	3.5	1.8
	Dental practices	0.5	0.3	0.3	1.2	0.4	1.2	0.4
	Agency and private midwives, nurses etc.	0.5	0.3	0.0	1.1	0.6	0.7	0.0
	TOTAL HEALTH SERVICE SECTOR	8.5	9.6	9.3	15.0	11.1	13.2	10.1
	Other sectors	42.1	52.4	51.7	58.0	56.2	61.4	49.1
	TOTAL ALL SECTORS	50.6	62.0	61.0	73.0	67.3	74.6	59.2

Source: Own calculations based on Labour Force Survey tapes.

Table 11.19
Sectoral distribution: all women employees with a nursing qualification by occupation, United Kingdom

(thousands)

Occupation	Sector	1983	1984	1985	1986	1987	1988	1989
Nursing	Hospitals, nursing homes etc.	256.7	239.6	261.9	274.8	274.6	283.7	278.9
	Other medical care institutions	50.6	53.5	56.0	55.6	47.8	38.4	40.5
	Medical practices	3.1	8.2	9.4	14.0	6.3	7.2	10.4
	Dental practices	1.6	2.0	2.5	1.1	1.4	0.5	1.5
	Agency and private midwives, nurses etc.	3.9	7.4	4.7	6.3	10.4	3.2	3.4
	TOTAL HEALTH SERVICE SECTOR	315.9	310.7	334.5	351.8	340.5	333.0	334.7
	Other sectors	22.8	30.8	21.4	22.5	55.8	60.5	56.1
	TOTAL ALL SECTORS	338.7	341.5	355.9	374.3	396.3	393.5	390.8
Other	Hospitals, nursing homes etc.	10.6	11.3	17.7	15.6	18.8	17.2	20.0
	Other medical care institutions	0.4	2.6	5.2	8.1	4.0	2.6	3.9
	Medical practices	1.5	3.0	4.2	2.8	4.6	4.5	2.7
	Dental practices	1.6	0.6	1.0	2.3	1.0	1.2	2.5
	Agency and private midwives, nurses etc.	1.2	0.7	0.7	2.5	2.0	1.1	1.0
	TOTAL HEALTH SERVICE SECTOR	15.3	18.2	28.8	31.3	30.4	26.6	30.1
	Other sectors	279.1	282.2	115.7	307.7	126.0	139.1	120.8
	TOTAL ALL SECTORS	294.4	300.4	144.5	339.0	156.4	165.7	150.9

Source: Own calculations based on Labour Force Survey tapes.

Appendix A
The Labour Force Survey: sampling procedure, interviewing methodolgy and relevant questions

This appendix draws heavily on Elias (1987). The Labour Force Survey is a large-sample national household survey which, until 1984, was conducted in the Spring at two-year intervals from 1973 on. Sampling strategies varied throughout this period and between the countries of the United Kingdom. From 1984, the 'small-user' sub-file of the Postcode Address File has been used as the sampling frame, stratified in various ways to facilitate efficient interviewing.

The survey is administered by interview. At each household sampled, the interviewer collects information on all household members usually present at that address. For the majority of respondents therefore, the information is provided by proxy.

In 1984 the LFS was placed on an annual basis and redesigned to contain two main elements; the quarterly survey, operated continuously throughout the year with a five-quarter rotating sampling frame and the 'boost' survey, an annual sample in March, April and May of each year designed to boost the quarterly survey in these months to a size large enough to meet the European Community requirement regarding the sample size. Fifteen thousand households were interviewed in each quarter, with three thousand households replaced in each successive quarter. To meet the European Community requirement, an additional sixty thousand households were interviewed in the Spring quarter. The five quarter rotating sample offers the opportunity of coding a longitudinal element to the analysis which in turn enables issues such as mobility to be addressed.

The data from which the tables shown in this report are drawn relate to this annual boost to the survey for the period 1984-89 inclusive and for the Spring surveys for all other years. As an illustration of the types of question used to derive information on the topic of interest in this report we refer to the 1984 LFS. The numbers given refer to their position in the 1984 survey schedule. The replies to these questions can be used to determine the distribution of persons with nursing qualifications by age group, sex, occupation, economic status, hours usually worked and industry.

For persons who performed any paid work in the seven days ending Sunday (date of previous Sunday) or who had a paid job that they were away from;

9.   What was your (main) occupation last week?
(a)   Enter job title
(b)   Describe fully work done

10. What does the firm/organization you work for actually make or do (at the place you work)?

11. Were you working as an employee or were you self-employed?

16. In that job, were you working full-time or part-time?

18. How many hours a week do you usually work in your (main) job/business that is excluding mealbreaks and any paid or unpaid overtime?

(if varies,take average over last four weeks)

(FOR MEN AGED 16-64 AND WOMEN AGED 16-59 ONLY)

98. Do you have any of these qualifications, or have you passed any of these examinations, of the types listed on this card (whether you are making use of them or not)?

CODE ALL THAT APPLY. 'SPECIFY' MEANS: GIVE TITLE OF COURSE OR QUALIFICATION IN FULL AND LIST SUBJECTS STUDIED.

Higher degree (SPECIFY)

First Degree (SPECIFY)

Other degree level qualification such as graduate membership of professional institute

BTEC or SCOTBTEC/BEC or SCOTBEC (National or General)/TEC or SCOTEC (National or general)/ONC, OND

Teaching Qualification:
    secondary
    primary

Nursing Qualifications (SPECIFY)

City and Guilds

'A' level or equivalent/SLC (Higher), SCE (Higher), SUPE (Higher)/Certificate of Sixth Year Studies

'O' level or equivalent (including CSE grade 1)/SLC (Lower), SCE (Ordinary), SUPE (Lower or Ordinary)

CSE (other than grade 1)

Any other professional/vocational qualification (SPECIFY)

None of these qualifications

Don't know

A review of the occupational codes and industrial categories chosen is in Section 11.2 of the main text.

Responses have been weighted to yield population estimates. Further information about sample structure, coding, editing and the weighting procedures are given in the published report of the 1983 and 1984 Labour Force Surveys, for example (OPCS, 1986).

Appendix B
Changes in mnemonics and technical characteristics/codings used in the Labour Force Surveys 1983-89

Mnemonics and codings LFS 1983-89

Year	1983	1984	1985	1986	1987	1988	1989

SEX: Gives sex of respondent, m=male, f=female.

Mnemonic	sex	sex	sex	sex	sex	sex	sex
Codes	m = 1 f = 2	m = 1 f = 2	m = 1 f = 2	m = 1 f = 2	m = 1 f = 2	m = 1 f = 2	m = 1 f = 2

AGE: Gives actual age of respondent in years.

Mnemonic	age	age	age	age	age	age	age
Recoded to (age groups)	yrs	yrs	yrs	yrs	yrs	yrs	yrs

ECONOMIC STATUS: Gives economic status of respondent.

Mnemonic	econpoe	econacrf	econacrg	earh	ecacj	ecara	ecarb
No. of Poss. Coded Responses	26	26	52	28	28	28	26
Recoding to 10 activities	status	status	status	status	status	status	status

QUALIFICATIONS: A maximum of three types of qualification can be recorded. (See Appendix A for range of replies.)

Mnemonic	qualonie qualtwie qualthie	quala qualb qualc	qualsm1 qualsm2 qualsm3	qualsm1 qualsm2 qualsm3	qualsm1 qualsm2 qualsm3	qualsm1 qualsm2 qualsm3	qualsm1 qualsm2 qualsm3
recoded into 3 groups	qual	qual	qual	qual	qual	qual	qual

Year	1983	1984	1985	1986	1987	1988	1989

HOURS USUALLY WORKED: Actual hours usually worked.

Mnemonic	hrsnomie	totushrs	totushrs	totushrs	totushrs	totushrs	totushrs
Recoded to (Groups of hrs)	hrs	hrs	hrs	hrs	hrs	hrs	hrs

RESIDENCE: Usual place of residence by region in UK.

Mnemonic	urescome	urescomf	urescomg	urescomh	urescomj	uresmca	uresmca
No of Regions	18	18	18	20	20	20	20

OCCUPATION: Occupational classification (350 possibities).

Mnenomic	kose	kosf	kosg	kosh	kosj	kosa	kosb
Codes							
Nurses	043	043	1600	1600	1600	1600	1600
Midwives	550	550	na	na	na	na	na
Recoded to	occ	occ	occ	occ	occ	occ	occ
Nurses	1	1	1	1	1	1	1
Midwives	2	2	-	-	-	-	-

INDUSTRY: Industrial classification (315 possibilities).

Mnenomic	inde	indf	indg	indh	indj	inda	indb
Codes	1-315	1-315	1-315	1-315	1-315	1-315	1-315

FULL-TIME/PART-TIME: Self-defined full-time/part-time, ft=full-time, pt=part-time.

Mnemonic	ftptwork	ftptwork	ftptwork	ftptwork	ftptwork	ftptwork	ftptwork
Codes	ft=1	ft=1	ft=1	ft=1	ft=1	ft=1	ft=1
	pt=3	pt=2	pt=2	pt=2	pt=2	pt=2	pt=2

12 Labour supply trends for selected regions: South East Thames and Trent RHAs

12.1 Regional disaggregation

The LFS can also provide labour supply data on a regional basis, for up to a maximum of 20 regions (prior to 1986 the data can be disaggregated into 18 regions). The LFS data refer to a person's usual place of residence (LFS code name = URESCOM or URESMCA). The method of matching Regional Health Authority (RHA) regions with LFS regions is illustrated in Table 12.1. As can be seen some of the Regional Health Authority (RHA) regions correspond well with the LFS regions. Indeed in some cases they match exactly whilst others require the simple combination of two separate LFS regions. RHA regions that can be identified in these ways include the Northern RHA, Yorkshire RHA, East Anglian RHA, and West Midlands RHA. It is also possible to distinguish Wales, Scotland and Northern Ireland.

However, differences in the way in which boundaries are drawn mean that the remaining RHA regions consist either of parts of the regions used by the LFS or combinations of those parts. For example, to construct estimates for the South West RHA, requires assumptions about what percentage share of labour supply comes from the South West LFS region, whilst for the Trent RHA one needs to know what percentage share of the East Midlands LFS region is needed.

The percentages used were obtained by comparing the population resident in RHA districts with LFS regions. Thus, referring to the examples above, 78.30 per cent of the population in the LFS South West region lived in districts served by the South West RHA whilst all of the population in the LFS Southern Yorkshire region and 85.64 per cent of the East Midlands LFS region lived in districts served by the Trent RHA. This method of calculation relies on a number of assumptions. First, that the population can be assumed evenly distributed within LFS regions. Second, that the place of usual residence of a respondent to the LFS can be taken as a reasonable proxy for the region of work of that resident. Third, that those moving from one region to another for the purpose of work approximately balance each other. This assumption is required as some individuals will work in a different RHA from their usual place of residence. Finally, the assumption that these proportions are relatively stable over time is required.

While it is doubtful if any of these assumptions holds strictly true, they are probably sufficiently close to reality to make the estimates presented here generally valid.

12.2 Results for South East Thames RHA and Trent RHA

South East Thames RHA and Trent RHA have been chosen for the purposes of illustrating the kind of information that can be developed for a regional comparison. This choice was somewhat arbitrary, but space considerations meant that it was not possible to cover all RHAs. Nevertheless, corresponding analyses could be conducted for all the other RHAs. The data, as noted above, need to be interpreted with some caution as the regional categories are broken down in terms of the usual place of residence of the individual answering the questionnaire rather than by place of work and thus there will be some individuals who cross regional boundaries from their place of residence to their place of work.

The region that encompasses Trent RHA had approximately 30 per cent more females in the sample in 1989 than SE Thames (1375 thousand compared to 1042). This mainly reflects the difference in population size between the regions and hence this ratio has remained fairly constant throughout the period. Both regions have seen population increases throughout the period from 1983-89 although there has been a marginally larger increase in the Trent region. A similar picture emerges for males with Trent RHA having 33-34 per cent more males in the sample than SE Trent.

Contrary to the national figures discussed in Chapter 11, both regions show declines in the total numbers of females, of all qualifications, employed full-time as nurses with the largest decline being experienced by the SE Thames region. The part-time situation is more or less in line with national figures for SE Thames which show an increase of 28 per cent (the national trend was 27½ per cent). This contrasts with an increase of 35 per cent in the number of females employed part-time in a nursing occupation for the Trent region.

The numbers of males employed in nursing occupations is small and thus interpretation of these data should be treated with extreme caution. However, from the reported data it can be seen that there has been a noticeable increase in the number of full-time males (all qualifications) employed as nurses in SE Thames (from 2.5 thousand to 3.2 thousand) whilst for Trent the numbers have been variable throughout the seven year period with relatively large recorded swings between years. These may simply reflect sampling variation.

In view of the small sample of males employed in nursing occupations in these regions the remainder of the discussion will concentrate on female employment. SE Thames shows a small growth (5 per cent over the period) in the number of females who have a nursing qualification whilst for Trent there has been a decline from 49 to 47 thousand. This compares to the national trend of a 7½ per cent increase.

Disaggregating these data further show similar patterns, with those females with nursing qualifications in full-time employment exhibiting little change over the period in SE Thames. The numbers rise from 13 thousand in 1983 to 14 thousand in 1984 and then decline to 13 thousand by 1989. Trent, in contrast, shows a steady decline from 18½ thousand to 16 thousand over the same period.

Part-time employment in nursing occupations for those females with nursing qualifications match the national trends with fairly substantial increases in both regions (48 per cent for SE Thames and 76 per cent for Trent compared to the UK growth of 50 per cent). Thus there appears to have been a greater tendancy within the Trent region to shift towards part-time employment in nursing occupations.

Considering those females with nursing qualifications who are employed in non-nursing occupations, it can be seen that there are substantial increases in full-time employment (around 20 per cent growth in both regions) whereas the situation for part-timers in non-nursing occupations is more variable with a growth in numbers only being sustained in the Trent region.

However, these numbers pale into insignificance when compared to those females with 'other' qualifications who are working in non-nursing occupations. In both regions there are very large increases in both full- and part-time employment. Unlike full-time employment in nursing which, as we have seen, shows little change over the period, non-nursing employment for those with other qualifications shows a growth of 33 per cent in Trent to 43 per cent in SE Thames whilst part-time employment in Trent RHA more than doubles with SE Thames not far behind. Nursing employment therefore lags well behind the growth in other areas of employment in both regions. Although the analysis has not focused on other RHAs, the implications of comparison with the national trends are that Trent and SE Thames have been much less successful than other areas in recruiting and retaining their nursing workforce.

In both regions there has also been a noticeable shift in the hours worked by full-time employees. For those employed as nurses, a decline in the numbers working 30-39 hours is almost matched by an increase in the numbers working 40-49 hours. For non-nursing occupations there have been increases in those working 40-49 hours in both regions and in the 30-39 hour range for Trent whilst SE Thames shows a decline in this latter category. In contrast no obvious trends emerge for part-time employment. The results for full-time nurses suggest that hours may have been increased to compensate for problems regarding numbers employed.

As far as the distribution of age is concerned, both regions show a clear decline in the proportion of females aged under 40 who are employed full-time in nursing occupations. This contrasts dramatically with part-time employment in nursing occupations for the Trent RHA for which there is an increase in the proportion of females aged under 40. For example, 63½ per cent of part-time employees in Trent RHA in nursing occupations were aged under 40 in 1989 compared to 56½ in 1983. There was a slight decline from 50 to 45 per cent in SE Thames over the same period.

Finally, considering the sectoral breakdown of those women employees who have a nursing qualification, the two regions exhibit similar characteristics to the UK data. Both regions show that around 90 per cent of all full-time females with a nursing qualification in nursing occupations are employed in the health service sector (a slightly higher share than for the UK) compared to around 20 per cent employed in the health service sector for those in other occupations. The situation for part-timers is very similar.

12.3 Conclusions

There is considerable similarity between the two regions examined. Both have experienced declines in the numbers of women employed full-time as nurses. This can be compared to the national trend which shows a marginal increase. When compared to the growth in other occupations (for *all* female employees regardless of qualification) the percentage of females employed as nurses has declined dramatically. Nursing employment therefore lags well behind the growth in employment in other areas of the economy. Clearly this conclusion needs to be interpreted with extreme care as it reflects both the growth in occuaptional opportunity available to women and hence increased female participation in 'non-traditional' areas of female employment.

Full-time nurses appear to have been working longer hours in 1989 when compared to 1983 and there also appears to be an increase in the average age of nurses working full-time in both regions with a growth in the proportion of over 40s who are emplyed as nurses. This contrasts to part-time employment which shows a growth in the emplyment of under 40s for Trent with almost two-thirds of part-time female nurses falling into this age category in 1989 compared to under half for SE Thames (a figure that has been declining).

Thus whilst the regional breakdown shows many similarities, some key differences do appear. It is important to repeat the health warning given at the start of Chapter 11, the regional dissagregation leads to relatively small numbers in the initial sample count and hence these numbers are subject to sampling fluctuations which are magnified when the appropriate weighting procedures are applied to bring them up to estimates of regional values. Nevertheless, it appears that the analysis of LFS data at this level can provide some useful indication of the labour market situation facing individual RHAs.

Table 12.1
RHAs defined in terms of LFS regions

1.	**Northern RHA**	01 Tyne & Wear		(whole)
		02 Rest of Northern Region		(whole)
2.	**Yorkshire RHA**	04 W. Yorks		(whole)
		05 Rest of Yorks & Humberside		(whole)
3.	**Trent RHA**	03 S. Yorks		(whole)
		06 E. Midlands		(part)
			included:	Derbys, Notts, Lincs, Leics.
			excluded:	Northants, (Oxford RHA)
4.	**East Anglia RHA**	07 East Anglia		(whole)
5.	**NW Thames RHA**	09 Outer London		(part)
			included:	Barnet, Ealing, Harrow, Hillingdon, Hounslow & Spelthorne (part)
		08 Inner London		(part)
			included:	Parkside, Riverside
		10 Rest of South East	included:	Herts, Beds, Surrey (part)
6.	**NE Thames RHA**	09 Outer London		(part)
			included:	Barking, Havering and Brentwood (pt), Enfield Hampstead, Redbridge, Waltham Forest
		08 Inner London		(part)
			included:	Bloomsbury, City & Hackney, Islington, Tower Hamlets, Haringey, Newham
		10 Rest of South East		(part)
			included:	Essex
			excluded:	Herts, Beds, Bucks, Berks, Oxon, Surrey, Hants, Sussex(E&W), Kent
7.	**SE Thames RHA**	09 Outer London		(part)
			included:	Bexley, Bromley, Camberwell,
Greenwich				
		08 Inner London		(part)
			included:	Lewisham, N.Southwark
		10 Rest of South East		(part)
			included:	Surrey, E.Sussex, Kent
			excluded:	W.Sussex, Hants,
Berks				
				Oxon, Bucks, Beds, Herts, Essex

Table 12.1 continued

8.	**SW Thames RHA**	09 Outer London		(part)
			included:	Croydon, Kingston & Esher, Merton & Sutton, Roehampton
		08 Inner London		(part)
			included:	Wandsworth
		10 Rest of South East		(part)
			included:	Surrey, W.Sussex
9.	**Wessex RHA**	10 Rest of South East		(part)
			included:	Hants
			excluded:	Kent, Essex, W.Sussex, E.Sussex, Surrey, Berks, Beds, Bucks, Herts, Oxon
		11 South West		(part)
			included:	Avon(part), Wiltshire, Dorset
			excluded:	Avon(largest part) Gloucs, Somerset, Devon, Cornwall
10.	**Oxford RHA**	10 Rest of South East		(part)
			included:	Bucks, Berks, Oxon
			excluded:	Surrey, Sussex (E&W), Kent, Herts, Beds, Essex
		06 East Midlands		(part)
			included:	Northants
			excluded:	Derbys, Notts, Lincs, Leics
11.	**South Western RHA**	11 South West		(part)
			included:	Avon(largest part) Gloucs, Cornwall, Devon, Somerset
			excluded:	Dorset, Wilts, Avon(part)
12.	**West Midlands RHA**	12 West Midlands		(whole)
		13 Rest of West Midlands		(whole)
13.	**Mersey RHA**	15 Merseyside		(whole)
		16 Rest of North West		(part)
			included:	Cheshire
			excluded:	Lancs
14.	**North Western RHA**	14 Greater Manchester		(whole)
		16 Rest of North West		(part)
			included:	Lancs
			excluded:	Cheshire Glossop in Derbyshire also excluded but is so small it has been ignored

15. **Wales, Scotland and Northern Ireland are as represented in the LFS regions.**

Note: Currently the weights used are assumed fixed. They are based on data for 1981. If the tables are to be extended beyond 1990 it will probably be advisable to reassess this assumption. The LFS codes are based on 1986-89 responses. There are minor changes for 1983-85.

Table 12.2
The distribution of females, with nursing qualifications, by occupation and economic status, SE Thames RHA

(thousands)

Economic status	Occupation	1983	1984	1985	1986	1987	1988	1989
Full-time employee	Nursing	12.9	13.0	13.7	13.4	13.0	13.2	12.7
	Midwifery	0.7	0.8	0.0	0.0	0.0	0.0	0.0
	Other	4.9	4.1	5.5	6.1	7.7	6.1	6.3
Part-time employee	Nursing	6.6	8.0	8.0	8.9	8.5	8.9	9.8
	Midwifery	0.7	0.1	0.0	0.0	0.0	0.0	0.0
	Other	2.8	3.8	3.6	3.7	3.9	3.5	2.8
Self employed		1.3	2.0	1.8	1.8	1.8	1.4	1.7
Employment status/time not stated		0.5	0.1	0.0	0.0	0.1	0.0	0.0
Government scheme		0.2	0.1	0.3	0.2	0.0	0.1	0.1
Unemployed actively seeking work		1.4	1.7	1.8	2.2	1.1	0.8	1.2
Unemployed - not seeking		1.3	1.6	1.9	1.9	2.0	1.8	1.5
Sick/holiday/disabled/retired		1.2	0.9	1.3	1.3	1.2	1.4	1.9
Student		0.5	0.4	0.5	0.3	0.4	0.7	0.3
Looking after home/family		6.8	5.1	6.2	5.9	5.8	4.9	5.7
TOTAL		41.8	41.7	44.6	45.7	45.5	42.8	44.0

Source: Own calculations based on Labour Force Survey tapes.
Note: The figures refer to persons of working age. Those under 16, men 65+ and women 60+ are excluded.

Table 12.3
The distribution of females, with other qualifications, by occupation and economic status, SE Thames RHA

(thousands)

Economic status	Occupation	1983	1984	1985	1986	1987	1988	1989
Full-time employee	Nursing	1.6	0.8	1.4	1.1	0.7	0.8	1.0
	Midwifery	0.1	0.0	0.0	0.0	0.0	0.0	0.0
	Other	83.8	85.8	95.4	94.9	96.5	102.1	120.1
Part-time employee	Nursing	0.4	0.1	0.3	0.5	0.6	0.3	0.5
	Midwifery	0.0	0.1	0.0	0.0	0.0	0.0	0.0
	Other	18.3	24.1	23.4	27.8	29.4	29.6	33.5
Self employed		9.2	13.2	12.5	15.6	13.8	12.8	18.2
Employment status/time not stated		1.2	0.1	0.0	0.3	0.3	0.0	0.1
Government scheme		1.8	0.1	0.4	0.6	0.7	1.2	0.7
Unemployed actively seeking work		6.9	9.8	8.5	9.5	8.2	6.7	6.3
Unemployed - not seeking		5.1	7.9	7.4	6.5	8.0	6.3	5.4
Sick/holiday/disabled/retired		1.7	2.0	1.5	2.9	2.6	2.7	3.3
Student		19.1	14.1	17.5	11.4	13.0	14.9	12.5
Looking after home/family		31.5	27.9	28.6	25.1	21.8	23.3	23.6
TOTAL		180.7	186.0	196.9	196.2	195.6	200.7	225.2

Source: Own calculations based on Labour Force Survey tapes.
Note: The figures refer to persons of working age. Those under 16, men 65+ and women 60+ are excluded.

Table 12.4
The distribution of females, with no qualifications, by occupation and economic status, SE Thames RHA

(thousands)

Economic status	Occupation	1983	1984	1985	1986	1987	1988	1989
Full-time employee	Nursing	6.5	6.0	4.6	3.9	3.9	4.7	5.1
	Midwifery	0.2	0.0	0.0	0.0	0.0	0.0	0.0
	Other	238.5	253.1	242.6	246.2	251.4	260.0	265.0
Part-time employee	Nursing	4.3	4.5	4.8	4.6	5.4	5.3	5.1
	Midwifery	0.0	0.0	0.0	0.0	0.0	0.0	0.0
	Other	152.8	181.4	178.9	186.1	190.4	193.8	189.3
Self employed		21.6	26.7	30.0	30.9	36.2	34.9	34.4
Employment status/time not stated		8.7	1.2	0.2	0.3	0.3	0.3	0.2
Government scheme		5.8	1.0	6.1	4.8	5.0	6.1	5.3
Unemployed actively seeking work		42.1	50.2	42.6	44.5	42.0	35.4	31.6
Unemployed - not seeking		33.7	41.7	47.3	45.5	51.6	49.3	39.4
Sick/holiday/disabled/retired		21.0	26.0	37.4	29.0	28.8	30.9	29.1
Student		43.6	27.2	42.7	23.0	22.7	19.7	21.8
Looking after home/family		209.0	171.5	166.9	172.6	158.7	155.9	146.8
TOTAL		787.8	790.5	804.1	791.4	796.4	796.3	773.1

Source: Own calculations based on Labour Force Survey tapes.
Note: The figures refer to persons of working age. Those under 16, men 65+ and women 60+ are excluded.

Table 12.5
The distribution of females, with all qualifications, by occupation and economic status, SE Thames RHA

(thousands)

Economic status	Occupation	1983	1984	1985	1986	1987	1988	1989
Full-time employee	Nursing	21.0	19.8	19.7	18.4	17.6	18.7	18.8
	Midwifery	1.0	0.8	0.0	0.0	0.0	0.0	0.0
	Other	327.2	343.0	343.5	347.2	355.6	368.2	391.4
Part-time employee	Nursing	11.3	12.6	13.1	14.0	14.5	14.5	15.4
	Midwifery	0.7	0.2	0.0	0.0	0.0	0.0	0.0
	Other	173.9	209.3	205.9	217.6	223.7	226.9	225.6
Self employed		32.1	41.9	44.3	48.3	51.8	49.1	54.3
Employment status/time not stated		10.4	1.4	0.2	0.6	0.7	0.3	0.3
Government scheme		7.8	1.2	6.8	5.6	5.7	7.4	6.1
Unemployed actively seeking work		50.4	61.7	52.9	56.2	51.3	42.9	39.1
Unemployed - not seeking		40.1	51.2	56.6	53.9	61.6	57.4	46.3
Sick/holiday/disabled/retired		23.9	28.9	40.2	33.2	32.6	35.0	34.3
Student		63.2	41.7	60.7	34.7	36.1	35.3	34.6
Looking after home/family		247.3	204.5	201.7	203.6	186.3	184.1	176.1
TOTAL		1010.3	1018.2	1045.6	1033.3	1037.5	1039.8	1042.3

Source: Own calculations based on Labour Force Survey tapes.
Note: The figures refer to persons of working age. Those under 16, men 65+ and women 60+ are excluded.

Table 12.6
The distribution of males, with nursing qualifications, by occupation and economic status, SE Thames RHA

(thousands)

Economic status	Occupation	1983	1984	1985	1986	1987	1988	1989
Full-time employee	Nursing	1.9	1.9	2.1	2.4	2.3	1.7	2.2
	Midwifery	0.0	0.0	0.0	0.0	0.0	0.0	0.0
	Other	1.1	0.8	1.9	1.6	0.6	2.1	0.9
Part-time employee	Nursing	0.0	0.0	0.0	0.0	0.0	0.0	0.1
	Midwifery	0.0	0.0	0.0	0.0	0.0	0.0	0.0
	Other	0.0	0.1	0.0	0.0	0.1	0.1	0.0
Self employed		0.2	0.2	0.4	0.2	0.3	0.4	0.1
Employment status/time not stated		0.0	0.0	0.0	0.0	0.0	0.0	0.0
Government scheme		0.0	0.0	0.0	0.0	0.0	0.0	0.0
Unemployed actively seeking work		0.0	0.1	0.1	0.5	0.2	0.2	0.1
Unemployed - not seeking		0.0	0.0	0.0	0.0	0.0	0.1	0.3
Sick/holiday/disabled/retired		0.2	0.2	0.2	0.2	0.2	0.3	0.4
Student		0.0	0.1	0.3	0.1	0.0	0.1	0.1
Looking after home/family		0.0	0.0	0.0	0.0	0.0	0.2	0.0
TOTAL		3.4	3.4	5.0	5.0	3.7	5.2	4.2

Source: Own calculations based on Labour Force Survey tapes.
Note: The figures refer to persons of working age. Those under 16, men 65+ and women 60+ are excluded.

Table 12.7

The distribution of males, with other qualifications, by occupation and economic status, SE Thames RHA

(thousands)

Economic status	Occupation	1983	1984	1985	1986	1987	1988	1989
Full-time employee	Nursing	0.3	0.3	0.4	0.3	0.1	0.3	0.2
	Midwifery	0.0	0.0	0.0	0.0	0.0	0.0	0.0
	Other	212.2	214.2	229.9	226.6	223.4	229.6	243.5
Part-time employee	Nursing	0.0	0.0	0.0	0.0	0.0	0.0	0.0
	Midwifery	0.0	0.0	0.0	0.0	0.0	0.0	0.0
	Other	3.2	5.7	3.5	4.0	7.0	7.5	7.6
Self employed		29.9	33.1	36.3	37.3	40.1	38.5	43.0
Employment status/time not stated		1.3	0.1	0.0	0.1	0.3	0.0	0.1
Government scheme		2.3	0.3	0.7	0.7	1.0	1.3	0.6
Unemployed actively seeking work		11.9	11.7	9.4	14.0	13.2	7.4	9.7
Unemployed - not seeking		3.6	3.6	3.9	4.2	2.8	3.2	2.9
Sick/holiday/disabled/retired		5.4	5.1	7.8	6.1	8.8	6.0	5.8
Student		23.9	18.2	22.6	18.2	18.4	16.1	16.6
Looking after home/family		0.3	0.2	0.2	0.4	0.2	0.1	0.3
TOTAL		294.3	292.5	314.7	311.9	315.3	310.0	330.3

Source: Own calculations based on Labour Force Survey tapes.
Note: The figures refer to persons of working age. Those under 16, men 65+ and women 60+ are excluded.

Table 12.8
The distribution of males, with no qualifications, by occupation and economic status, SE Thames RHA

(thousands)

Economic status	Occupation	1983	1984	1985	1986	1987	1988	1989
Full-time employee	Nursing	0.3	0.4	0.2	1.1	0.5	0.7	0.8
	Midwifery	0.0	0.0	0.0	0.0	0.0	0.0	0.0
	Other	523.6	533.6	508.5	506.7	491.9	506.7	489.4
Part-time employee	Nursing	0.0	0.1	0.0	0.0	0.1	0.0	0.1
	Midwifery	0.0	0.0	0.0	0.0	0.0	0.0	0.0
	Other	6.8	18.8	9.6	19.2	20.5	24.9	22.2
Self employed		89.1	102.2	107.4	104.4	122.5	132.1	142.0
Employment status/time not stated		3.1	1.8	0.3	0.7	1.0	0.2	0.4
Government scheme		7.4	1.8	7.5	8.8	9.2	8.9	9.4
Unemployed actively seeking work		71.3	72.5	65.1	69.6	64.1	53.3	40.5
Unemployed - not seeking		17.6	16.8	18.1	21.7	19.4	14.6	13.8
Sick/holiday/disabled/retired		36.3	39.3	52.7	40.7	46.3	41.0	44.9
Student		43.2	27.2	42.9	27.6	26.6	23.8	26.1
Looking after home/family		2.6	2.4	3.7	3.2	3.0	3.5	2.7
TOTAL		801.3	816.9	816.0	803.7	805.1	809.7	792.3

Source: Own calculations based on Labour Force Survey tapes.
Note: The figures refer to persons of working age. Those under 16, men 65+ and women 60+ are excluded.

Table 12.9
The distribution of males, with all qualifications, by occupation and economic status, SE Thames RHA

(thousands)

Economic status	Occupation	1983	1984	1985	1986	1987	1988	1989
Full-time employee	Nursing	2.5	2.6	2.7	3.8	2.9	2.7	3.2
	Midwifery	0.0	0.0	0.0	0.0	0.0	0.0	0.0
	Other	736.9	748.6	740.3	734.9	715.9	738.4	733.8
Part-time employee	Nursing	0.0	0.1	0.0	0.0	0.1	0.0	0.2
	Midwifery	0.0	0.0	0.0	0.0	0.0	0.0	0.0
	Other	10.0	24.6	13.1	23.2	27.6	32.5	29.8
Self employed		119.2	135.5	144.1	141.9	162.9	171.0	185.1
Employment status/time not stated		4.4	1.9	0.3	0.8	1.3	0.2	0.5
Government scheme		9.7	2.1	8.2	9.5	10.2	10.2	10.0
Unemployed actively seeking work		83.2	84.3	74.6	84.1	77.5	60.9	50.3
Unemployed - not seeking		21.2	20.4	22.0	25.9	22.2	17.9	17.0
Sick/holiday/disabled/retired		41.9	44.6	60.7	47.0	55.3	47.3	51.1
Student		67.1	45.5	65.8	45.9	45.0	40.0	42.8
Looking after home/family		2.9	2.6	3.9	3.6	3.2	3.8	3.0
TOTAL		1099.0	1112.8	1135.7	1120.6	1124.1	1124.9	1126.8

Source: Own calculations based on Labour Force Survey tapes.
Note: The figures refer to persons of working age. Those under 16, men 65+ and women 60+ are excluded.

Table 12.10
Distribution of hours worked: full-time women employees with a nursing qualification by occupation, SE Thames RHA

(thousands)

Occupation	Usual hours worked per week	1983	1984	1985	1986	1987	1988	1989
Nursing	Less than 10	0.0 (0.0)	0.0 (0.0)	0.0 (0.0)	0.1 (0.7)	0.1 (0.8)	0.0 (0.0)	0.0 (0.0)
	10 to 19	0.1 (0.7)	0.0 (0.0)	0.0 (0.0)	0.0 (0.0)	0.0 (0.0)	0.0 (0.0)	0.0 (0.0)
	20 to 29	0.3 (2.2)	0.1 (0.7)	0.1 (0.7)	0.1 (0.7)	0.1 (0.8)	0.0 (0.0)	0.0 (0.0)
	30 to 39	7.2 (53.3)	6.2 (44.6)	5.7 (41.9)	7.3 (54.5)	6.3 (48.5)	5.3 (40.2)	3.5 (27.3)
	40 to 49	5.2 (38.5)	6.4 (46.0)	7.0 (51.5)	5.1 (38.1)	5.8 (44.6)	6.6 (50.0)	0.9 (7.0)
	50 and over	0.7 (5.2)	1.2 (8.6)	0.8 (5.9)	0.8 (6.0)	0.7 (5.4)	1.3 (9.8)	0.1 (0.8)
	Not stated	0.0 (0.0)	0.0 (0.0)	0.0 (0.0)	0.0 (0.0)	0.0 (0.0)	0.0 (0.0)	8.3 (64.8)
	TOTAL	13.5 (100.0)	13.9 (100.0)	13.6 (100.0)	13.4 (100.0)	13.0 (100.0)	13.2 (100.0)	12.8 (100.0)
Other	Less than 10	0.0 (0.0)	0.0 (0.0)	0.0 (0.0)	0.1 (1.6)	0.0 (0.0)	0.0 (0.0)	0.0 (0.0)
	10 to 19	0.0 (0.0)	0.1 (2.4)	0.0 (0.0)	0.0 (0.0)	0.0 (0.0)	0.0 (0.0)	0.0 (0.0)
	20 to 29	0.3 (6.1)	0.2 (4.8)	0.1 (1.9)	0.0 (0.0)	0.1 (1.3)	0.1 (1.6)	0.0 (0.0)
	30 to 39	2.4 (49.0)	2.5 (59.5)	2.5 (46.3)	2.7 (43.5)	2.9 (37.7)	2.5 (41.0)	2.5 (40.3)
	40 to 49	1.7 (34.7)	1.1 (26.2)	2.2 (40.7)	2.9 (46.8)	3.1 (40.3)	2.7 (44.3)	0.1 (1.6)
	50 and over	0.5 (10.2)	0.3 (7.1)	0.6 (11.1)	0.5 (8.1)	1.5 (19.5)	0.7 (11.5)	0.2 (3.2)
	Not stated	0.0 (0.0)	0.0 (0.0)	0.0 (0.0)	0.0 (0.0)	0.1 (1.3)	0.1 (1.6)	3.4 (54.8)
	TOTAL	4.9 (100.0)	4.2 (100.0)	5.4 (100.0)	6.2 (100.0)	7.7 (100.0)	6.1 (100.0)	6.2 (100.0)

Note: Percentage values are given in parentheses.

Source: Own calculations based on Labour Force Survey tapes.

Table 12.11

Distribution of hours worked: part-time women employees with a nursing qualification by occupation, SE Thames RHA

(thousands)

Occupation	Usual hours worked per week	1983	1984	1985	1986	1987	1988	1989
Nursing	Less than 10	0.3 (4.1)	0.5 (6.1)	0.4 (5.1)	0.9 (10.1)	0.5 (5.8)	0.6 (6.8)	0.4 (4.1)
	10 to 19	1.7 (23.3)	2.2 (26.8)	1.8 (22.8)	2.0 (22.5)	2.0 (23.3)	2.4 (27.3)	1.1 (11.2)
	20 to 29	3.6 (49.3)	3.9 (47.6)	3.8 (48.1)	3.5 (39.3)	3.7 (43.0)	3.2 (36.4)	2.2 (22.4)
	30 to 39	1.5 (20.5)	1.4 (17.1)	1.7 (21.5)	2.2 (24.7)	2.2 (25.6)	2.1 (23.9)	1.6 (16.3)
	40 to 49	0.1 (1.4)	0.0 (0.0)	0.2 (2.5)	0.3 (3.4)	0.1 (1.2)	0.5 (5.7)	0.0 (0.0)
	50 and over	0.1 (1.4)	0.2 (2.4)	0.0 (0.0)	0.0 (0.0)	0.1 (1.2)	0.0 (0.0)	0.0 (0.0)
	Not stated	0.0 (0.0)	0.0 (0.0)	0.0 (0.0)	0.0 (0.0)	0.0 (0.0)	0.0 (0.0)	4.5 (45.9)
	TOTAL	7.3 (100.0)	8.2 (100.0)	7.9 (100.0)	8.9 (100.0)	8.6 (100.0)	8.8 (100.0)	9.8 (100.0)
Other	Less than 10	0.4 (14.3)	0.9 (23.7)	0.6 (16.2)	0.7 (19.4)	0.9 (23.7)	0.9 (27.3)	0.7 (25.9)
	10 to 19	0.9 (32.1)	1.3 (34.2)	1.6 (43.2)	1.1 (30.6)	1.3 (34.2)	1.1 (33.3)	0.7 (25.9)
	20 to 29	1.0 (35.7)	1.0 (26.3)	1.2 (32.4)	1.3 (36.1)	1.3 (34.2)	0.8 (24.2)	0.3 (11.1)
	30 to 39	0.4 (14.3)	0.5 (13.2)	0.2 (5.4)	0.5 (13.9)	0.3 (7.9)	0.5 (15.2)	0.0 (0.0)
	40 to 49	0.0 (0.0)	0.1 (2.6)	0.0 (0.0)	0.0 (0.0)	0.0 (0.0)	0.0 (0.0)	0.0 (0.0)
	50 and over	0.1 (3.6)	0.0 (0.0)	0.0 (0.0)	0.0 (0.0)	0.0 (0.0)	0.0 (0.0)	0.0 (0.0)
	Not stated	0.0 (0.0)	0.0 (0.0)	0.1 (2.7)	0.0 (0.0)	0.0 (0.0)	0.0 (0.0)	1.0 (37.0)
	TOTAL	2.8 (100.0)	3.8 (100.0)	3.7 (100.0)	3.6 (100.0)	3.8 (100.0)	3.3 (100.0)	2.7 (100.0)

Note: Percentage values are given in parentheses.

Source: Own calculations based on Labour Force Survey tapes.

Table 12.12

Distribution of hours worked: all women employees with a nursing qualification by occupation, SE Thames RHA

(thousands)

Occupation	Usual hours worked per week	1983	1984	1985	1986	1987	1988	1989
Nursing	Less than 10	0.3 (1.4)	0.5 (2.3)	0.4 (1.9)	1.0 (4.5)	0.6 (2.8)	0.6 (2.7)	0.4 (1.8)
	10 to 19	1.8 (8.5)	2.2 (10.0)	1.8 (8.4)	2.0 (9.0)	2.0 (9.3)	2.4 (10.9)	1.1 (4.9)
	20 to 29	4.0 (19.0)	4.0 (18.1)	3.9 (18.1)	3.6 (16.1)	3.8 (17.6)	3.2 (14.5)	2.2 (9.7)
	30 to 39	8.9 (42.2)	7.6 (34.4)	7.4 (34.4)	9.5 (42.6)	8.5 (39.4)	7.4 (33.6)	5.1 (22.6)
	40 to 49	5.3 (25.1)	6.4 (29.0)	7.2 (33.5)	5.4 (24.2)	5.9 (27.3)	7.1 (32.3)	0.9 (4.0)
	50 and over	0.8 (3.8)	1.4 (6.3)	0.8 (3.7)	0.8 (3.6)	0.8 (3.7)	1.3 (5.9)	0.1 (0.4)
	Not stated	0.0 (0.0)	0.0 (0.0)	0.0 (0.0)	0.0 (0.0)	0.0 (0.0)	0.0 (0.0)	12.8 (56.6)
	TOTAL	21.1 (100.0)	22.1 (100.0)	21.5 (100.0)	22.3 (100.0)	21.6 (100.0)	22.0 (100.0)	22.6 (100.0)
Other	Less than 10	0.4 (5.2)	0.9 (11.3)	0.6 (6.6)	0.8 (8.2)	0.9 (7.8)	0.9 (9.6)	0.7 (7.9)
	10 to 19	0.9 (11.7)	1.4 (17.5)	1.6 (17.6)	1.1 (11.2)	1.3 (11.3)	1.1 (11.7)	0.7 (7.9)
	20 to 29	1.3 (16.9)	1.2 (15.0)	1.3 (14.3)	1.3 (13.3)	1.4 (12.2)	0.9 (9.6)	0.3 (3.4)
	30 to 39	2.8 (36.4)	3.0 (37.5)	2.7 (29.7)	3.2 (32.7)	3.2 (27.8)	3.0 (31.9)	2.5 (28.1)
	40 to 49	1.7 (22.1)	1.2 (15.0)	2.2 (24.2)	2.9 (29.6)	3.1 (27.0)	2.7 (28.7)	0.1 (1.1)
	50 and over	0.6 (7.8)	0.3 (3.8)	0.6 (6.6)	0.5 (5.1)	1.5 (13.0)	0.7 (7.4)	0.2 (2.2)
	Not stated	0.0 (0.0)	0.0 (0.0)	0.1 (1.1)	0.0 (0.0)	0.1 (0.9)	0.1 (1.1)	4.4 (49.4)
	TOTAL	7.7 (100.0)	8.0 (100.0)	9.1 (100.0)	9.8 (100.0)	11.5 (100.0)	9.4 (100.0)	8.9 (100.0)

Source: Own calculations based on Labour Force Survey tapes.

Note: Percentage values are given in parentheses.

Table 12.13
Age distribution: full-time women employees with a nursing qualification by occupation, SE Thames RHA

(thousands)

Occupation	Age group	1983	1984	1985	1986	1987	1988	1989
Nursing	16 to 19	0.0 (0.0)	0.1 (0.7)	0.0 (0.0)	0.2 (1.5)	0.0 (0.0)	0.0 (0.0)	0.1 (0.8)
	20 to 29	5.4 (40.0)	4.5 (32.6)	4.8 (35.0)	5.4 (40.3)	5.2 (40.0)	4.3 (32.8)	4.7 (37.0)
	30 to 39	3.8 (28.1)	3.4 (24.6)	3.7 (27.0)	3.2 (23.9)	3.0 (23.1)	2.8 (21.4)	2.5 (19.7)
	40 to 49	2.4 (17.8)	3.7 (26.8)	3.4 (24.8)	2.7 (20.1)	3.3 (25.4)	3.7 (28.2)	3.7 (29.1)
	50 to 59	1.9 (14.1)	2.1 (15.2)	1.8 (13.1)	1.9 (14.2)	1.5 (11.5)	2.3 (17.6)	1.7 (13.4)
	TOTAL	13.5 (100.0)	13.8 (100.0)	13.7 (100.0)	13.4 (100.0)	13.0 (100.0)	13.1 (100.0)	12.7 (100.0)
Other	16 to 19	0.0 (0.0)	0.2 (4.9)	0.0 (0.0)	0.1 (1.6)	0.2 (2.6)	0.2 (3.3)	0.1 (1.6)
	20 to 29	1.5 (30.6)	0.8 (19.5)	2.3 (41.8)	1.9 (31.1)	3.0 (39.0)	1.6 (26.2)	2.5 (39.1)
	30 to 39	1.0 (20.4)	0.8 (19.5)	1.3 (23.6)	1.9 (31.1)	1.7 (22.1)	1.5 (24.6)	1.6 (25.0)
	40 to 49	1.5 (30.6)	1.2 (29.3)	1.4 (25.5)	1.2 (19.7)	2.0 (26.0)	1.5 (24.6)	1.0 (15.6)
	50 to 59	0.9 (18.4)	1.1 (26.8)	0.5 (9.1)	1.0 (16.4)	0.8 (10.4)	1.3 (21.3)	1.2 (18.8)
	TOTAL	4.9 (100.0)	4.1 (100.0)	5.5 (100.0)	6.1 (100.0)	7.7 (100.0)	6.1 (100.0)	6.4 (100.0)

Source: Own calculations based on Labour Force Survey tapes.
Note: Percentage values are given in parentheses.

Table 12.14
Age distribution: part-time women employees with a nursing qualification by occupation, SE Thames RHA

(thousands)

Occupation	Age group	1983	1984	1985	1986	1987	1988	1989
Nursing	16 to 19	0.1 (1.4)	0.0 (0.0)	0.0 (0.0)	0.0 (0.0)	0.0 (0.0)	0.0 (0.0)	0.0 (0.0)
	20 to 29	1.0 (13.9)	0.8 (9.8)	1.4 (17.5)	1.2 (13.6)	1.6 (18.8)	1.5 (16.9)	1.4 (14.3)
	30 to 39	2.6 (36.1)	3.5 (42.7)	2.7 (33.8)	2.7 (30.7)	3.6 (42.4)	3.6 (40.4)	3.0 (30.6)
	40 to 49	2.2 (30.6)	2.9 (35.4)	2.6 (32.5)	3.0 (34.1)	2.0 (23.5)	2.4 (27.0)	3.8 (38.8)
	50 to 59	1.3 (18.1)	1.0 (12.2)	1.3 (16.3)	1.9 (21.6)	1.3 (15.3)	1.4 (15.7)	1.6 (16.3)
	TOTAL	7.2 (100.0)	8.2 (100.0)	8.0 (100.0)	8.8 (100.0)	8.5 (100.0)	8.9 (100.0)	9.8 (100.0)
Other	16 to 19	0.0 (0.0)	0.0 (0.0)	0.0 (0.0)	0.0 (0.0)	0.0 (0.0)	0.0 (0.0)	0.0 (0.0)
	20 to 29	0.3 (10.7)	0.5 (12.8)	0.2 (5.4)	0.1 (2.7)	0.3 (7.7)	0.5 (14.3)	0.4 (14.8)
	30 to 39	0.8 (28.6)	1.7 (43.6)	1.1 (29.7)	1.6 (43.2)	1.5 (38.5)	0.7 (20.0)	0.9 (33.3)
	40 to 49	1.1 (39.3)	0.9 (23.1)	1.6 (43.2)	1.1 (29.7)	1.0 (25.6)	1.8 (51.4)	1.1 (40.7)
	50 to 59	0.6 (21.4)	0.8 (20.5)	0.8 (21.6)	0.9 (24.3)	1.1 (28.2)	0.5 (14.3)	0.3 (11.1)
	TOTAL	2.8 (100.0)	3.9 (100.0)	3.7 (100.0)	3.7 (100.0)	3.9 (100.0)	3.5 (100.0)	2.7 (100.0)

Source: Own calculations based on Labour Force Survey tapes.
Note: Percentage values are given in parentheses.

Table 12.15
Age distribution: all women employees with a nursing qualification by occupation, SE Thames RHA

(thousands)

Occupation	Age group	1983	1984	1985	1986	1987	1988	1989
Nursing	16 to 19	0.1 (0.5)	0.1 (0.5)	0.0 (0.0)	0.2 (0.9)	0.0 (0.0)	0.0 (0.0)	0.1 (0.4)
	20 to 29	6.4 (30.5)	5.3 (24.1)	6.2 (28.6)	6.6 (29.7)	6.8 (31.6)	5.8 (26.4)	6.1 (27.1)
	30 to 39	6.6 (31.4)	6.9 (31.4)	6.4 (29.5)	5.9 (26.6)	6.6 (30.7)	6.4 (29.1)	5.5 (24.4)
	40 to 49	4.7 (22.4)	6.6 (30.0)	6.0 (27.6)	5.7 (25.7)	5.3 (24.7)	6.1 (27.7)	7.5 (33.3)
	50 to 59	3.2 (15.2)	3.1 (14.1)	3.1 (14.3)	3.8 (17.1)	2.8 (13.0)	3.7 (16.8)	3.3 (14.7)
	TOTAL	21.0 (100.0)	22.0 (100.0)	21.7 (100.0)	22.2 (100.0)	21.5 (100.0)	22.0 (100.0)	22.5 (100.0)
Other	16 to 19	0.0 (0.0)	0.2 (2.5)	0.0 (0.0)	0.1 (1.0)	0.2 (1.7)	0.2 (2.1)	0.1 (1.1)
	20 to 29	1.8 (23.4)	1.3 (16.3)	2.5 (27.2)	2.0 (20.4)	3.3 (28.4)	2.1 (21.9)	2.9 (31.9)
	30 to 39	1.8 (23.4)	2.5 (31.3)	2.4 (26.1)	3.5 (35.7)	3.2 (27.6)	2.2 (22.9)	2.5 (27.5)
	40 to 49	2.6 (33.8)	2.1 (26.3)	3.0 (32.6)	2.3 (23.5)	3.0 (25.9)	3.3 (34.4)	2.1 (23.1)
	50 to 59	1.5 (19.5)	1.9 (23.8)	1.3 (14.1)	1.9 (19.4)	1.9 (16.4)	1.8 (18.8)	1.5 (16.5)
	TOTAL	7.7 (100.0)	8.0 (100.0)	9.2 (100.0)	9.8 (100.0)	11.6 (100.0)	9.6 (100.0)	9.1 (100.0)

Source: Own calculations based on Labour Force Survey tapes.
Note: Percentage values are given in parentheses.

Table 12.16
Sectoral distribution: full-time women employees with a nursing qualification by occupation, SE Thames RHA

(thousands)

Occupation	Sector	1983	1984	1985	1986	1987	1988	1989
Nursing	Hospitals, nursing homes etc.	10.2	9.3	10.1	10.1	9.0	10.0	9.7
	Other medical care institutions	2.0	2.3	3.0	1.8	1.7	1.5	1.4
	Medical practices	0.0	0.0	0.2	0.5	0.2	0.1	0.1
	Dental practices	0.4	0.2	0.1	0.1	0.1	0.0	0.2
	Agency and private midwives, nurses etc.	0.1	0.6	0.1	0.2	0.4	0.0	0.1
	TOTAL HEALTH SERVICE SECTOR	12.7	12.4	13.5	12.7	11.4	11.6	11.5
	Other sectors	1.1	1.5	0.6	0.9	2.0	1.6	1.4
	TOTAL ALL SECTORS	13.8	13.9	14.1	13.6	13.4	13.2	12.9
Other	Hospitals, nursing homes etc.	0.3	0.3	0.8	0.8	1.3	0.6	0.8
	Other medical care institutions	0.0	0.1	0.2	0.4	0.3	0.1	0.5
	Medical practices	0.0	0.1	0.1	0.0	0.1	0.2	0.1
	Dental practices	0.1	0.0	0.0	0.2	0.0	0.0	0.1
	Agency and private midwives, nurses etc.	0.0	0.0	0.0	0.1	0.4	0.0	0.1
	TOTAL HEALTH SERVICE SECTOR	0.4	0.5	1.1	1.5	2.1	0.9	1.6
	Other sectors	4.9	4.1	5.1	5.4	6.2	5.9	5.7
	TOTAL ALL SECTORS	5.3	4.6	6.2	6.9	8.3	6.8	7.3

Source: Own calculations based on Labour Force Survey tapes.

Table 12.17
Sectoral distribution: part-time women employees with a nursing qualification by occupation, SE Thames RHA

(thousands)

Occupation	Sector	1983	1984	1985	1986	1987	1988	1989
Nursing	Hospitals, nursing homes etc.	5.4	5.1	5.2	5.9	5.7	5.6	7.0
	Other medical care institutions	1.1	1.1	0.9	1.5	1.1	1.0	0.8
	Medical practices	0.2	0.7	0.4	0.8	0.2	0.5	0.9
	Dental practices	0.0	0.0	0.1	0.0	0.0	0.0	0.1
	Agency and private midwives, nurses etc.	0.4	0.5	0.5	0.6	0.8	0.2	0.1
	TOTAL HEALTH SERVICE SECTOR	7.1	7.4	7.1	8.8	7.8	7.3	8.9
	Other sectors	0.6	1.1	0.9	0.5	1.1	1.8	1.1
	TOTAL ALL SECTORS	7.7	8.5	8.0	9.3	8.9	9.1	10.0
Other	Hospitals, nursing homes etc.	0.4	0.7	0.4	0.4	0.4	0.5	0.7
	Other medical care institutions	0.0	0.0	0.0	0.3	0.1	0.0	0.0
	Medical practices	0.2	0.1	0.2	0.0	0.3	0.2	0.1
	Dental practices	0.0	0.0	0.1	0.1	0.0	0.0	0.0
	Agency and private midwives, nurses etc.	0.0	0.1	0.0	0.1	0.0	0.0	0.0
	TOTAL HEALTH SERVICE SECTOR	0.6	0.9	0.7	0.9	0.8	0.7	0.8
	Other sectors	2.8	4.2	4.0	3.3	3.5	3.2	2.5
	TOTAL ALL SECTORS	3.4	5.1	4.7	4.2	4.3	3.9	3.3

Source: Own calculations based on Labour Force Survey tapes.

Table 12.18
Sectoral distribution: all women employees with a nursing qualification by occupation, SE Thames RHA
(thousands)

Occupation	Sector	1983	1984	1985	1986	1987	1988	1989
Nursing	Hospitals, nursing homes etc.	15.9	14.4	15.3	16.0	14.7	15.6	16.7
	Other medical care institutions	3.1	3.4	3.9	3.3	2.8	2.5	2.2
	Medical practices	0.2	0.7	0.6	1.3	0.4	0.6	1.0
	Dental practices	0.4	0.2	0.2	0.1	0.1	0.0	0.3
	Agency and private midwives, nurses etc.	0.5	1.1	0.6	0.8	1.2	0.2	0.2
	TOTAL HEALTH SERVICE SECTOR	20.1	19.8	20.6	21.5	19.2	18.9	20.4
	Other sectors	1.7	2.6	1.5	1.4	3.1	3.4	2.5
	TOTAL ALL SECTORS	21.8	22.4	22.1	22.9	22.3	22.3	22.9
Other	Hospitals, nursing homes etc.	0.7	1.0	1.2	1.2	1.7	1.1	1.5
	Other medical care institutions	0.0	0.1	0.2	0.7	0.4	0.1	0.5
	Medical practices	0.2	0.2	0.3	0.0	0.4	0.4	0.2
	Dental practices	0.1	0.0	0.1	0.3	0.0	0.0	0.1
	Agency and private midwives, nurses etc.	0.0	0.1	0.0	0.2	0.4	0.0	0.1
	TOTAL HEALTH SERVICE SECTOR	1.0	1.4	1.8	2.4	2.9	1.6	2.4
	Other sectors	18.9	18.1	9.1	20.4	9.7	9.1	8.2
	TOTAL ALL SECTORS	19.9	19.5	10.9	22.8	12.6	10.7	10.6

Source: Own calculations based on Labour Force Survey tapes.

Table 12.19
The distribution of females, with nursing qualifications, by occupation and economic status, Trent RHA

(thousands)

Economic status	Occupation	1983	1984	1985	1986	1987	1988	1989
Full-time employee	Nursing	18.6	15.2	17.5	17.5	19.4	17.4	16.2
	Midwifery	0.9	2.1	0.0	0.0	0.0	0.0	0.0
	Other	4.9	4.2	5.5	6.4	3.6	6.6	6.2
Part-time employee	Nursing	7.5	9.5	10.0	8.6	12.3	10.5	13.2
	Midwifery	0.3	0.6	0.0	0.0	0.0	0.0	0.0
	Other	3.2	4.0	5.6	5.5	4.1	7.1	4.1
Self employed		1.3	0.9	1.3	1.4	2.1	2.1	1.9
Employment status/time not stated		0.7	0.0	0.0	0.0	0.0	0.0	0.0
Government scheme		0.0	0.0	0.0	0.0	0.0	0.0	0.0
Unemployed actively seeking work		1.5	3.1	1.3	1.6	1.0	1.7	1.2
Unemployed - not seeking		1.1	1.6	2.2	2.7	1.9	1.1	1.2
Sick/holiday/disabled/retired		1.7	1.3	0.3	0.3	0.7	1.1	1.3
Student		0.5	0.0	0.3	0.0	0.3	0.4	0.0
Looking after home/family		6.8	5.7	6.9	7.4	5.1	3.5	2.0
TOTAL		49.0	48.2	50.9	51.4	50.5	51.5	47.3

Source: Own calculations based on Labour Force Survey tapes.
Note: The figures refer to persons of working age. Those under 16, men 65+ and women 60+ are excluded.

Table 12.20
The distribution of females, with other qualifications, by occupation and economic status, Trent RHA

(thousands)

Economic status	Occupation	1983	1984	1985	1986	1987	1988	1989
Full-time employee	Nursing	0.2	0.7	1.7	1.7	1.7	1.3	1.7
	Midwifery	0.0	0.0	0.0	0.0	0.0	0.0	0.0
	Other	65.3	70.6	73.5	78.5	78.4	80.9	88.4
Part-time employee	Nursing	0.0	0.3	0.3	0.9	0.3	0.0	0.2
	Midwifery	0.0	0.0	0.0	0.0	0.0	0.0	0.0
	Other	17.6	18.6	22.1	28.8	26.1	27.8	36.4
Self employed		4.7	5.2	5.5	7.0	7.1	5.2	11.5
Employment status/time not stated		1.1	0.3	0.0	0.0	0.0	0.0	0.0
Government scheme		1.1	0.0	0.7	1.1	0.5	1.5	0.6
Unemployed actively seeking work		5.1	9.1	6.4	7.7	6.6	6.5	5.3
Unemployed - not seeking		2.7	5.7	7.0	4.7	5.8	3.8	5.5
Sick/holiday/disabled/retired		0.2	1.5	2.3	3.0	2.2	1.4	3.9
Student		14.3	8.0	11.3	4.6	11.6	11.4	12.2
Looking after home/family		25.8	25.5	17.5	19.9	17.9	20.2	13.8
TOTAL		138.1	145.5	148.3	157.9	158.2	160.0	179.5

Source: Own calculations based on Labour Force Survey tapes.
Note: The figures refer to persons of working age. Those under 16, men 65+ and women 60+ are excluded.

223

Table 12.21
The distribution of females, with no qualifications, by occupation and economic status, Trent RHA

(thousands)

Economic status	Occupation	1983	1984	1985	1986	1987	1988	1989
Full-time employee	Nursing	8.0	7.9	4.5	4.1	4.4	5.2	8.6
	Midwifery	0.0	0.0	0.0	0.0	0.0	0.0	0.0
	Other	288.2	295.8	280.0	282.7	281.2	308.6	313.1
Part-time employee	Nursing	8.6	8.4	4.2	7.9	8.7	6.9	8.8
	Midwifery	0.0	0.4	0.0	0.0	0.0	0.0	0.0
	Other	246.7	286.2	282.6	312.6	298.2	306.9	318.4
Self employed		35.6	37.0	36.2	38.0	40.3	48.8	43.1
Employment status/time not stated		17.5	1.3	0.0	0.6	0.8	0.7	0.9
Government scheme		14.8	3.1	10.3	14.2	16.5	21.5	21.7
Unemployed actively seeking work		70.6	81.6	74.0	84.4	84.7	68.8	59.1
Unemployed - not seeking		47.4	78.9	96.8	70.9	80.6	70.9	55.2
Sick/holiday/disabled/retired		32.1	42.5	54.2	45.4	47.9	56.5	55.9
Student		50.4	33.9	50.0	29.0	25.9	27.0	30.7
Looking after home/family		317.7	262.2	264.9	253.9	260.7	240.5	232.5
TOTAL		1137.6	1139.2	1157.7	1143.7	1149.9	1162.3	1148.0

Source: Own calculations based on Labour Force Survey tapes.
Note: The figures refer to persons of working age. Those under 16, men 65+ and women 60+ are excluded.

Table 12.22
The distribution of females, with all qualifications, by occupation and economic status, Trent RHA

(thousands)

Economic status	Occupation	1983	1984	1985	1986	1987	1988	1989
Full-time employee	Nursing	26.8	23.8	23.7	23.3	25.5	23.9	26.5
	Midwifery	0.9	2.1	0.0	0.0	0.0	0.0	0.0
	Other	358.4	370.6	359.0	367.6	363.2	396.1	407.7
Part-time employee	Nursing	16.1	18.2	14.5	17.4	21.3	17.4	22.2
	Midwifery	0.3	1.0	0.0	0.0	0.0	0.0	0.0
	Other	267.5	308.8	310.3	346.9	328.4	341.8	358.9
Self employed		41.6	43.1	43.0	46.4	49.5	56.1	56.5
Employment status/time not stated		19.3	1.6	0.0	0.6	0.8	0.7	0.9
Government scheme		15.9	3.1	11.0	15.3	17.0	23.0	22.3
Unemployed actively seeking work		77.2	93.8	81.7	93.7	92.3	77.0	65.6
Unemployed - not seeking		51.2	86.2	106.0	78.3	88.3	75.8	61.9
Sick/holiday/disabled/retired		34.0	45.3	56.8	48.7	50.8	59.0	61.1
Student		65.2	41.9	61.6	33.6	37.8	38.8	42.9
Looking after home/family		350.3	293.4	289.3	281.2	283.7	264.2	248.3
TOTAL		1324.7	1332.9	1356.9	1353.0	1358.6	1373.8	1374.8

Source: Own calculations based on Labour Force Survey tapes.
Note: The figures refer to persons of working age. Those under 16, men 65+ and women 60+ are excluded.

Table 12.23
The distribution of males, with nursing qualifications, by occupation and economic status, Trent RHA

(thousands)

Economic status	Occupation	1983	1984	1985	1986	1987	1988	1989
Full-time employee	Nursing	3.2	4.1	2.7	4.1	4.2	2.5	2.1
	Midwifery	0.0	0.0	0.0	0.0	0.0	0.0	0.0
	Other	2.3	1.2	1.7	1.6	0.7	1.2	0.6
Part-time employee	Nursing	0.0	0.0	0.0	0.0	0.3	0.0	0.4
	Midwifery	0.0	0.0	0.0	0.0	0.0	0.0	0.0
	Other	0.0	0.0	0.0	0.0	0.0	0.0	0.0
Self employed		0.2	0.0	0.0	0.0	0.7	0.4	0.0
Employment status/time not stated		0.0	0.0	0.0	0.0	0.0	0.0	0.0
Government scheme		0.0	0.0	0.0	0.0	0.0	0.0	0.0
Unemployed actively seeking work		0.3	0.0	0.4	0.6	0.0	0.0	0.0
Unemployed - not seeking		0.0	0.0	0.0	0.0	0.0	0.0	0.0
Sick/holiday/disabled/retired		0.3	0.6	0.7	0.3	0.9	0.6	0.3
Student		0.0	0.0	0.0	0.0	0.0	0.0	0.0
Looking after home/family		0.0	0.0	0.0	0.0	0.0	0.0	0.0
TOTAL		6.3	5.9	5.5	6.6	6.8	4.7	3.4

Source: Own calculations based on Labour Force Survey tapes.
Note: The figures refer to persons of working age. Those under 16, men 65+ and women 60+ are excluded.

Table 12.24
The distribution of males, with other qualifications, by occupation and economic status, Trent RHA

(thousands)

Economic status	Occupation	1983	1984	1985	1986	1987	1988	1989
Full-time employee	Nursing	0.3	0.4	0.0	0.4	0.8	0.3	0.7
	Midwifery	0.0	0.0	0.0	0.0	0.0	0.0	0.0
	Other	183.3	208.0	199.1	194.6	182.8	221.1	215.8
Part-time employee	Nursing	0.0	0.0	0.4	0.0	0.0	0.0	0.0
	Midwifery	0.0	0.0	0.0	0.0	0.0	0.0	0.0
	Other	2.1	1.9	0.7	4.9	6.5	5.6	6.0
Self employed		14.7	16.3	24.4	25.5	30.4	35.8	35.1
Employment status/time not stated		0.4	0.4	0.0	0.0	0.0	0.0	0.0
Government scheme		2.1	0.0	1.5	1.2	1.6	2.3	0.7
Unemployed actively seeking work		12.2	12.1	13.1	14.2	9.7	8.3	7.6
Unemployed - not seeking		3.4	3.2	3.1	4.5	2.1	2.3	1.6
Sick/holiday/disabled/retired		6.0	6.1	1.8	6.0	8.3	4.8	4.6
Student		20.6	13.3	15.1	18.6	18.3	16.8	18.4
Looking after home/family		0.2	0.0	0.0	0.0	0.3	0.3	0.0
TOTAL		245.3	261.7	259.2	269.9	260.8	297.6	290.5

Source: Own calculations based on Labour Force Survey tapes.
Note: The figures refer to persons of working age. Those under 16, men 65+ and women 60+ are excluded.

Table 12.25
The distribution of males, with no qualifications, by occupation and economic status, Trent RHA

(thousands)

Economic status	Occupation	1983	1984	1985	1986	1987	1988	1989
Full-time employee	Nursing	0.9	2.1	0.4	0.9	0.7	0.2	1.5
	Midwifery	0.0	0.0	0.0	0.0	0.0	0.0	0.0
	Other	773.2	763.3	733.6	756.6	737.5	727.5	747.3
Part-time employee	Nursing	0.0	0.0	0.0	0.0	0.0	0.0	0.0
	Midwifery	0.0	0.0	0.0	0.0	0.0	0.0	0.0
	Other	8.3	27.2	11.6	23.2	26.2	27.3	28.0
Self employed		111.9	116.4	120.6	114.8	127.0	137.6	149.8
Employment status/time not stated		4.5	2.4	0.0	0.0	0.4	0.0	0.3
Government scheme		19.4	4.7	26.2	26.8	28.5	32.9	31.9
Unemployed actively seeking work		123.9	134.0	130.1	131.1	133.5	114.2	99.1
Unemployed - not seeking		32.7	40.6	55.0	57.0	51.5	37.1	29.3
Sick/holiday/disabled/retired		81.9	79.3	114.2	83.5	90.7	96.1	96.0
Student		49.7	34.7	50.8	26.4	35.9	33.3	29.6
Looking after home/family		3.9	7.6	5.8	7.7	5.9	9.6	6.8
TOTAL		1210.3	1212.3	1248.3	1228.0	1237.8	1215.8	1219.6

Source: Own calculations based on Labour Force Survey tapes.
Note: The figures refer to persons of working age. Those under 16, men 65+ and women 60+ are excluded.

228

Table 12.26

The distribution of males, with all qualifications, by occupation and economic status, Trent RHA

(thousands)

Economic status	Occupation	1983	1984	1985	1986	1987	1988	1989
Full-time employee	Nursing	4.4	6.6	3.1	5.4	5.7	3.0	4.3
	Midwifery	0.0	0.0	0.0	0.0	0.0	0.0	0.0
	Other	958.8	972.5	934.4	952.8	921.0	949.8	963.7
Part-time employee	Nursing	0.0	0.0	0.4	0.0	0.3	0.0	0.4
	Midwifery	0.0	0.0	0.0	0.0	0.0	0.0	0.0
	Other	10.4	29.1	12.3	28.1	32.7	32.9	34.0
Self employed		126.8	132.7	145.0	140.3	158.1	173.8	184.9
Employment status/time not stated		4.9	2.8	0.0	0.0	0.4	0.0	0.3
Government scheme		21.5	4.7	27.7	28.0	30.1	35.2	32.6
Unemployed actively seeking work		136.4	146.1	143.6	145.9	143.2	122.5	106.7
Unemployed - not seeking		36.1	43.8	58.1	61.5	53.6	39.4	30.9
Sick/holiday/disabled/retired		88.2	86.0	116.7	89.8	99.9	101.5	100.9
Student		70.3	48.0	65.9	45.0	54.2	50.1	48.0
Looking after home/family		4.1	7.6	5.8	7.7	6.2	9.9	6.8
TOTAL		1461.9	1479.9	1513.0	1504.5	1505.4	1518.1	1513.5

Source: Own calculations based on Labour Force Survey tapes.
Note: The figures refer to persons of working age. Those under 16, men 65+ and women 60+ are excluded.

Table 12.27

Distribution of hours worked: full-time women employees with a nursing qualification by occupation, Trent RHA

(thousands)

Occupation	Usual hours worked per week	1983	1984	1985	1986	1987	1988	1989
Nursing	Less than 10	0.0 (0.0)	0.0 (0.0)	0.0 (0.0)	0.4 (2.3)	0.0 (0.0)	0.0 (0.0)	0.0 (0.0)
	10 to 19	0.0 (0.0)	0.0 (0.0)	0.0 (0.0)	0.0 (0.0)	0.0 (0.0)	0.0 (0.0)	0.0 (0.0)
	20 to 29	0.0 (0.0)	0.0 (0.0)	0.0 (0.0)	0.0 (0.0)	0.0 (0.0)	0.0 (0.0)	0.0 (0.0)
	30 to 39	13.8 (70.4)	9.5 (54.3)	8.0 (46.0)	9.9 (56.6)	11.7 (60.0)	9.9 (56.9)	5.3 (32.7)
	40 to 49	5.4 (27.6)	6.8 (38.9)	8.8 (50.6)	6.6 (37.7)	7.6 (39.0)	7.2 (41.4)	1.7 (10.5)
	50 and over	0.4 (2.0)	1.2 (6.9)	0.6 (3.4)	0.6 (3.4)	0.2 (1.0)	0.3 (1.7)	0.7 (4.3)
	Not stated	0.0 (0.0)	0.0 (0.0)	0.0 (0.0)	0.0 (0.0)	0.0 (0.0)	0.0 (0.0)	8.5 (52.5)
	TOTAL	19.6 (100.0)	17.5 (100.0)	17.4 (100.0)	17.5 (100.0)	19.5 (100.0)	17.4 (100.0)	16.2 (100.0)
Other	Less than 10	0.0 (0.0)	0.0 (0.0)	0.0 (0.0)	0.0 (0.0)	0.0 (0.0)	0.0 (0.0)	0.0 (0.0)
	10 to 19	0.0 (0.0)	0.4 (9.5)	0.0 (0.0)	0.0 (0.0)	0.0 (0.0)	0.3 (4.5)	0.0 (0.0)
	20 to 29	0.7 (14.3)	0.0 (0.0)	0.0 (0.0)	0.5 (7.7)	0.0 (0.0)	0.0 (0.0)	0.0 (0.0)
	30 to 39	2.2 (44.9)	1.9 (45.2)	2.1 (38.2)	2.1 (32.3)	2.7 (75.0)	3.2 (48.5)	2.0 (32.3)
	40 to 49	1.3 (26.5)	1.6 (38.1)	3.0 (54.5)	2.1 (32.3)	0.5 (13.9)	2.3 (34.8)	0.8 (12.9)
	50 and over	0.7 (14.3)	0.3 (7.1)	0.4 (7.3)	1.8 (27.7)	0.4 (11.1)	0.8 (12.1)	0.0 (0.0)
	Not stated	0.0 (0.0)	0.0 (0.0)	0.0 (0.0)	0.0 (0.0)	0.0 (0.0)	0.0 (0.0)	3.4 (54.8)
	TOTAL	4.9 (100.0)	4.2 (100.0)	5.5 (100.0)	6.5 (100.0)	3.6 (100.0)	6.6 (100.0)	6.2 (100.0)

Note: Percentage values are given in parentheses.

Source: Own calculations based on Labour Force Survey tapes.

Table 12.28

Distribution of hours worked: part-time women employees with a nursing qualification by occupation, Trent RHA

(thousands)

Occupation	Usual hours worked per week	1983	1984	1985	1986	1987	1988	1989
Nursing	Less than 10	0.0 (0.0)	0.0 (0.0)	0.3 (3.0)	0.3 (3.5)	1.8 (14.6)	1.5 (14.3)	2.0 (15.2)
	10 to 19	1.4 (17.9)	3.0 (29.7)	1.4 (14.0)	1.5 (17.4)	2.0 (16.3)	2.7 (25.7)	0.0 (0.0)
	20 to 29	3.0 (38.5)	4.6 (45.5)	5.0 (50.0)	3.7 (43.0)	5.5 (44.7)	2.5 (23.8)	3.8 (28.8)
	30 to 39	3.1 (39.7)	2.5 (24.8)	3.0 (30.0)	2.8 (32.6)	2.7 (22.0)	3.5 (33.3)	0.8 (6.1)
	40 to 49	0.0 (0.0)	0.0 (0.0)	0.3 (3.0)	0.0 (0.0)	0.3 (2.4)	0.0 (2.9)	0.0 (0.0)
	50 and over	0.3 (3.8)	0.0 (0.0)	0.0 (0.0)	0.3 (3.5)	0.0 (0.0)	0.0 (0.0)	0.0 (0.0)
	Not stated	0.0 (0.0)	0.0 (0.0)	0.0 (0.0)	0.0 (0.0)	0.0 (0.0)	0.0 (0.0)	6.6 (50.0)
	TOTAL	7.8 (100.0)	10.1 (100.0)	10.0 (100.0)	8.6 (100.0)	12.3 (100.0)	10.5 (100.0)	13.2 (100.0)
Other	Less than 10	0.0 (0.0)	1.0 (25.0)	0.6 (10.7)	0.9 (16.7)	1.2 (29.3)	1.6 (22.2)	1.2 (28.6)
	10 to 19	0.9 (29.0)	2.7 (67.5)	1.3 (23.2)	2.4 (44.4)	1.8 (43.9)	2.6 (36.1)	0.9 (21.4)
	20 to 29	1.2 (38.7)	0.3 (7.5)	3.0 (53.6)	1.5 (27.8)	1.1 (26.8)	2.1 (29.2)	1.1 (26.2)
	30 to 39	0.8 (25.8)	0.0 (0.0)	0.7 (12.5)	0.3 (5.6)	0.0 (0.0)	0.6 (8.3)	0.0 (0.0)
	40 to 49	0.0 (0.0)	0.0 (0.0)	0.0 (0.0)	0.3 (5.6)	0.0 (0.0)	0.3 (4.2)	0.0 (0.0)
	50 and over	0.2 (6.5)	0.0 (0.0)	0.0 (0.0)	0.0 (0.0)	0.0 (0.0)	0.0 (0.0)	0.0 (0.0)
	Not stated	0.0 (0.0)	0.0 (0.0)	0.0 (0.0)	0.0 (0.0)	0.0 (0.0)	0.0 (0.0)	1.0 (23.8)
	TOTAL	3.1 (100.0)	4.0 (100.0)	5.6 (100.0)	5.4 (100.0)	4.1 (100.0)	7.2 (100.0)	4.2 (100.0)

Source: Own calculations based on Labour Force Survey tapes.   Note: Percentage values are given in parentheses.

Table 12.29
Distribution of hours worked: all women employees with a nursing qualification by occupation, Trent RHA

(thousands)

Occupation	Usual hours worked per week	1983	1984	1985	1986	1987	1988	1989
Nursing	Less than 10	0.2 (0.7)	0.0 (0.0)	0.3 (1.1)	0.7 (2.7)	1.8 (5.7)	1.5 (5.4)	2.0 (6.8)
	10 to 19	1.6 (5.7)	3.0 (10.9)	1.4 (5.1)	1.5 (5.7)	2.0 (6.3)	2.7 (9.7)	0.0 (0.0)
	20 to 29	3.2 (11.4)	4.6 (16.7)	5.0 (18.2)	3.7 (14.2)	5.5 (17.3)	2.5 (9.0)	3.8 (12.9)
	30 to 39	16.9 (60.4)	12.0 (43.5)	11.0 (40.1)	12.7 (48.7)	14.4 (45.3)	13.4 (48.0)	6.1 (20.7)
	40 to 49	5.4 (19.3)	6.8 (24.6)	9.1 (33.2)	6.6 (25.3)	7.9 (24.8)	7.5 (26.9)	1.7 (5.8)
	50 and over	0.7 (2.5)	1.2 (4.3)	0.6 (2.2)	0.9 (3.4)	0.2 (0.6)	0.3 (1.1)	0.7 (2.4)
	Not stated	0.0 (0.0)	0.0 (0.0)	0.0 (0.0)	0.0 (0.0)	0.0 (0.0)	0.0 (0.0)	15.1 (51.4)
	TOTAL	28.0 (100.0)	27.6 (100.0)	27.4 (100.0)	26.1 (100.0)	31.8 (100.0)	27.9 (100.0)	29.4 (100.0)
Other	Less than 10	0.0 (0.0)	1.0 (12.2)	0.6 (5.4)	0.9 (7.6)	1.2 (15.6)	1.6 (11.6)	1.2 (11.5)
	10 to 19	0.9 (11.3)	2.7 (32.9)	1.3 (11.7)	2.4 (20.2)	1.8 (23.4)	2.6 (18.8)	0.9 (8.7)
	20 to 29	1.9 (23.8)	0.7 (8.5)	3.0 (27.0)	2.0 (16.8)	1.1 (14.3)	2.4 (17.4)	1.1 (10.6)
	30 to 39	3.0 (37.5)	1.9 (23.2)	2.8 (25.2)	2.4 (20.2)	2.7 (35.1)	3.8 (27.5)	2.0 (19.2)
	40 to 49	1.3 (16.3)	1.6 (19.5)	3.0 (27.0)	2.4 (20.2)	0.5 (6.5)	2.6 (18.8)	0.8 (7.7)
	50 and over	0.9 (11.3)	0.3 (3.7)	0.4 (3.6)	1.8 (15.1)	0.4 (5.2)	0.8 (5.8)	0.0 (0.0)
	Not stated	0.0 (0.0)	0.0 (0.0)	0.0 (0.0)	0.0 (0.0)	0.0 (0.0)	0.0 (0.0)	4.4 (42.3)
	TOTAL	8.0 (100.0)	8.2 (100.0)	11.1 (100.0)	11.9 (100.0)	7.7 (100.0)	13.8 (100.0)	10.4 (100.0)

Source: Own calculations based on Labour Force Survey tapes.

Note: Percentage values are given in parentheses.

Table 12.30
Age distribution: full-time women employees with a nursing qualification by occupation, Trent RHA

(thousands)

Occupation	Age group	1983	1984	1985	1986	1987	1988	1989
Nursing	16 to 19	0.0 (0.0)	0.0 (0.0)	0.0 (0.0)	0.0 (0.0)	0.0 (0.0)	0.0 (0.0)	0.0 (0.0)
	20 to 29	10.2 (52.0)	7.9 (45.7)	6.4 (36.6)	7.7 (44.0)	10.6 (54.4)	9.0 (51.7)	3.3 (20.5)
	30 to 39	2.4 (12.2)	3.2 (18.5)	2.8 (16.0)	3.2 (18.3)	3.3 (16.9)	3.2 (18.4)	5.4 (33.5)
	40 to 49	4.1 (20.9)	3.8 (22.0)	4.3 (24.6)	4.9 (28.0)	4.5 (23.1)	3.3 (19.0)	5.0 (31.1)
	50 to 59	2.9 (14.8)	2.4 (13.9)	4.0 (22.9)	1.7 (9.7)	1.1 (5.6)	1.9 (10.9)	2.4 (14.9)
	TOTAL	19.6 (100.0)	17.3 (100.0)	17.5 (100.0)	17.5 (100.0)	19.5 (100.0)	17.4 (100.0)	16.1 (100.0)
Other	16 to 19	0.2 (4.0)	0.0 (0.0)	0.0 (0.0)	0.0 (0.0)	0.0 (0.0)	0.3 (4.6)	0.0 (0.0)
	20 to 29	2.1 (42.0)	1.3 (31.0)	1.3 (23.6)	1.8 (28.1)	0.9 (25.0)	1.6 (24.6)	1.5 (24.2)
	30 to 39	1.3 (26.0)	0.3 (7.1)	1.8 (32.7)	1.9 (29.7)	1.0 (27.8)	1.1 (16.9)	2.0 (32.3)
	40 to 49	0.9 (18.0)	1.7 (40.5)	1.1 (20.0)	1.2 (18.8)	1.1 (30.6)	2.0 (30.8)	2.4 (38.7)
	50 to 59	0.5 (10.0)	0.9 (21.4)	1.3 (23.6)	1.5 (23.4)	0.6 (16.7)	1.5 (23.1)	0.3 (4.8)
	TOTAL	5.0 (100.0)	4.2 (100.0)	5.5 (100.0)	6.4 (100.0)	3.6 (100.0)	6.5 (100.0)	6.2 (100.0)

Source: Own calculations based on Labour Force Survey tapes.
Note: Percentage values are given in parentheses.

Table 12.31
Age distribution: part-time women employees with a nursing qualification by occupation, Trent RHA

(thousands)

Occupation	Age group	1983	1984	1985	1986	1987	1988	1989
Nursing	16 to 19	0.0 (0.0)	0.0 (0.0)	0.0 (0.0)	0.0 (0.0)	0.0 (0.0)	0.0 (0.0)	0.0 (0.0)
	20 to 29	2.2 (28.2)	2.3 (22.8)	2.6 (26.0)	0.7 (8.1)	2.3 (18.9)	1.2 (11.4)	3.0 (22.9)
	30 to 39	2.2 (28.2)	3.2 (31.7)	3.3 (33.0)	2.4 (27.9)	3.7 (30.3)	5.6 (53.3)	5.3 (40.5)
	40 to 49	1.9 (24.4)	2.6 (25.7)	2.8 (28.0)	4.1 (47.7)	3.7 (30.3)	1.3 (12.4)	2.0 (15.3)
	50 to 59	1.5 (19.2)	2.0 (19.8)	1.3 (13.0)	1.4 (16.3)	2.5 (20.5)	2.4 (22.9)	2.8 (21.4)
	TOTAL	7.8 (100.0)	10.1 (100.0)	10.0 (100.0)	8.6 (100.0)	12.2 (100.0)	10.5 (100.0)	13.1 (100.0)
Other	16 to 19	0.0 (0.0)	0.0 (0.0)	0.0 (0.0)	0.0 (0.0)	0.0 (0.0)	0.0 (0.0)	0.0 (0.0)
	20 to 29	0.3 (9.4)	0.7 (17.5)	0.3 (5.4)	0.7 (12.7)	1.9 (45.2)	0.9 (12.5)	0.0 (0.0)
	30 to 39	0.9 (28.1)	1.1 (27.5)	1.6 (28.6)	1.8 (32.7)	1.7 (40.5)	4.0 (55.6)	1.9 (46.3)
	40 to 49	1.3 (40.6)	1.9 (47.5)	2.0 (35.7)	2.1 (38.2)	0.3 (7.1)	1.7 (23.6)	1.6 (39.0)
	50 to 59	0.7 (21.9)	0.3 (7.5)	1.7 (30.4)	0.9 (16.4)	0.3 (7.1)	0.6 (8.3)	0.6 (14.6)
	TOTAL	3.2 (100.0)	4.0 (100.0)	5.6 (100.0)	5.5 (100.0)	4.2 (100.0)	7.2 (100.0)	4.1 (100.0)

Source: Own calculations based on Labour Force Survey tapes.
Note: Percentage values are given in parentheses.

Table 12.32
Age distribution: all women employees with a nursing qualification by occupation, Trent RHA

(thousands)

Occupation	Age group	1983	1984	1985	1986	1987	1988	1989
Nursing	16 to 19	0.0 (0.0)	0.0 (0.0)	0.0 (0.0)	0.0 (0.0)	0.0 (0.0)	0.0 (0.0)	0.0 (0.0)
	20 to 29	12.6 (45.0)	10.2 (37.2)	9.0 (32.7)	8.4 (32.2)	12.9 (40.7)	10.2 (36.6)	6.3 (21.6)
	30 to 39	4.8 (17.1)	6.4 (23.4)	6.1 (22.2)	5.6 (21.5)	7.0 (22.1)	8.8 (31.5)	10.7 (36.6)
	40 to 49	6.0 (21.4)	6.4 (23.4)	7.1 (25.8)	9.0 (34.5)	8.2 (25.9)	4.6 (16.5)	7.0 (24.0)
	50 to 59	4.6 (16.4)	4.4 (16.1)	5.3 (19.3)	3.1 (11.9)	3.6 (11.4)	4.3 (15.4)	5.2 (17.8)
	TOTAL	28.0 (100.0)	27.4 (100.0)	27.5 (100.0)	26.1 (100.0)	31.7 (100.0)	27.9 (100.0)	29.2 (100.0)
Other	16 to 19	0.2 (2.4)	0.0 (0.0)	0.0 (0.0)	0.0 (0.0)	0.0 (0.0)	0.3 (2.2)	0.0 (0.0)
	20 to 29	2.4 (29.3)	2.0 (24.4)	1.6 (14.4)	2.5 (21.0)	2.8 (35.9)	2.5 (18.2)	1.5 (14.6)
	30 to 39	2.2 (26.8)	1.4 (17.1)	3.4 (30.6)	3.7 (31.1)	2.7 (34.6)	5.1 (37.2)	3.9 (37.9)
	40 to 49	2.2 (26.8)	3.6 (43.9)	3.1 (27.9)	3.3 (27.7)	1.4 (17.9)	3.7 (27.0)	4.0 (38.8)
	50 to 59	1.2 (14.6)	1.2 (14.6)	3.0 (27.0)	2.4 (20.2)	0.9 (11.5)	2.1 (15.3)	0.9 (8.7)
	TOTAL	8.2 (100.0)	8.2 (100.0)	11.1 (100.0)	11.9 (100.0)	7.8 (100.0)	13.7 (100.0)	10.3 (100.0)

Source: Own calculations based on Labour Force Survey tapes.
Note: Percentage values are given in parentheses.

235

Table 12.33

Sectoral distribution: full-time women employees with a nursing qualification by occupation, Trent RHA

(thousands)

Occupation	Sector	1983	1984	1985	1986	1987	1988	1989
Nursing	Hospitals, nursing homes etc.	14.3	14.5	13.0	11.7	14.4	13.4	11.7
	Other medical care institutions	3.5	2.2	3.8	2.9	3.5	2.4	3.1
	Medical practices	0.4	0.0	0.3	1.5	0.0	0.3	0.3
	Dental practices	0.0	0.0	0.0	0.3	0.0	0.0	0.0
	Agency and private midwives, nurses etc.	0.0	0.0	0.0	0.0	0.0	0.0	0.0
	TOTAL HEALTH SERVICE SECTOR	18.2	16.7	17.1	16.4	17.9	16.1	15.1
	Other sectors	1.3	0.6	0.7	1.2	1.5	1.7	1.0
	TOTAL ALL SECTORS	19.5	17.3	17.8	17.6	19.4	17.8	16.1
Other	Hospitals, nursing homes etc.	0.7	0.3	1.3	0.9	0.9	0.5	0.6
	Other medical care institutions	0.0	0.6	0.7	0.3	0.0	0.4	0.0
	Medical practices	0.0	0.0	0.0	0.4	0.3	0.0	0.5
	Dental practices	0.0	0.0	0.0	0.0	0.0	0.0	0.0
	Agency and private midwives, nurses etc.	0.0	0.0	0.0	0.0	0.0	0.0	0.4
	TOTAL HEALTH SERVICE SECTOR	0.7	0.9	2.0	1.6	1.2	0.9	1.5
	Other sectors	5.3	3.5	4.2	5.9	3.6	6.9	5.7
	TOTAL ALL SECTORS	6.0	4.4	6.2	7.5	4.8	7.8	7.2

Source: Own calculations based on Labour Force Survey tapes.

Table 12.34
Sectoral distribution: part-time women employees with a nursing qualification by occupation, Trent RHA

(thousands)

Occupation	Sector	1983	1984	1985	1986	1987	1988	1989
Nursing	Hospitals, nursing homes etc.	7.0	7.4	7.5	6.8	9.2	7.2	8.1
	Other medical care institutions	0.8	1.2	1.7	1.3	0.9	0.6	2.8
	Medical practices	0.0	0.0	0.3	0.0	1.0	0.7	0.3
	Dental practices	0.0	0.3	0.0	0.0	0.0	0.0	0.0
	Agency and private midwives, nurses etc.	0.0	0.0	0.3	0.3	0.0	0.0	0.0
	TOTAL HEALTH SERVICE SECTOR	7.8	8.9	9.8	8.4	11.1	8.5	11.2
	Other sectors	0.0	1.1	0.5	0.6	1.2	2.0	2.0
	TOTAL ALL SECTORS	7.8	10.0	10.3	9.0	12.3	10.5	13.2
Other	Hospitals, nursing homes etc.	0.0	0.3	0.3	0.0	0.3	0.5	0.8
	Other medical care institutions	0.2	0.3	0.3	0.0	0.3	0.3	0.0
	Medical practices	0.2	0.0	0.3	0.3	0.0	0.3	0.0
	Dental practices	0.2	0.0	0.0	0.0	0.0	0.0	0.0
	Agency and private midwives, nurses etc.	0.0	0.0	0.0	0.0	0.0	0.0	0.0
	TOTAL HEALTH SERVICE SECTOR	0.6	0.6	2.0	0.9	0.6	1.1	0.8
	Other sectors	2.7	4.1	3.9	4.6	4.4	6.6	4.2
	TOTAL ALL SECTORS	3.3	4.7	5.9	5.5	5.0	7.7	5.0

Source: Own calculations based on Labour Force Survey tapes.

Table 12.35
Sectoral distribution: all women employees with a nursing qualification by occupation, Trent RHA

(thousands)

Occupation	Sector	1983	1984	1985	1986	1987	1988	1989
Nursing	Hospitals, nursing homes etc.	22.0	21.9	20.5	18.5	23.6	20.6	19.8
	Other medical care institutions	4.3	3.4	5.5	4.2	4.4	3.0	5.9
	Medical practices	0.4	0.0	0.6	1.5	1.0	1.0	0.6
	Dental practices	0.0	0.3	0.0	0.3	0.0	0.0	0.0
	Agency and private midwives, nurses etc.	0.0	0.0	0.3	0.3	0.0	0.0	0.0
	TOTAL HEALTH SERVICE SECTOR	26.7	25.6	26.9	24.8	29.0	24.6	26.3
	Other sectors	1.3	1.7	1.2	1.8	2.7	3.7	3.0
	TOTAL ALL SECTORS	28.0	27.3	28.1	26.6	31.7	28.3	29.3
Other	Hospitals, nursing homes etc.	0.7	0.6	2.7	1.5	1.2	1.0	1.4
	Other medical care institutions	0.2	0.9	1.0	0.3	0.3	0.7	0.0
	Medical practices	0.2	0.0	0.3	0.7	0.3	0.3	0.5
	Dental practices	0.2	0.0	0.0	0.0	0.0	0.0	0.0
	Agency and private midwives, nurses etc.	0.0	0.0	0.0	0.0	0.0	0.0	0.4
	TOTAL HEALTH SERVICE SECTOR	1.3	1.5	4.0	2.5	1.8	2.0	2.3
	Other sectors	19.6	19.2	8.1	22.5	8.0	13.5	9.9
	TOTAL ALL SECTORS	20.9	20.7	12.1	25.0	9.8	15.5	12.2

Source: Own calculations based on Labour Force Survey tapes.

13 Mothers as student nurses

13.1 The context: the demographic crisis and the equal opportunities' imperative

In recent years there has been growing concern that the decline in the numbers of eighteen year old female school leavers, who have traditionally been seen as the typical nurse trainee, would lead to a crisis in nurse recruitment, at a time when the demand for health care was projected to increase in line with a rise in the number of elderly people. This prompted Government, professional bodies and nurse representatives to urge the nursing profession to widen its intake of students from other segments of the population. This, as discussed in Chapter 2, has taken place against a backdrop of rising female activity rates especially amongst mature women wishing to work part-time.

In May 1988 John Moore, then Secretary of State for Social Services, wrote to the Chairman of the United Kingdom Central Council for Nursing, Midwifery and Health Visiting (UKCC) giving the Government's response to the Council's proposals for the reform of nurse education and training. Amongst his comments were a number of references to mature entrants:

> We attach great importance, in view of future demographic trends, to the work being done by the Council and Boards in examining the ways in which... there can be greater access to nurse training for recruits of all ages... It is essential that we should safeguard our ability to recruit and retain enough staff to meet service needs (Moore 1988).

This proposition was in line with policies of the UKCC (UKCC, 1987b) and the Royal College of Nursing (Hancock, 1989), and added impetus was given to this by the publication in 1991 of an Equal Opportunities Commission (EOC) Report which accused the NHS of widely practised discrimination against women, citing (p.5) amongst many other points that:

Most Health Authorities are not adequately facilitating the recruitment and retention of women with family responsibilities through flexible working and training arrangements...

* 53 per cent do not offer any training opportunities on a part-time basis.

* 61 per cent of Health Authorities have taken no positive action measures to improve the position of women and married people.

This is in spite of the fact that, as Nazarko of the Working Mothers' Association had recently pointed out, with only 53 per cent of NHS nurses working full-time, the service is now heavily dependent upon part-time nurses. She called upon the English National Board for Nursing, Midwifery and Health Visiting (the ENB) which is responsible for validating training programmes:

to provide more accessible educational opportunities for all those with caring responsibilities. Women are often forced to delay their education and to make great sacrifices in order to avail themselves of educational opportunities. Nurse education must rise to the challenge of providing ongoing education for those with caring responsibilities (Nazarko, 1991).

From this it becomes clear that there has been a wide measure of agreement that older entrants to nursing have an important contribution to make to the provision of patient care. Moreover it has been recognised that their successful recruitment and retention will require adjustments to the *status quo*, including the removal of barriers to their employment and modifications to the patterns of training. In this context the introduction of part-time pre-registration nurse training programmes geared specifically to meet the needs of those with domestic responsibilities may be seen as one example of Colleges of Nursing and Health Authorities acting to implement declared national policy.

This chapter examines the provision of part-time Registered General Nurse (RGN) training courses for mature entrants in England. Such courses are designed to provide training for students with domestic commitments, and the study considers the origins of such courses and comments on their likely future in the context of current changes in nurse education. It also explores whether courses of this kind attract recruits who would not otherwise have entered nurse training or who would have commenced at a later date. In the process it addresses the likely enhanced lifetime participation of such recruits and their value as a training investment.

The research was carried out over a period of five months at the end of 1991 and involved interviewing part-time and some full-time mature students at different stages of their training and also recruitment and allocation officers, course tutors and college principals at four of the sixteen institutions known to have been offering part-time RGN places at sometime during the last three to five years. Copies of a working research brief were sent at the outset to a senior nurse educator who agreed to facilitate the data collection (see Appendix A in Bond, 1992, for further information). More details about the participants are shown in Table 13.1.

Research sites were selected to include larger and smaller Colleges of Nursing which were geographically spread across England. One was in an inner city, one in an ethnically mixed conurbation, one in a dormitory town and one in a rural area. The institutions chosen included ones at different stages of site amalgamations, Project 2000 implementation and the exploration of the introduction of Trust status. Work was also done at a fifth city site in a region where only full-time pre-registration courses are available.

The research was undertaken by means of interview and questionnaire (Bond, 1992). Additional information was sought by letter and in telephone interviews from the seventeen other institutions thought to be offering part-time RGN courses (five incorrectly as it turned out). Thus contact was made with a quarter of all English colleges and with staff in five Regional Health Authorities.

The English National Board was approached for statistical information and a policy statement. National and local recruitment materials and some course documentation were examined as well as relevant literature from the nursing press. Finally, information provided by the appropriate Training and Enterprise Councils and local authority Economic Development Units about the five local labour markets was analysed to provide a context within which the interview data and nurse staffing figures could be understood.

13.2 Part-time courses and student numbers

Obtaining basic information

It has proved remarkably difficult to arrive at figures for the part-time places available and the number of students in training or even to discover the whereabouts of Colleges offering such courses.

The Department of Health and the Central Office of Information produce a series of Health Service Careers factsheets. These are widely

Table 13.1
Participant's list

Site	Students		Education staff	Service staff	RHA	Additional interviews
	P/T[a]	F/T[b]				
1	16	4	5	1	No response	1 potential applicant
2	1	2	8	1	Information provided	4 potential applicants 1 College of F.E. lecturer
3	15	7	7	3	1	
4	20	4	3	1	1	
5	0	1	2	0	1	5 Access students 2 College of F.E. lecturers 1 local education authority careers officer 1 crèche worker

Notes:

(a) P/T - on a part-time (i.e. extended) course.
(b) F/T - on a full-time course.

Table 13.2
Institutions offering part-time training courses

College	First intake Date	No	ENB BC7 8/90	12/90	5/91	EMB 7/91 Hand book^a	ENB BC7 10/91	ENB per communic. 21.10.91 Approv. inst.	Nos. training	1991 intake	1992 intake √/X/?
Airedale	1989	12		√	√	I/T	√			√	?
Avon	1988	11	√			T	√P2000	√	21	√	√
Bath	1989	10	√	√				√	5		X
Bloomsbury	1989	6	√					√	5		X
Bolton	1989	12	√					√	0		X
Carshalton	1989	9	√				√P2000	√	6	√	√
Dorset	1987	15	√					√	0		X
Sussex	1988	12	√	√	√	I/T	√	√	25		?
Mid-Trent	1988	10	√					√	7	√	√
Norfolk	1990	10	√				√^b	√	9	√	X
Normanby	1989	12	√								X
NE Essex	1989	12	√			T	√P2000	√	21	√	√
N London	1990	12	√	√	√	I/T	√	√	17	√	√(last)
NW London	1987	9	√								X
Solent	1970	12	√					√		√	√
Thames	1988	15	√	√					9	√	?

Notes:
(a) Handbook entry in index (I) and/or text (T).
(b) College reported ENB course approbal already expired.
(c) √ - Yes; X - no; ? - Unknown.

243

available from careers information points and provide basic information on nursing careers. The most recently available factsheet on becoming a qualified nurse HSC 2 (December 1990) includes the following paragraph about 'mature applicants':

There is no defined upper age limit for becoming a nurse. Different Schools have different views on the subject. There is an increasing number of courses available on a part-time basis, particularly designed to meet the needs of mature students with family commitments. Details of these will be included in the NCCH[1] handbook.

This handbook (ENB, 1991a) was described in a 1991 ENB Careers Service information pack for prospective applicants as providing:

comprehensive information on all the training institutions in England offering courses leading to registration as a nurse or midwife. It shows which courses each institution offers; when they start; what their entry requirements are and also gives a summary of what each institution and its locality has to offer.

The July 1991 Handbook under the index heading of RGN part-time courses listed only three courses (Table 13.2). Enquiries in September 1991 revealed that none had firm plans at that time to accept a further annual intake beyond the one just accepted (E Sussex/W Kent in June 1991) or for which they were currently recruiting (Airedale in October 1991 and North London in March 1992). An examination of the eighty four college entries revealed a further two courses (Avon and NE Essex) that were available within Project 2000 programmes. In fact it was discovered that there were four more colleges offering modified Project 2000 courses - Portsmouth (Solent), the longest running and most well-known, Carshalton and Croydon, Mid-Trent and Thames. It is possible there may be others because as one nurse recruitment officer said:

We don't advertise our part-time course in the Handbook because we would only get people wanting to come from a distance. That kind of recruitment is inappropriate - what's the point if they have to live away from home for much of the time, or have to spend hours every day travelling miles to get to and from College, home and their clinical placements?

It seems therefore that confusing and sometimes conflicting information is being provided for potential applicants and their advisers who enquire at different information points about the availability of part-time courses.

Whilst it is recognised that the dynamic nature of course provision creates difficulties for administrators charged with the provision of accurate, timely information, nevertheless it is a source of some concern that, as Table 13.2 illustrates, different arms of the ENB were at the same time drawing upon differing and, in some cases, outdated facts. Presumably this at least in part explains why the Board, which approves courses and now runs the centralised nurse trainee applicant clearing house system in Bristol, was unable when asked to provide reliable figures on part-time training places. Appendix 5 of the Board's Annual report for 1989/90 states that twenty one training institutions were offering pre-registration RGN training courses for entry to Part 1 of the Professional Register as at 31 March 1990. Requests for further elucidation of this produced in October 1991 a list of eleven Colleges with one hundred and twenty students in training (Table 13.2). But enquiries at these revealed that the list and the numbers of students in training were both inaccurate, a point highlighted by the omission of Portsmouth (Solent), the only well-known and well-established course in the country.

This situation seems unlikely to improve because the ENB's Clearing House, which generates key national statistics, is not coding part-time programmes separately from full-time ones within Project 2000 courses. Once traditional courses have been phased out, students entering on a part-time basis will therefore be lost in the mass of full-time applicants.

In the past, Health Authorities in general have not maintained basic workforce databases and in particular have not routinely collected statistics linking, for example, age and part-time/full-time status. The recent report by the EOC (1991) highlighted not just how primitive these information systems are but also how little use has been made of the figures collected. Moreover, part-timers have often been rendered invisible within NHS workforce statistics by the long-standing and widespread use of the concept of 'whole-time equivalent' numbers of staff.

Falling numbers

Although it has been impossible to obtain accurate figures of the number of part-time RGN courses available, of the number of places on offer at each intake and of the number of students in training, it is clear that nationally there are very few part-time training places. Indeed the number appears to be falling. Writing on the role of part-timers in nursing Buchan (1989) observed that while 'one in three nursing and midwifery staff in the NHS works part-time... in 1986 only 260 out of 64,650 learner nurses in England were classified as part-time - only 0.4 per cent of the total.'

Drawing on the Department of Health's 1989 'NHS Workforce in England' statistics Buchan added that the part-time learner nurse figure:

> has not increased in recent years, and is markedly lower than the number of part-time learners being trained in the mid 1970s. Numerically more (state enrolled i.e. SEN) pupil nurses than (RGN) student nurses have been trained part-time, but with the phasing out

of second level training, the number of pupil nurses training part-time has fallen from 1,393 in 1975 to 102 in 1986[2].

If the one hundred and two pupil nurses were to be excluded from the 1986 part-time learner total of two hundred and sixty, it would leave a figure of one hundred and fifty eight to account for part-time student nurses. This figure is fifty three more than the one used in 1990 by the General Secretary of the RCN who was reported as saying:

> A service which provides child care facilities for less than half a per cent of its staff, offers part-time training positions for only 105 mature entrants among 45,000 nursing students, has only a minimal number of part-time senior posts, and routinely refuses to offer part-time contracts to would-be returners, cannot hope to deliver the NHS reforms to which the Government has committed it (Nursing Standard, 1990).

The findings of the present study are that the number of training places on offer in 1992 is probably about one hundred in five Colleges, with the possibility of a further few places being available in two other colleges. There may be around five hundred students currently in training, including those at Colleges which have discontinued their extended courses (Table 13.2)[3]. This decline in the number of courses available and the failure to increase the numbers of part-time RGN students in training have occurred despite policy pronouncements to the contrary. Reasons for this are discussed below in the context of changing nurse recruitment patterns in the NHS and the introduction of Project 2000.

13.3 Course origins and definitions

Of the sixteen part-time courses identified as having been in existence since 1987 (Table 13.2) all but two have been set up in the area of the country south of a line drawn between the Wash and the Bristol Channel and east of a line between Bristol and Portsmouth. That is to say, most of them are in areas characterised until very recently by high levels of employment which might therefore have been expected to have difficulty in attracting new recruits from the 'traditional' age group.

However, such courses were not set up as part of a co-ordinated national 'top down' initiative[4]. The findings of this research are that they were developed by pioneering and sometimes championing nurse educators often acting in response to an expressed local demand for such programmes from women seeking entry to training with reduced working hours spread over an extended period.

Part-time courses designed with the mature entrant in mind have several key features in common. Working hours are reduced, to about thirty a week, and leave is timetabled to be taken during the major school holidays. In addition students are given some flexibility to negotiate their working hours whilst in clinical placements. The courses are extended in order to enable students to complete the required number of hours in training. Intakes have been smaller than those for full-time courses and on an annual basis rather than several times a year. The documentation from one 'Mature Entrants Part-Time Course' typically sets out eligibility criteria as follows. 'Anyone 25 years to 45 years of age who by reason of their domestic responsibilities is prevented from following a normal 3 year full-time course.' The descriptions 'mature' student and 'part-time' course are by no means unproblematic as also emerged in a study by Gobbi (1989) of older entrants to full and part-time training programmes. One student, approaching the end of her extended training, voiced the views of other students and tutors when she commented:

Working for thirty hours a week on the wards or in College is scarcely less than full-time. People think that because you're part-time you're no use to them. The term has caused us real problems because staff on the wards think we're never going to be there. But in fact on the days when we're in, we often work normal shifts and stay late if necessary to help out. And the word 'mature' is often misused by other members of staff who've said things like 'Here come the crumblies'. Some staff think we're more experienced nurses than we are and then use us to give bad news or to cope with very distressed children.

In practice, the term 'mature' is used to denote someone who has domestic responsibilities and stands in opposition to the 'traditional' recruit who has come into nursing in her late teens after taking examinations at school or College of Further Education. However, one College has accepted a nineteen year old single parent and other Colleges indicated that an applicant over fifty would receive individual consideration, although there was concern that with women being able to retire at sixty, entry so late in life may not allow for a sufficient return on any investment in training.

Reference is made in some course literature to married and single parents 'with children in full-time compulsory education' and to those with 'dependent parents'. Academic requirements are the same as for full-time RGN courses including a score of fifty one or above in the UKCC-approved DC Educational test (DC test).

In practice those who enter via the part-time route are women[5] with children living at home, the majority of whom have partners. A study of part-time courses for mature students is therefore a study of student mothers with dual role responsibilities within the home and as trainees. Colleges have apparently not managed to recruit mothers from black and minority ethnic groups on to these extended courses. Commenting on the failure of the NHS in general to put comprehensive equal opportunities policies into practice, the EOC (1991) remarks on the extent to which

247

women from black and minority ethnic groups and women with disabilities experience discrimination, for example in obtaining training and promotion. In particular it points out that the neglect of such issues:

is having its own impact. Applications from black groups for nursing are declining rapidly...(which will) be a key factor in whether service providers, who are striving to identify and meet the service needs of the black and minority ethnic communities are able to deliver equality in service provision (p.39-40).

13.4 The educational qualifications and working backgrounds of students entering part-time courses

Educational qualifications

Some of the fifty or so students contacted had entered part-time training without any formal educational qualifications on the basis of an acceptable score in the DC Test. Other women declared a handful of 'O' level/CSE/GCSE passes and/or vocational qualifications in such subjects as typing, business and banking, catering, and hairdressing and wig-making, enabling them to meet the minimum academic requirements for entry to nurse training. Some had been achieved years earlier at school/College of Further Education, others had been collected piecemeal as an adult.

Although it was clear that passing a DC test gave access to a number of applicants who thereby avoided having to gain from scratch, or top-up existing, formal qualifications in order to reach the minimum entry requirements, nevertheless both students and tutors expressed concern at the high failure rates in such tests. These tests have been criticised by Darcy (1988) as being 'designed from an English cultural and educational background' and Goode observed that they were designed:

specifically for sixteen to eighteen year olds... (but are) being offered to mature candidates....(They show) that the successful candidates are seventeen to twenty-four years of age and not, if I may use the term for those of twenty-five and over, the 'mature' candidate. It also emerges that the degree of failure increases on a par with the increase in age (Goode, 1988).

At one site attempts were made to direct potential candidates towards sources of help to prepare for taking this test, whilst at another (where only full-time courses are available), its use was about to be discontinued, on the grounds that it was disproportionately expensive to run. With no shortage of qualified applicants coming forward, those older people who need to gain minimum entry qualifications and who have not done any studying for a while are now being advised that they would do better to pursue an access course designed specifically for mature entrants to the caring professions. Some students reported that such a preparation had served to increase their confidence in their abilities to return to studying, to cope with academic work and to combine these with continuing to fulfil their domestic responsibilities. One twenty-six year old with five 'O' levels obtained ten years previously, said that lacking such preparation, she was finding 'the studying for nursing and the exams in school tough'.

Amongst the students interviewed from part-time intakes were two graduates. One woman, now nearly forty, had left school with eight 'O' levels and three 'A' levels and gone into vocational education, to gain a Higher National Certificate in applied science. Once at home with young children, she had pursued an Open University course over five years, to gain an Arts degree.

The eighteen mature students interviewed on full-time courses had between them a range of entry qualifications similar in all respects to those outlined above and this picture of a wide mix of achievement amongst both part and full-time students fits with the findings of Dodd's (1987) sample study of direct entrants to general nurse training.

Work histories

Many of the interviewees had had very varied working lives which had often led from full to part-time posts associated with their changing status from single woman to married mother. The majority of them included in their lists people-orientated occupations, many within the caring and public sectors. An unexpected number of the mature students were on a nurse training course for the second time in their lives.

At one College, amongst their most recent intake of twelve part-time students, ranging in age from twenty-eight to forty-one, six women mentioned a previous unsuccessful attempt at nurse training on a full-time basis. Five of these had subsequently worked part-time as a nursing auxiliary and/or as a care assistant. The sixth had been a child-minder full-time.

Of the remaining six students, two had worked part-time as care assistants, another had had a full-time job as a nursery carer, and a fourth had been a police cadet and then a police-woman before moving into part-time employment as a dental nurse and shop assistant. The fifth woman had managed a shop full-time, then been a kitchen assistant and a welfare assistant part-time before returning to work full-time as a special needs assistant. The sixth woman mentioned, first, full-time employment as a telephonist, followed by part-time work initially as a school meals assistant and then as a telephonist/receptionist.

All these women described themselves as being 'primarily responsible for children' in the period immediately before starting their current course eight weeks earlier.

Analysis of the work histories of another set of ten students eighteen months into their part-time course showed similar patterns, except that employment in the manufacturing and agriculture sectors featured more frequently than that in catering and retailing, reflecting the different employment opportunities available to women in that locality.

Looking at the work histories of the mature students interviewed from full-time courses, there is some evidence of people in full-time work making career changes. Again, there were recruits from the health and social care sectors - a part-time doctor's receptionist, two auxiliary nurses (one full-time) and two care assistants, one of whom had recently given up an established career in marketing to become a full-time care assistant in a mental hospital. This move may have been a step along the way for someone who wanted to discover the validity of an incipient shift in career orientation. As Gobbi (1989) points out, the presence of those with significant previous experience in health and social care clearly raises the question of whether they should be viewed not as novices but as 'advanced beginners' in some aspects of their nurse training programmes.

In conclusion, it seems that the acceptance of mature people into nurse training allows some to realise a previous ambition and others to make a career change. Part-time courses, in particular, offer part-time women workers an opportunity to continue to care for their families whilst consolidating their vocational direction. Those who enter these courses are clearly already very experienced at combining their paid and unpaid roles. It seems that full-time workers and those from other sectors will be unlikely to switch directly to part-time nurse training. But the evidence presented here suggests that part-time courses offer a much sought after opportunity for existing unqualified and erstwhile learner nurses to gain a professional qualification.

13.5 Juggling the personal and the professional

Working as a nurse entails in many respects the paid performance of activities which wives, mothers and daughters undertake unpaid with and for dependent relatives in their own homes. Nursing is often seen as the embodiment of good womanhood (Simnett, 1986). It is likely therefore that mothers who are recruited into nurse training, partly on the basis of their commitment and caring, will continue to display these attitudes in relation to their growing families.

Those who set up the innovatory course at Portsmouth in early 1970 specifically recognised this in that they were targeting for recruitment 'married women who are deeply committed to their family as well as to nursing' (Hooper, 1975). Therefore, it was acknowledged from the outset that 'the course would need to take full account of the students' domestic situations, and the hours and conditions should cause the least conflict between their dual roles as mother and student' (Watts, 1984).

In spite of their well-established track histories as managers of the work/home divide, mothers who enter full-time nurse training continually worry about their ability to 'cope' with what they see as the many legitimate but conflicting demands upon their time and energies (McVey, 1991). According to very many of those students interviewed for this research, the provision of part-time nurse training helps those who enrol 'to juggle' more successfully with the complexities of being a wife, a mother, a student and a worker. When describing the advantages of doing a part-time as opposed to a full-time course a single parent with four children wrote 'With school aged children I work when they are at school. I can see them out to school in the morning and am there on their return. It is the only way I can combine nurse training and motherhood.'

Many similar comments were made by the interviewees, but what also emerged over and over again in discussions with students was that in many respects they still felt they were 'constantly on a knife edge. ' Even if nothing went wrong, as wives, mothers and part-time student nurses they were still engaged in a juggling, 'a plate-spinning' act. A thirty six year old married woman with a four and a half year old child summed up the worst aspects of this as 'constant stress over managing family/working life, being too tired to do study once (your) child is in bed, guilt at leaving a sick child with a friend, problems with rushing to finish ward duty to get home on time.'

A key source of stress for many of these women seemed to come from sorting out the whereabouts and well-being of their families and then trying 'to fit' (a much used term) their own commitments into the spaces left behind. Many women had to make complicated arrangements for child care taking into account that predictable and unexpected changes could occur on all fronts. The following comment was typical:

I don't pay for child care in money but do child care for friends in exchange. For example, when I next do a late shift I will deliver my eight and eleven year olds and my friends' children to their different schools. Two friends will pick them up from school. One will deliver them to grandma's, then my spouse will pick them up and care for them till the end of my shift.

Analysis of the data highlights the over-riding importance for mothers of feeling that they can 'cope' successfully with the demands upon them. The more they assume several roles - as wives and mothers, housewives and students, nurses and wage earners - the more they are faced with meeting the basic expectations within each in reduced time slots. In such situations their ability to have some sense of control over the timing of the demands likely to be made upon them is crucial.

To the extent that College staff and service managers place a recognition of this at the centre of course planning and timetabling, they will increase the ability of women to manage the logistical challenges associated with their multiple roles. As Gobbi (1989) also discovered from the mature students she interviewed, this means taking into account the fine grain detail of these students' lives by for example, notifying them in advance of the exact pattern and whereabouts of their training and legitimising their right to negotiate the timing of their clinical placement

251

hours. But too often the students were made to feel awkward and demanding, by senior staff and their full-time student colleagues.

A number of students pointed out that there was a significant difference for them between a 9 a.m. - 4 p.m. working day and one that instead began at 9.15/9.30 a.m. after they had taken children to school and finished at 3.00/3.30 p.m. in time for them to meet their children after school. Given this, it is perhaps not surprising that one college, which has apparently preserved a 9.30 a.m. - 3 p.m. day within an extended Project 2000 course has such a pool of suitable and successful applicants that it is now recruiting for its October 1994 intake.

By contrast, at another Project 2000 site the part-time students' leave allocation within the forthcoming school summer holidays has recently been reduced to three weeks. Concern has been expressed by at least one educator at the impact which this decision is likely to have on mothers already in training who could not have anticipated it and on future recruitment.

13.6 An untapped pool of labour

Demand for part-time courses

The ENB does not keep national statistics on the numbers of enquiries which its Careers Service receives about part-time courses. However, College tutors and those concerned specifically with recruitment reported that demand outstripped the places available, by factors of between four and eight (ratios of application forms received to available places). Since most applicants apply to a local school only, this figure is not subject to correction on account of multiple applications.

The only College which reported any recruitment difficulties found that demand shot up once staff began routinely to include details of their extended course in mailings to all enquirers and set up two recruitment days. They received a hundred enquiries and eighteen women subsequently sat the DC test, of whom fifty per cent passed. These nine candidates were successful at interview and made up three quarters of the next part-time intake.

The existence of a considerable pool of untapped labour was further confirmed in interviews in two other parts of the country with tutors at Colleges of Further Education running Access courses for mature students aiming to enter the caring professions. Where such courses are directly linked to the local part-time RGN course mothers apparently 'come in droves'.

Finally, staff at Colleges of Nursing reported that when courses are advertised, potential students from some distance away often declare an interest, partly because, in rural areas, the College is their nearest course but, more significantly, because their local College does not offer training on a part-time basis. Even when they face round trips of two hours or more, some mature students in training and potential applicants attending a

252

recruitment session said that the travelling costs and time involved were outweighed by the prospect of gaining enhanced control over their working hours, without which 'full-time training as a mother with children to care for is simply out of the question'.

A good training investment

Mothers recruited on to extended nurse training courses not only represent an extra resource to the NHS because they come from a scarcely tapped pool of labour, but in addition they may prove to be a particularly good training investment.

Mothers as good students and nurses

There was unanimity in this study amongst nurse educators and service managers that, generally speaking mothers make committed students and good nurses.

College staff commented upon the strong feelings of purposefulness, commitment and shared identity amongst the all-mother groups of part-timers which were missing in mixed age and gender groups of full-timers. There was evidence that they flourished in the small sets characteristic of part-time courses where their life experiences could be taken into account in the teaching. They had a sense of 'all being in this together' and of 'helping each other through'. Tutors reported that they set high standards for themselves and their teachers and that they were keen and challenging students who behaved proactively rather than passively. Examples were given of the women bringing about improvements in the way their extended courses were run, thus demonstrating their abilities to meet the profession's aspirations of training reflective practitioners who will act as advocates on their patients' behalf.

Commitment, as Fogg (1988) and Whyte (1988) also found in their research, was a recurring topic in interviews with the students themselves who referred to the investment which they and their families have in a successful outcome to their studies. Some had to 'cox and box' with spouses to cover school holidays to such an extent that they were never able to be on holiday together throughout the length of the course. Some had given up jobs and taken a drop in salary in order to enter training and others were incurring additional travelling and child care costs to the extent that they were barely breaking even on their student wage. Some single mothers reported serious financial hardship ameliorated in one or two cases by the payment of maintenance or the claiming of family credit.[6] A number had previously dropped out of nurse training in their late teens and early twenties and like their peers on these extended courses were now determined to succeed. They saw the course as their only chance of having a career and in many cases of realising a long-standing ambition to qualify as a nurse. The following is a typical comment: 'I chose the part-time course because I desperately want to gain the RGN qualification. However, due to my family, travelling, study time etc. I was not sure that I would cope with this while working full-time. I did not want to start the full-time course and 'drop out' again.'

Most extended courses have not been running long enough to provide much evidence on examination successes and wastage during training. Indeed few Colleges have yet seen a whole cohort through training. However, there is evidence of consistently high success rates from the Portsmouth part-time course which has run for over twenty years. Heywood Jones (1986) spelt out the measure of its achievements: 'Among entrants who have completed their families, with school-age children, there has been consistently low student wastage, significantly low sickness, absenteeism and unpaid leave, combined with above national average pass rates in final exams.'

Gobbi (1989) drawing attention to the low wastage rate there of eight per cent, remarked too on 'the exceptionally high pass rate of one hundred per cent at the first attempt in the final examination during the period 1982-88' (p.28).

Other evidence of academic achievements amongst part-time mature entrants is provided by Bailey (1988) who found in one College that over a ten year period the part-time registered mental nurse students had scored 'significantly higher' in the intermediate and final examinations than their full-time counterparts.

The low wastage rates reported at Portsmouth were confirmed by some figures obtained for the present study (Bond, 1992, Table 3). In those three Colleges where students had completed their extended courses thirteen out of fifteen, nine out of ten, and eight out of eleven mothers qualified i.e. six out of a combined intake of thirty six left prematurely, giving an average attrition rate of fifteen per cent. For students who, by the end of 1991 had reached the mid-point of their extended training periods, the number of those remaining were fifteen out of sixteen, eleven out of twelve, ten out of twelve (with one of the two who left transferring to a full-time course) and sixteen out of twenty two from a fourth institution (here spread over two 1989 intakes in the same institution). Excluding the student who transferred and was therefore not lost to nursing, these figures indicate a loss of only a single student at each of the first three colleges i.e. an attrition rate on average of seven and a half per cent. However, if the loss of the six students from the two sets at the fourth College is also included in the calculation there was an overall attrition rate of nine students from a combined intake of sixty two i.e. fourteen and a half per cent.

Clearly these numbers are very small and must be treated with great caution. But it would appear that these attrition rates compare favourably with those for full-time students on pre-Project 2000 courses where according to the literature those dropping out and failing to register have been twenty per cent or more (Lindop, 1988; Vousden, 1988; and Nursing Standard, 1989a and 1989b). These extended course figures are also comparable to those cited (Jowett *et al.*, 1991 with similar caveats) for the first year of Project 2000 intakes at six demonstration schemes which ranged from two per cent to sixteen per cent.

Absence figures for students during training proved even more difficult to obtain than the numbers of women who left these part-time courses before qualifying. However, at one site some 1988 intake statistics were made available comparing the sickness rates of eight mothers who had recently qualified from a part-time course with the sickness rates for twenty two students who were within ten days of completing their full-time course. The latter ranged in age from eighteen to twenty four on entry and three of the twenty one women were married. None was thought to have children. Excluding additional 'special leave' these full-time students had taken on average 34.6 days of sickness against a built-in allowance of twenty one days each for the three years' training period. Such figures were described here as 'reasonably typical'. By contrast, during their extended course which lasted three years and eight month's, the eight mothers, all in their thirties and forties and including some single parents, had taken a mere 11.8 days each, in other words only half their built-in sickness allowance. Moreover, figures for the next part-time (January 1989) set of students indicated that over a period of two years nine months, the eleven mothers had taken between them only forty five days off sick (i.e. an average of only four days each) with only a quarter of their extended course still to run.

These figures confirmed what tutors and students said here and elsewhere about student mothers who went to great lengths to fulfil the expectations of a part-time course, only taking time off if it was unavoidable and always making up any lost hours as quickly as possible. It is interesting that 'part-time' women, who are frequently stereotyped by employers as being unreliable workers because of their mothering responsibilities emerge from these statistics as rather more reliable, albeit within the reduced working hours of their contracts, than full-time student nurses. As College staff so often spontaneously remarked, mothers on extended courses are 'very dedicated students'.

Extended working lives

The provision of part-time training courses may increase the post-qualifying working life of nurses, which Grocott (1989) has estimated to be on average twelve years[7]. This is through two mechanisms. First, evidence emerged from this study that many student mothers entering full-time nurse training would have started sooner had a part-time course been available locally. Of 25 students asked specifically about this, fourteen would have liked to have begun their part-time training earlier, and in some cases up to ten years earlier.

For the majority it emerged that the option of nurse training would have been an attractive proposition at the point when her youngest child entered primary school. This coincides with a potential entry point mentioned in the literature on womens' paid working patterns (Martin and Roberts, 1984) and also in some of the publicity materials for these extended courses. 'The married or single parent with children in full-time compulsory education, and a strong desire to do something more, can now begin training for this highly prized qualification.' In this connection it is interesting to note that Moores *et al.* (1982) found that of the reasons for qualified nurses' non-participation in the labour force it was the existence of a young family which so dominated the working/not working decision that it 'swamped' attitudinal differences picked up by their study. For older women wishing to gain their RGN there is a further complication, in that entry requirements may specify an upper age limit. The timing of their application, acceptance and entry to nurse education is therefore important.

Second, there is evidence to suggest that once qualified, such part-time trainees will continue as practising members of the nursing workforce. It is not, of course, certain that mature women coming in on part-time training programmes will work until they retire, but in discussion many women saw themselves as at last embarking on a career. Some talked of hoping to move from part-time training to full-time work after qualifying because by then their children would be older and more independent. Others talked of wanting to do further part or full-time post-qualifying training for which they would first need some staff nurse experience. Two women in their early fifties, who were interviewed just before they sat their finals, said that the prospect of working until they were sixty five years old seemed only too short, and between them the women mentioned earlier potentially offered many additional years of service.

As Heywood Jones (1986) put it five years ago, 'It may seem uneconomical to offer training to students in their middle years, but a woman with a grown-up family is an equal bet to a 21 year old, with the probability of a 7-10 year child rearing gap ahead - and no guarantee of her return'. The economics of investing resources in training older women on part-time courses was specifically addressed in a review of the Portsmouth course. 'It was decided that it was reasonable and cost effective to accept an individual who would be able to give ten years' service in nursing on completion of a course of this duration' (Watts, 1984).

A stable local workforce

Furthermore there is evidence that, once qualified, such students are highly likely to remain working in the area where they trained. Nessling and Boyle (1990a and 1990b) recently reported on a major study in the North West Thames Regional Health Authority which challenged the received wisdom that nursing is a high wastage profession to which leavers do not return.

Using the UKCC to mail 22,127 questionnaires to locally resident RGN-qualified nurses, the North West Thames RHA research team analysed

7,566 replies (a 34.19 per cent response rate) and came up with some interesting findings:

> Nurses who lived in the North West Thames region had a high probability of having trained in that region or one of the Thames regions. Those who took subsequent nursing qualifications were likely to do so in North West Thames. Examination of career patterns revealed 61 per cent of nurses not changing jobs in a year and this figure was fairly consistent over an 18-year period. Just over a quarter (26 per cent) of nurses moved from one NHS job to another, again consistent over the same period. The flow out of NHS nurses averaged 8 per cent while the flow in was 5.2 per cent a year resulting in an overall loss of 2.8 per cent. The picture that emerged is of a relatively stable nursing workforce, which because it is largely female (96 per cent in North West Thames) could be expected to take breaks in service to raise a family. This notion of a stable workforce has not been explored in the relatively few studies of the nursing labour market because they have concentrated on turnover and mobility (Nessling and Boyle, 1990b).

The analysis of the North Hertfordshire data within the North West Thames RHA study leads to this comment;

> Pregnancy is by far the largest cause for breaks in service (and) this phenomenon has been identified in other countries....(The) evidence reflects a predictable pattern for women's careers. Over 60 per cent of the workforce take a break in service, and 47 per cent believed there was a possibility they would do so in the future (Nessling and Boyle, 1990a, p.17).

These figures are especially interesting in that they are drawn from an area which as a whole had 'low unemployment rates and a fairly buoyant economy' (*ibid* p.3). Far from being attracted into the locally expanding spheres of new technology, distribution, hotel, catering, scientific and business services, the women continued to be part of a mature and settled workforce well attached to the NHS locally. Qualified nurses were largely married women with family commitments, a higher than average percentage of whom were employed on a part-time basis.

This research suggests that whilst acquisition of a nursing qualification may provide some nurses with a passport to enhanced mobility, for the majority here it seemed to be associated with attachment to a locality which was then further reinforced by marital and/or child care and housing commitments. These findings are of relevance to the consideration of the provision of part-time nurse training opportunities because local mothers who enter such courses may be more likely than most other students to seek stability not mobility of employment, and to pursue their long awaited and much prized careers locally. In terms of life-cycles, those interviewed for this study were older than the 'traditional' nursing recruits and since in many cases they saw themselves as having completed their families, any (career) move on their part would have to take account of financial costs, changes in housing and schooling, and often in a partner's job. Many also talked of having significant kinship links in the locality: since many are 'in and of' the local community, nurse training is more likely to reinforce rather than to weaken this.

All these factors tend to suggest that mothers who qualify as nurses after completing their families are more likely to remain employed within their area of training than those who qualify at an earlier stage in their life-cycle. Most part-time courses have not been running long enough to test this hypothesis fully but the findings of other studies lend support to this line of argument. Hutt's (1983) research into the career patterns of Registered Sick Children's Nurses indicated that mature adult learners were more likely than their younger colleagues to stay in their parent hospital after completing their training. Waite *et al.* (1990) in their study of the career patterns of Scotland's qualified nurses calculated that, compared with younger entrants, 'mature entrants (to normal training courses) in fact gave back more total working years to the NHS in return for the training effort invested in them' (p.153). Also as mentioned earlier, at Portsmouth the part-time course 'proved good value to the health authority which retained a high proportion of these qualified nurses, many opting for full-time employment and staying in the area because of fixed home arrangements' (Heywood Jones, 1986).

This tendency of part-time students to seek employment locally is confirmed by information gathered from one study site which indicated that within three months of qualifying all their first part-time set had gone into posts in the two course-sponsoring Health Authorities and students elsewhere expressed the hope of obtaining full but in some cases part-time work in their immediate localities. Indeed it was a source of concern to some of them that since entering training there had been a marked reduction in nurse vacancies in their locality.

A note on the comparative costs of full and part-time training

In their paper on nurse substitution and training, Hartley and Shiell (1988) estimated that on the basis of several 'heroic' assumptions it cost the Exchequer at 1985/6 prices £10,000 and £4,400 respectively to train each registered and enrolled nurse. But they acknowledged that lack of evidence in a number of significant areas - for example, on whether RGN qualified staff were more inclined to leave or about whether they offered qualitatively better patient care - prevented them from reaching any firm conclusions.

Some information did emerge in the course of the present study that extended courses, at least when planned as small scale additional initiatives, may be more expensive in the short-term, and may be 'problematic' for those who run them. For example, where only one or two part-time sets had been admitted on an experimental basis a year apart, tutors sometimes referred to such courses as disproportionately expensive because the groups were smaller than the standard, more frequent, full-time intakes and took up tutor time over a longer period. Sometimes they generated extra work because they were an additional intake and they contributed to bottle-necks in clinical placements. Sometimes they 'caused trouble' because they replaced a full-time intake and ward nursing teams, whose hours were not made up in recognition of a shortfall in student hours, complained to allocation officers about the problems of students 'privileged to work flexible hours'. On occasion such comments were also associated with criticisms that part-time students were poorly placed to pay attention to the professional issue of continuity of care-giving to patients. Here it seemed that little recognition was given to the fact that even full-timers at best are usually only available to patients for seven and a half out of twenty four hours on five out of seven days of any week. As Bailey (1988) says, 'Evidence also suggests that continuity of care is not significantly affected when a learner works 30 hours a week instead of 37.5. The use of part-time learners in nursing suggests that the anxieties of nurse managers are more imaginary than real, and the judicious use of part-time staff can provide an effective service.'

It is clear from the material presented so far that any study which sought to assess the comparative costs and benefits of training students on standard and extended courses would have to look at factors such as student wastage rates on each type of course, success rates in examinations, post-qualifying wastage rates and the students' subsequent contributions as practising nurses. On all these counts, such evidence as there is from traditional courses suggests that extended courses would compare favourably with full-time training. Furthermore, such students, with a clear run ahead of them in career terms are unlikely to take up places later on 'return to learn' courses. Against this would have to be offset any extra costs incurred in running extended programmes as additions to mainstream patterns of training, but these costs are likely to be less for established than for experimental and short-lived courses.

13.7 The future for part-time training

Given the arguments and policy pronouncements set out at the beginning of this chapter in favour of recruiting more mothers into nursing through the part-time training route, and given the evidence above regarding their worth, the question arises as to why so few courses have been established and remain in existence.

Changing nurse recruitment patterns in a changed labour market

The short answer is that the predicted recruitment crisis has failed, so far, to materialise and this fact has over-ridden any motivation to initiate and sustain such courses on equal opportunity grounds. The reasons why nursing has, to date, not experienced the recruitment crisis that was widely anticipated, and which is discussed in detail in Chapter 2 above, seems to be a combination of the changing external environment and changing recruitment patterns within the NHS. Rising labour market participation by women generally, combined with the recession has meant that external labour market conditions have, temporarily at least, eased as far as the NHS is concerned. Furthermore, it appears that the NHS has already begun to redirect its recruitment away from the traditional young, female school leaver.

Looking at student recruitment patterns, national figures broken down by age and sex are only now becoming available so it is difficult to comment on trends. However, the Personnel Director in Trent Regional Health Authority, draws attention to the 'drop in entrants to nurse education of around a third nationally over the last decade', whilst activity rates for women in general and qualified nurses in particular continued to rise. Not only are the learner to qualified to unqualified staff proportions changing, but:

> what does seem clear is that even before the economy went into recession and despite continuing adverse publicity the NHS was widening its appeal to potential recruits. In my own health region, 16 per cent of new entrants to nurse education are now male compared with a workforce which is only 10 per cent male. In 1986-7, 11 per cent of the 1,249 new entrants were aged over 25; only two years later in 1988-9 this had risen to 29 per cent (406 out of 1,382). Put another way, in 1986-7 we took around 16 per cent of eligible female school leavers, by 1988-9 we had reduced this to 11 per cent (Rogers, 1991).

Figures supplied by the ENB for 1 April 1990 - 31 March 1991 on new entrants to first level general nursing (RGN) courses show that twenty nine per cent were over twenty five, of whom eighty three per cent were women. This trend towards the recruitment of more mature entrants, predominantly women, to a virtually static nurse labour force with fewer openings for new entrants due to financial cutbacks and a decline in employee wastage (Grocott, 1989) is confirmed by figures obtained from East Anglian Regional Health Authority.

Here, where the nursing workforce was the smallest in the country, the planned requirement by the Health Service for new learners for March 1991 was fifteen per cent lower than the March 1989 actual figures (Department of Health, 1991, Table A1.4). With wastage from training expected to fall, colleges in the Region anticipated recruiting a reduced proportion of the local eligible female school leaver population.

Overall the picture is one of a nationally shrinking demand for trainee nurses, which is increasingly being met by older women and some men, in a context of growing numbers of mothers entering a general labour market still hit by recession and in which qualified school leavers are facing 'a dearth of jobs' (Edwards-Jones, 1991). In other words a more than sufficient supply of appropriately qualified recruits has been forthcoming without the provision of part-time courses. As one regional workforce planner put it 'We do not at present have a problem with recruitment. The proportion of mature entrants is increasing all the time, but this is happening naturally without any effort.'

Given the above, it is not surprising that of the sixteen colleges which have been identified as offering nurse training places on a part-time basis in recent years, only five (Table 13.2) are actively recruiting for future intakes. (A sixth has no plans beyond its already fully subscribed last traditional course.) All of these colleges have moved over to Project 2000 which they have adapted to a greater or lesser extent to take account of the needs of student mothers.

The main reasons given for the demise of courses were the lack of any recruitment imperative and the belief that Project 2000 will accommodate mature entrants with dependents, with only minor, if any, adjustments to the timetable. When asked about the current impact of demographic changes locally the typical response of staff at different levels of the nurse education system and in different places was 'Demographic timebomb?, What demographic timebomb?' One senior nurse educator echoed the views of others in saying 'The move to student status with learners being supernumerary, able more freely to negotiate their clinical placements and spending more time in the College and the Poly - well it's more like part-time training for everybody isn't it?' In one case, in the apparent absence of any very strong commitment to part-time training on ideological grounds, the 'trouble' caused to staff by the extra organizational requirements of the part-time options seems to have been influential in determining the future of the extended course.

At a time when nurse educators and service providers are already stretched to the limit by the impact of legislative and organizational changes in the NHS, the introduction of Project 2000 courses and increased pressure to run enrolled nurse conversion courses seem to have swallowed up some part-time programmes, with staff energy going into implementing more mainstream changes to the neglect of the extended courses. With no recruitment imperative and with approximately half the Colleges in the country now offering Project 2000 programmes, and given the widespread amalgamation and rationalisation of schools of nursing combined with the impending transfer of funding and key education planning responsibilities to regional level, it seems that the odds are stacked against the preservation of these essentially small scale local initiatives. Nationally there is no means of identifying the level of expressed demand for such courses because the ENB does not collect statistics on the number of enquiries for them and is not retaining for Project 2000 courses a separate coding for candidates pursuing an extended programme. It is difficult to avoid the interpretation that this is yet another example of the way in which these part-time initiatives have failed to make any real impact on the mainstream of pre-registration nurse training. Indeed in the newly published ENB Annual Report for 1990-1991 (ENB, 1991b) they have been rendered invisible: there is not a single reference to any part-time pre-registration courses.

Given the declared policy and increasing practice of recruiting more older candidates into nurse training and in the light of the EOC (1991) criticisms of the NHS's treatment of women in the service, the failure to sustain and further extend these small scale initiatives are grounds for serious concern. Many senior nurses seem to accept that in the absence of any recruitment crisis, economic arguments will outweigh any 'moral imperative' in the new look NHS. As one person at the RCN said:

> With the increase in unemployment, applications for nurse training have gone up. Project 2000 courses are proving extremely popular so on the supply side, things are adequate. Staff turnover is also down so that has reduced the demand for new recruits. At the same time there have been fewer dropouts from Project 2000 courses so the problems of recruitment are fewer. Whilst recognising that individuals need part-time courses and courses need students, this is the context in which you have to set part-time courses which are seen as a lot of trouble anyway.

Part-time courses and Project 2000

Given that the implementation of Project 2000 was in its early stages when this study was conceived, the focus necessarily has been upon the provision of extended courses within the traditional model of general nurse training. However, by placing the views and performance of students at the centre of this research, it has been possible to explore those features of such courses which they, their tutors and service managers perceive as significant in meeting the needs of mothers in training. The findings therefore provide both a lens through which to view developments within Project 2000 now that no new courses will be started along traditional lines, and also provide a yardstick against which to measure the potential of such programmes for enabling mature entrants with dependents to succeed as student nurses. It is clear that in so far as educators and managers ensure that parenting and nursing are not conflicting interests, to that extent will they draw into the student nursing workforce able and committed mothers and promote their retention. Such an approach has implications for the educational model adopted and for the manner in which it is put into practice.

In theory Project 2000 courses are 'mature student friendly' in their avowed commitment to adult centred, self-directed educational practices. In addition they have higher education college working days and holidays which to some extent mesh with school hours. However, such features alone may not be sufficient to attract and retain the sort of student mothers who have sought training on extended courses explicitly designed to meet their needs.

One of the first evaluative reports from the Project 2000 demonstration districts (Jowett *et al.*, 1991) draws attention to the effect of replacing the frequent smaller student intakes of the past with fewer larger influxes. This 'has militated against the student-centred approaches advocated for the new course. The necessity for formal lectures to such large groups and the difficulties of taking account of individual students' past experience and education when arranging placements are obvious manifestations' (p 21). Block treatment, as research by Fogg (1988) indicated, was a contributory factor to the loss of older learners from the mixed groups of full-time students which he studied on traditional courses.

Other aspects of the new programmes may militate against the continuation and extension of 'family friendly' courses. The indication that annual leave may be arranged in advance to be co-terminous with school holidays clearly cannot apply to all holidays, since children have more weeks out of school than their student parents have entitlements to annual leave, and concern has been expressed at one College that mothers have recently been told that their forthcoming summer break has been reduced to three weeks. It seems therefore that the practice of giving student mothers extended summer holidays may be constrained by the introduction of Project 2000, which in some places also seems to be associated with college days running from 9 a.m. - 4 p.m or longer (Gallagher, 1990). This seems to ignore the needs of mothers taking children to and from school for whom a variation of as little as half an hour at each end of a day can be crucial. Moreover, the amalgamation of Colleges of Nursing and their linking with higher education establishments, combined with the introduction of enhanced periods of community-based learning, have increased the peripatetic nature of nurse training under Project 2000. This may create additional problems for student mothers who frequently function within tight child care deadlines. Some women may therefore need the scope to work foreshortened hours throughout their course not just within the final rostered element of their training, which some Colleges are permitting them to extend.

The existence of an element of flexibility is also presumed to enable all Project 2000 students to negotiate education rather than service-led clinical placements throughout their training. However, as one College lecturer in this study said of their experiences of introducing a part-time traditional course and then Project 2000:

> It can be problematic for individuals to have to negotiate their way round the rota. Do full-timers fit around part-timers or part-timers round full-timers? Students have faced resistance from ward staff to doing modified hours and have had snide remarks made about them. This is a key issue.

Elkan and Robinson (1991) also noted the problems for students of managing such negotiations in their recent study of the implementation of Project 2000 in one health authority. Such difficulties have considerable implications for service managers and educators undertaking to provide training for mothers, whose low status as students inevitably disempowers them in such individualised exchanges. In addition their requirement for part-time hours may leave them feeling that they are asking for favours rather than acting upon their entitlements within the terms of an extended training course. The lack of control which this implies and its consequences for their time management may lead some mothers to opt out of nurse training and may discourage others from entering.

Finally, there are indications that under Project 2000 the level of bursaries may be such that mothers who do not have access to free child care and single parents especially, who have to be self-supporting, may not be able to cope with the costs of training. More worrying still was the observation of one nurse educator who suggested that with students over twenty six and/or with dependents attracting enhanced rates, there may be a built-in financial disincentive to the recruitment of mature candidates. In addition the three year rolling programmes for funding nurse education may militate against the extending of students' courses into a fourth year to accommodate reduced working weeks.

In spite of this somewhat bleak picture there is evidence of continuing attempts within some Colleges to respond to the needs of working mothers. In one, students on a part-time option are all allocated to the same tutorial group in which their life skills can be recognised and their particular needs addressed. At another, students' taught hours in College have been reduced in favour of more self-directed study in their own time. Most encouragingly it seems that where extended courses are run alongside mainstream programmes there is scope for students to move between them in either direction. This suggests that working reduced hours at the outset may allow some women to discover that full-time studying is within their capacity and they may therefore use the part-time option as a springbboard into full-time training. On the other hand part-time courses can offer a safety net for those overwhelmed by the demands of full-time studying and mothering, and as such they may serve to reduce wastage from Project 2000 courses.

The development of flexible modules within Project 2000 programmes are still in their early stages and it is therefore unwise to jump to premature conclusions about their success in accommodating the needs of working parents. However, given the increase in mature entrants to nursing and the concerns expressed here, there is an urgent need to examine the extent to which mothers with domestic responsibilities may be disadvantaged by the new arrangements which in theory may seem geared to meet their needs, but which in practice may be falling short of this. A revival in the economy could turn this issue into a pressing problem and if the pool of able and committed mothers identified in this chapter needed to be fully tapped in the future, courses would have to be designed which explicitly and fully took into account the needs of women caring for dependents. Even if demographic necessity does not impose it, equal opportunities considerations may make it imperative to increase the number of extended courses and to make them more responsive to the needs of dual role women workers. Indeed the recruitment of more mothers into nurse training may prove to be good value for money for the NHS. As one person with wide experience of the nurse workforce planning scene nationally put it 'if we could get recruitment and retention right for part-time women, we'd be getting it right for everyone else as well.'

Notes

1   The ENB's Nurses and Midwives Central Clearing House

2   In recent months SEN courses have ceased recruiting altogether.

3   The latest Department of Health (1991) NHS staffing figures for England indicate that part-time learners including district nurse, health visitor and midwifery students numbered 630 or 1 per cent of the total NHS nursing workforce at the end of September 1989.

4   In the case of enrolled nurse conversion courses, recent promptings by the ENB were apparently instrumental in obtaining an increase on this front (Nursing Times News, 1989).

5   One man was reported as having been recruited.

6   Family credit is a means tested state benefit payable to low earners with children. Evidence of student nurses bringing up children in poverty may be found elsewhere (Blackburn, 1991).

7   Hancock (1989) has suggested that an average nurse's working life is only eight and a half years including training.

14 Summary points from each chapter

Chapter 1. Introduction, aims and objectives

■   The demand for health care services will substantially increase over the next 25 years as the number of the very elderly rises.

■   The supply of young females to become nurses, radiographers, laboratory workers etc. will fall up to the turn of the century because of lower birth rate levels in the 1970s, but the numbers of older women of working age who are economically active will rise.

■   The effect on the NHS of the fall in supply of young females has been masked by the economic recession.

■   The NHS currently employs some 25 per cent of females who leave education with a minimum of 5 GCSEs. Since the size of this pool will continue to shrink, unless the NHS changes its recruitment patterns it will soon need to catch about 45 per cent of those available, in a market where other employers may become even more competitive.

■   The question is raised whether rising NHS budgets and the plentiful labour of the 1970s and early 1980s led to inefficient labour practices.

■   Many of the Professions Allied to Medicine, especially nurses, are driving towards a greater professionalisation of their status independently of market conditions. Nursing is newly subject to two somewhat inconsistent pressures - if RGNs become more expert (and better paid), they should, according to management theory, devolve more of the relatively unskilled care to less well paid support workers. But the new professional model is toward holistic nursing, where only a small number of jobs which do not involve patient contact can be done by unqualified staff.

- The introduction of NHS Trusts is likely to increase competition in the labour market over the 1990s.

- Flexibility will be the key to success for employers in the 1990s. The NHS must examine its own methods of producing health care, to see whether each service is produced with the optimum mix of resources. Equally, it must be flexible in the way in which it is prepared to employ staff, in terms of pay, benefits and conditions of employment.

- A number of key areas where further research is needed are identified most notably dealing with issues of substitution, wastage and recruitment.

Chapter 2.   The general labour supply picture

- Between 1980 and 1995 the number of school leavers in the United Kingdom will drop by about 260 thousand or 35 per cent. This drop is entirely in social classes III-V; a drop of some 40 per cent, whereas the (much smaller) numbers in social classes I and II will actually increase by about 20 per cent.

- Numbers staying in post-compulsory education may well rise by even more than the DES predicts, further reducing the pool of early school leavers.

- However, the total labour force will grow, by up to 800 thousand, most of whom will be female in the 25-44 age group.

- Changes in the numbers of 16 year olds vary by region, from a 29 per cent drop in Scotland and 27 per cent in the West Midlands to a 15 per cent fall in the South West over the 1988-2000 period.

- Ethnic minorities have a different age structure and will provide more, rather than fewer, 16 year olds in 1995.

- Projections of students in higher education are being continuously revised upwards. From 676 thousand in 1987 the number is expected to reach at least 805 thousand by 1999 and 816 thousand by 2000, but the most recent estimate suggests that the 805 thousand figure will be reached by 1993.

- Numbers of first degree graduates may drop slightly between 1992 and 1998, before recovering to about 130 thousand by the turn of the century.

Chapter 3.   The demand for skills from other employers

- After the recession of the early 1990s is over, real incomes are expected to grow at about 2.25 per cent, with 4 per cent inflation.

- Overall the demand for labour will increase by 730 thousand jobs between 1990 and 2000 than 1990 although many of these will be part-time. Considerable falls are expected in agriculture, mining and much of manufacturing, especially areas such as food and textiles where competition from abroad increases pressures for higher productivity.

- Business and other services will expand employment, particularly in leisure and tourism. Some growth, in line with GDP, is also expected in health, education, and public administration.

- Self employment and part-time employment, especially among females, will increase. The number of full-time wage earners will fall.

- Unemployment is expected to fall back from just under 3 million around 1993 to levels modestly above those of the first half of 1990 by the turn of the century.

- Job opportunities will improve for professional and managerial occupations, worsen for industrial operatives and unskilled workers, but remain much the same for craft, skilled manual and clerical workers, and sales staff.

- The demand for highly qualified staff will increase, by over a million jobs by 2000. The NHS currently employs a much higher proportion than average of the highly qualified, it could therefore face increasing competition.

Chapter 4.   The balance of labour supply and demand in the 1990s

- The tightest labour market will be that for new graduates. This is likely to be felt most in non-medical recruitment, because medical salaries are likely to remain relatively high.

- More recruitment channels will be necessary to keep up the inflow of persons with intermediate qualifications, chiefly nurses.

- Few shortages of clerical or secretarial staff are expected.

- Shortages of craftsmen, the numbers of whom are diminishing, probably reflect a lack of demand and the decline in apprenticeships/training opportunities rather than a reduction in the number of potential new entrants.

- There will be few problems in recruiting staff for services such as hotels and catering especially to part-time posts.

- It is difficult to predict post 1992 intra-EEC migration. Although health professionals are relatively low paid in the UK there are many informal barriers to movement.

- Employers who are likely to be successful in filling vacancies for the highly qualified will be those who offer imaginative overall career packages, including sponsorship and structured promotion prospects.

Chapter 5. Conditions of employment and career aspirations

- There remains scope for more detailed research comparing pay, and especially fringe benefits and pensions, within the NHS, with the private sector.

- Conditions of employment have changed dramatically throughout the whole economy in the 1970s and 1980s. Generally speaking these changes have been improvements.

- Throughout the economy working hours have remained quite stable over the past two decades. Manual males' hours at normal rates have decreased slightly, and at overtime rates increased slightly less; non-manual males' and all females' hours have remained the same.

- Average holiday entitlements have risen from 2.6 weeks to 4.6 weeks since 1970.

- Shift working has generally increased, with a wage premium of between 20 and 50 per cent. NHS unsocial hours premia may well be lower than their competitors in the labour market.

- Self employment is increasing rapidly outside the NHS at least in part due to demands from individuals for more control over their work. Family doctors are self employed and there may be increasing pressure from other NHS staff to offer labour services in this way.

Chapter 6. Labour supply and the NHS in the 1990s

■   Expected recruitment difficulties can be met by improving retention, increasing productivity or retargeting recruitment. However, given the importance of females in the NHS workforce, factors influencing their labour supply are of crucial importance.

■   Economic analysis of labour supply focuses on the family rather than the individual, and can provide a good explanation of women's work supply decisions.

■   In addition to economic factors, female labour supply is affected by changing social attitudes - more jobs are now considered suitable for women.

■   Increasing family aspirations put a premium on continuity of employment which is associated with higher income, and this factor is now applying to females as well as males.

■   Nevertheless, women still shoulder most of the domestic burden.

■   More women, and more employers, prefer part-time employment.

■   Comparing 1980 and 2000, 2¼ million more women will be economically active.

■   The empirical evidence suggests that wage increases do not increase the numbers of hours worked by males in employment, because they generally appear to prefer to take such gains in the form of more leisure. Wage increases may, however, be particularly useful in attracting new young males.

■   Wage increases do increase the numbers of hours offered by women in general, whether already in a particular employment or new to that employment. This is also true of nurses. The effect is stronger for full-time than part-time female employees.

■   The needs to look after young children restrains women from working, but the presence of teenage children (who need more money spent on them) tends to encourage women to work.

■   Child care facilities (unsurprisingly) or the subsidization of childcare increases female participation in the workforce.

Chapter 7.   Demand and supply within the NHS: general issues

- *Willingness to pay* for labour is the conventional measure of demand. The NHS has been a dominant buyer (in economics terminology a monopsonist). Since labour shortages have appeared in the last five years, the NHS has argued that it can solve particular shortages by a targeted response.

- Unions claim that since the NHS is a monopsonist, wages should be *fair.* The DoH tends to sidestep this argument, basing its evidence to the Review body on its estimates of the responsiveness of recruitment to changes in payments.

- Estimates of the quantity of labour demanded are derived either from *top down* modelling - such as a nurse/bed ratio - or *bottom-up* modelling, based upon an aggregation and translation of tasks and times to required staff.   Little emphasis is placed on the possibilities of substitution, 'fixed coefficients' or labour input ratios are generally assumed.

- Nevertheless, skill mix is increasingly recognised as important in nursing and all PAMs.   *Labour substitutability* is one of the most important, and politically one of the hottest, current issues.

- The British theoretical work being used to approach the issue of skill mix, and labour demand in general, is very basic and takes advantage of few sophisticated techniques.   There are few good studies in this area.

- *Performance indicators* have been developed to assess relative cost-effectiveness - or, how to get staff levels down.   They are still not very useful, since the available outcome measures are so limited.

Chapter 8.   Demand and supply within the NHS: supply issues

- Despite conventional wisdom the available evidence suggests that nurses are like other female workers - they respond, possibly strongly, to changes in wage rates.

- Despite the importance of women in the workforce, non-pay measures, such as child care vouchers, are given only lip service, and career prospects in the NHS are not as good for female employees as for males.

- Workforce planning models are being developed, based upon extrapolation of historic trends such as wastage rates and participation rates.   These models are an advance on what has been done previously, but they fail to get behind the observed patterns in an attempt to *explain*

271

them. More sophisticated behavioural analysis is needed in order to achieve this.

■ Project 2000 will reduce the service contribution of learners, especially since many schools of nursing may be closed. Existing SENs may be marginalised.

■ Estimates have been made of the costs of Project 2000 training in comparison with the traditional type. These estimates are based upon very preliminary data on drop-out rates. Although the cost per qualifier may be higher under Project 2000, it is not impossible that the cost of achieving a target workforce may be less.

■ Past wage levels offered by competitive employers for fairly well educated school leavers may well increase in the future, so the level of the Project 2000 bursary may not be high enough.

Chapter 9. Labour turnover within the NHS

■ Four factors determine the supply of qualified staff to the NHS: employment of newly trained staff; the quit rate; the return rate; and finally, the number of hours per week worked.

■ Turnover studies are hampered because they usually measure leaving and joining a particular DHA, not the NHS as a whole. The new Körner methods of collecting workforce data are better, but unfortunately many of the data returns use the permitted entry 'not known' for leavers' destinations.

■ Turnover is higher the younger the staff, and the less well qualified they are. Full-time nurses show the same pattern as part-time nurses, but part-time P&T are the most mobile of all qualified staff.

■ Turnover rates for nurses vary across the country by between about 12 per cent and 30 per cent. But as suggested below some 8 per cent to 15 per cent of leavers are transferring to other DHAs. Turnover over the age of 40 is down to about 7 per cent.

■ Individual Health Regions have been given special responsibility for workforce studies of particular staff groups. The Trent studies in Physiotherapy staffing have shown that over *half* of leavers were going to other NHS jobs - which confirms that the overall turnover rates are over estimates of the loss rate to the NHS as a whole.

■ Attitude surveys to find why nurses, in particular, leave their job, have elicited reasons such as stress and frustration and 'dropping morale'. The drawback of these sociological studies is that they are not well designed to assess the significance of the most likely *a priori* reason for leaving - low relative pay. Economic studies based on observing what people do rather than what they say suggest that this is a key factor although not necessarily the only one.

■ Observed behaviour surveys, based upon statistical methods, are few and, so far, either inconclusive or unsatisfactory. Some results of studies for DoH are eagerly awaited.

Chapter 10. Manpower planning in the NHS: a critical review

■ This chapter pulls together the manpower planning themes of Chapters Nine and Ten. Despite the predominance of women in the NHS workforce and the fact that 50 per cent of intake into medical schools are now female the term 'manpower' remains in use. This appears increasingly inappropriate.

■ Manpower or workforce planning is important and useful, but it must always be remembered that it depends upon the continuation of past relationships between key indicators, and if these relationships change predictions will be wrong.

■ NHS workforce planning has generally been fairly unsophisticated, partly because the data have not been very suitable or reliable.

■ Supply models for nurses are either centred upon the existing workforce, and extrapolate observed leaving and joining rates, or are centred upon the qualified population and extrapolate participation rates. These models are better in the short than the long term, because joining, leaving and participation rates all change in response to changes in the overall economic situation. There is a need for a strong behavioural content in such models.

■ In assessing demand, 'bottom up' approaches have been more popular, but such systems have been designed mainly to assist in ward or unit level decision making. They may have been *systematic* but they have not usually been *scientific*. In general they ignore labour substitutability and cost-outcome trade offs - largely because there is almost no evidence about the latter. This remains a major gap in existing knowledge.

■ Models have been developed separately for doctors and other groups, partly because they are intended to fulfil different ends. There is a case for linking them together.

Chapter 11. The supply of nursing skills:evidence from the LFS

■   The Labour Force Survey (LFS) is one of the most important sources of information about the supply of labour skills. This chapter focuses on the situation in the UK as a whole.

■   The LFS collects information about qualifications held by the population. Ninety-five per cent of nurses report that their nursing qualification is their highest qualification.

■   The number of females with a nursing qualification has increased from 633,000 in 1983 to 680,000 in 1989. Their participation in nursing has increased from 51½ per cent in 1983 to 57 per cent in 1989, explained by return to employment. Part-time working has increased by 38 per cent, full-time by 7½ per cent.

■   The number of males whose highest reported qualification was in nursing has declined from 66,000 to 55,000 over the same period. Sixty per cent of such males are employed as full-time nurses, compared with 32½ per cent of females. The number of males employed as nurses has increased by 14 per cent over the same period.

■   'Part-time' in nursing means considerably more hours than in non-nursing, for females with nursing qualifications.

■   More nurses than non-nurses work in excess of 40 hours per week - 50 per cent against 46-47 per cent - and this has increased over the five years from 1983-1988.

■   Of women with nursing qualifications, younger women have tended to move out of nursing, but older women have returned to full-time nursing.

■   An increasing number of females with a nursing qualification are working in non-nursing, health service jobs, such as administrators or managers.

Chapter 12. Labour supply trends for selected regions: South East Thames and Trent RHAs

■   It is possible to produce LFS figures for most Health Regions, despite a few problems due to lack of coterminosity with LFS regions and small sample numbers. Two examples, SE Thames and Trent are given.

■   Both regions show a decline in women employed full time as nurses, contrary to the national figures. Part-timers have increased by about the national average (28 per cent) in SE Thames, and more (35 per cent) in Trent.

- In both regions the trends are for full-time nurses to work longer hours, and for the proportion aged over 40 to rise.

- The employment of young part-timers is greater in Trent than in SE Thames, and this is rising in Trent but falling in SE Thames.

- The most important overall comparison with national figures is possibly that both Regions have seen their *qualified but non-nursing* female labour force rise dramatically, in contrast to the relatively static employment situation in the local health services.

- The tabulation illustrate the potential of the LFS for providing a broad overview of the labour supply avialable for a particular region.

Chapter 13. Mothers as student nurses

- By 1989 all nursing authorities and bodies were agreed that more mature entrants to nursing should be encouraged.

- One form of response was the development for mature entrants of part-time RGN training courses, designed around the constraints of the working mother.

- There is no reliable central information upon the numbers of part-time courses, or the numbers of students. But it is very small and falling, because in the past more SENs have been trained part-time, and SEN training is stopping. There are perhaps about 100 places on offer for 1992, and some 500 nurses in part-time training.

- An interview study established that applicants had usually had a job with a caring content, and many had previously tried a full-time nursing training course unsuccessfully.

- Existing part-time courses are 'only just' part-time (unlike, for example, day release or OU courses) and the students still feel very stressed by their dual roles.

- All existing courses are heavily oversubscribed.

- Part-time trainees are generally more committed to their training, and make good nurses. Low wastage rates make their training cost-effective.

■ The failure of educators to extend this type of training is due to three factors; traditional reliance on full-time courses (ie. inertia), the concentration of effort on starting up Project 2000 courses, and the apparent failure of the demographic timebomb to explode (thus far at least).

■ Project 2000 courses, although theoretically suited to part-time training, are not, in all cases, being developed sympathetically, and the relatively low level of the training bursary acts as a disincentive, especially for mature entrants with children.

References and bibliography

Abrams, M. (1973). 'Subjective Social Indicators', *Social Trends*, 4, 35-50.

Advisory Committee for Medical Manpower Planning (1989). *Report of the Second Advisory Committee*, Department of Health, HMSO, London.

Agassi, J.B. (1979). *Women on the Job*, Lexington, Lexington Books.

Ahamad, B. and M. Blaug (eds.) (1973). *The Practice of Manpower Forecasting*, Elsevier, Amsterdam.

Aiken, H. (1984). 'The Nurse Labour Market', *Journal of Nursing Administration*, January, 18-23.

All Wales Nurse Manpower Planning Committee (1985). *First Report*, Welsh Office, Cardiff.

Arrufat, J. and A. Zabalza (1986). 'Female Labour Supply with Taxation, Random Preferences and Optimization Errors', *Econometrica*, 54, 47-64.

Ashworth, J. and D. Ulph (1981). 'Estimating Labour Supply with Piecewise Budget Constraints' in C. Brown (ed.), *Taxation and Labour Supply*.

Association of University Teachers (1983). *'The Real Demand for Student Places'*, AUT, London.

Atkinson, J. (1989). 'Four Stages of Adjustment to the Demographic Downturn', *Personnel Management*, August, 20-4.

Audit Commission for England and Wales (1990). *The Pathology Services; A Management Review*, HMSO, London.

Audit Commission for England and Wales (1991). *The Virtue of Patients; Making Best Use of Ward Nursing Resources*, HMSO, London.

Bagust, A., J. Prescott and A. Smith (1988). 'Numbering the Nurses', *Health Service Journal*, 98, no.5108, 766-7.

Bailey, C. (1988). 'Different, not Worse', *Nursing Times*, 84, 17, 36-7.

Ball, J.A., K. Hurst, M.R. Booth and R. Franklin (1989). *... But Who Will Make the Beds?* Report of the Mersey Region project on assessment of nurse staffing and support worker requirements for acute general hospitals, Nuffield Institute for Health Services Studies/Mersey RHA.

Bankowski, Z. and A. Mejia (1987). 'Health Manpower out of Balance: conflicts and prospects, conference papers, conclusions and recommendations', XX CIOMS Conference, Acapulco, Mexico, CIOMS, Geneva.

Barr, A. (1964). 'Measuring Nursing Care', in G. McLachlan (ed.) *Problems and Progress in Medical Care*, Nuffield Provincial Hospital Trust/Oxford University Press.

Barry, J.T., K.L. Soothill and B.J. Francis (1989). 'Nursing the statistics: a demonstration study of nurse turnover and retention', *Journal of Advanced Nursing*, 14, 528-35.

Beardshaw, V. and R. Robinson (1990). *New for Old? Prospects for Nursing in the 1990s*, Research Report no.8, Kings Fund Institute, London.

Beaumont, K. (1988). *The Trent Nurse Supply Model: User Guide*, Trent RHA, Sheffield.

Beaumont, K., J. Thornton and H. Sleney (1989). *Physiotherapy: An examination of demand and supply issues*, Trent RHA, Sheffield.

Benham, L. (1971). 'The Labour Market for Registered Nurses: a three equation model', *Review of Economics and Statistics*, 53, 246-52.

Bevan, S., J. Buchan, S. Hayday (1989). *Women in Hospital Pharmacy*, Institute of Manpower Studies, report no.182, IMS, Brighton.

Binnie, A. (1987). 'Primary nursing: structural changes', *Nursing Times*, 83, 39.

Birch, S., A. Maynard and A. Walker (1986). 'Doctor Manpower Planning in the United Kingdom: Problems arising from Myopia in Policy Making', Centre for Health Economics, Discussion Paper 18, University of York, York.

Blackburn, C. (1991). *Poverty and Health: Working with Families*, OUP, Milton Keynes.

Blundell, R. and I. Walker (1982). 'Modelling the Joint Determination of Household Labour Supplies and Commodity Demands' *Economic Journal*, 351-64.

Blundell, R., J. Ham and C. Meghir (1987). 'Unemployment and Labour Supply', *Economic Journal*, S44-65.

Boganno, M, J. Hixson and J. Jeffers (1974). 'The Short Run Supply of Nurses Time', *Journal of Human Resources*, 80-94.

Bond, M. (1992). 'Mothers as Student Nurses', Occasional Paper no.3. Health Services Research Unit, University of Warwick, Coventry.

Borrill, C. (1988). 'Cultivating an interest in nursing', *Nursing Times*, 84, no.50, 44-5.

Bosanquet, N. and K. Gerard (1985). 'Nursing Manpower: recent trends and policy options', Discussion Paper 9, Centre for Health Economics, University of York.

Bosanquet, N. and L. Goodwin (1986). *Nurses and Higher Education: the cost of change*, discussion paper no.13, Centre for Health Economics, University of York.

Bosanquet, N. and R. Jeavons (1989). *The Future Structure of Nurse Education: an appraisal of policy options at the local level*, Centre for Health Economics, University of York, discussion paper no.54.

279

Bosworth, D.L. (1989). *Duration of Unemployment; An Analysis of the Labour Force Survey*, Project Report, Institute for Employment Research, University of Warwick, Coventry.

Bosworth, D.L. and P.J. Dawkins (1980). 'Compensation for Workers Disutility: Time of Day, Length of Shift and Other Features of Work Patterns', *Scottish Journal of Political Economy*, 27, no.1, 80-96.

Bosworth, D.L., P.C. Taylor and R.A Wilson (1989). *Projecting the Labour Market for the Highly Qualified'*, Training Agency Project Report, January 1989, Institute for Employment Research, University of Warwick, Coventry.

Bosworth, D.L. and P. Warren (1990a). 'Disequilibrium, Base Wage Rigidity and Adjustment', *Journal of Employment and Productivity*. (forthcoming).

Bosworth, D.L. and P. Warren (1990b). *Labour Markets: Operation and Failure*, Gower Press, Aldershot.

Bosworth, D.L. and R.A. Wilson (1989). 'The Pay of Scientists and Engineers: Evidence from Surveys Conducted by the Professional Institutes', Institute for Employment Research, University of Warwick, Coventry.

Bosworth, D.L. and R.A. Wilson (1990). 'Hours of Work and Pay Developments: Evidence from the New Earnings Survey', In M. Gregory and A. Thompson (eds.), *Pay Developments in the 1970s*, Oxford U.P. Oxford.

Boussofiane, A., E. Thonassoulis and R.G. Dyson (1991). 'Using Data Envelopment Analysis to Assess the Efficiency of Perinatal Care Provision in England', Warwick Business School Research Paper no.5, University of Warwick, Coventry.

Braverman, H. (1974). *Labour and Monopoly Capital*, Monthly Review Press, New York.

Brindle, D. (1989). 'Number of new nurses 13% down', *The Guardian*, 26th April.

Brinkworth, K. and E. Snape (1989). The Law as Gamekeeper? Skills Poaching and Training in the UK, Employment Research Unit, Cardiff Business School, UWCC, Cardiff.

Briscoe, G. and R. Wilson (1991). 'Explanations of the Demand for Labour in the United Kingdom Engineering Sector'. *Applied Economics*, 23, 913-26.

Briscoe, G. and R. Wilson (1992). 'Forecasting Economic Activity Rates', *International Journal of Forecasting*, (forthcoming).

Brook, L., R. Jowell and S. Witherspoon (1989). 'Recent Trends in Social Attitudes', *Social Trends*, 19, 13-22.

Brown, C., E. Levin and D. Ulph (1976). 'Estimates of Labour Hours Supplied Married Male Workers in Great Britain, '*Scottish Journal of Political Economy*, 261-77.

Brown, C., E. Levin, P. Rosa, P. Ruffell and D. Ulph (1983). 'Direct Taxation and Labour Supply', HM Treasury Project. Working Papers 10-11, University of Stirling.

Brown, C. (1985). 'Military Enlistments: What Can We Learn From Geographic Variation', *American Economic Review*, 75, 1, 228-34.

Buchan, J. (1989). 'Policy Notes', *Nursing Standard*, 4, 5, 46-47.

Buchan, J. (1989). 'Open all Hours', *Nursing Standard*, 4, 24, 46.

Buchan, J. and G. Pike (1989). PAMS into the 1990s - Professions Allied to Medicine: the wider labour market context, IMS Report no.175.

Buchan, J., S. Bevan and J. Atkinson (1988). Costing Labour Wastage in the National Health Service, Institute of Manpower Studies report no.175, IMS, Brighton.

Cairncross, A. (1969). 'Economic Forecasting', *Economic Journal*, December, 79, 797-812.

Campaign, (1989). 'Straight from the Client's Mouth', Campaign Twenty One, London.

Carr-Hill, R., P. Dixon, M. Griffiths, M. Higgins, D. McCaughan and K. Wright (1991). A Selective Review of the Literature on Skill Mix, *Journal of Advanced Nursing*, 16, 242-49.

Cavanagh, S.J. (1989). 'Nursing Turnover: literature review and methodological critique', *Journal of Advanced Nursing*, 14, no.7, Oxford, 587-96.

Central Statistical Office (1974). 'Social Commentary: Men and Women', *Social Trends*, 5. 8-25.

Central Statistical Office (1989). *Social Trends*, 19, HMSO, London.

Cohen, H.A. (1972). 'Monopsony and Discriminating Monopsony in the Nursing Market', *Applied Economics*, 4, 41-50.

Colclough, C. (1990). 'How can the manpower planning debate be resolved?' in R. Amjad, C. Colclough, N. Garcia, M. Hopkins, R. Infante and G. Rodgers (eds.), *Quantitative Techniques in Employment Planning*, International Labour Office, Geneva.

Commission of the European Communities (1979). 'Women and Men in Europe in 1978', Supplement 3 to *Women of Europe*, CEC, Brussels.

Commission of the European Communities (1984). *Summary of a Survey about Socio-Political Attitudes in the Countries of the European Community*, CEC, Brussels.

Commission of the European Communities (1987). *European Barometer*, no.27. June, CEC, Brussels.

Commission of the European Communities (1988). 'Men and Women of Europe in 1987', Supplement 26 to *Women of Europe*, CEC, Brussels.

Commission of the European Communities (1990). *Employment in Europe 1990*, Directorate General for Employment Industrial Relations and Social Affairs, Office for Official Publications, Brussels.

Committee of Public Accounts (1981). *Financial Control and Accountability in the NHS*, 17th Report of Session 80/81, House of Commons Paper 255.

Committee of Public Accounts (1982). *Financial Control and Accountability in the NHS*, 17th Report of Session 81/82, HC Paper 375.

Committee of Public Accounts (1984). *Manpower Control, Accountablity and Other Matters Relating to the NHS*, 16th Report of Session 83/84, HC Paper 113.

Committee of Public Accounts (1986). *NHS: Control of Nursing Manpower*, 14th Report of Session 85/86, HC Paper 98.

Committee of Public Accounts (1987). *Control of NHS Manpower*, 11th Report of Session 86/87, HC Paper 213.

Confederation of British Industry (1989). *'Attitudes of Young People to Training Careers and Employment - Survey Results'*, CBI, London .

Conroy, M. and M. Stidston, (1988). *2001 - The Black Hole: An examination of labour market trends in relation to the NHS*, NHS Regional Manpower Planners' Group.

Council for Professions Supplementary to Medicine (1981). *Annual Report 1980/81*, CPSM, London.

Cree, J. (1978). 'The Manpower Contribution to Strategic Planning: a possible approach', *Health Service Manpower Review*, 4, 1.

Darcy, P. (1988). 'Time to Mature?', *Nursing Times*, 84, no.35, 43-4.

Dawson, C., V. Barrett and J. Ross (1990). 'A Case of Financial Approach of Manpower Planning in the NHS', *Personnel Review*, 19, no.4, 16-25.

Dean, D.J. (1987). *Manpower Solutions*, Scutari Projects Ltd. for the RCN.

Delamothe, T. (1988a). 'Nursing Grievances I: Voting with their feet', *British Medical Journal*, 296, 2nd. Jan, 25-8.

Delamothe, T. (1988b). 'Nursing Grievances II: Pay', *British Medical Journal*, 296, 9th Jan, 120-23.

Delamothe, T. (1988c). 'Nursing Grievances III: Conditions', *British Medical Journal*, 296, 16th Jan, 182-85.

Delamothe, T. (1988d). 'Nursing Grievances IV: Not a profession, not a career', *British Medical Journal*, 296, 23rd Jan, 271-74.

Delamothe, T. (1988e). 'Nursing Grievances V: Women's Work', *British Medical Journal*, 296, 30th Jan, 345-47.

Department of Education and Science (1986). *'Projections of Demand for Higher Education in Great Britain 1986-2000'*, HMSO, London.

Department of Education and Science (1987). *Higher Education: Meeting the Challenge*, April, HMSO, London.

Department of Education and Science (1990). 'Young People Leaving School', *Employment Gazette,* August, 382-89.

Department of Education and Science (1990). *Highly Qualified People: Supply and Demand,* Report of an Interdepartmental Review, HMSO, London.

Department of Education and Science (1991). *Higher Education a New Framework,* Cmnd.1541, HMSO, London.

Department of Employment (1986). 'Training Provided by the Armed Forces'. *Employment Gazette,* May, 153-60, HMSO, London.

Department of Employment (1988). 'New Entrants to the Labour Market in the 1990s', *Employment Gazette,* May, 267-74, HMSO, London.

Department of Employment (1989). 'Labour Force Outlook to the Year 2000', *Employment Gazette,* April, 159-72, HMSO, London.

Department of Employment (1990). 'Regional Labour Force Outlook to the year 2000', *Employment Gazette,* January, 9-19, HMSO, London.

Department of Employment, *Employment Gazette,* HMSO, London.

Department of Employment, *New Earnings Survey,* HMSO, London.

Department of Health (1989). *NHS Workforce in England,* Department of Health, Crown Copyright, London.

Department of Health (1991). *NHS Workforce in England,* Department of Health, Crown Copyright, London.

Department of Health and Central Office of Information (1990). *Health Service Careers Factsheet 2,* HMSO, London.

Department of Health and Social Services/Operational Research Service (Jessup N.E.) (1980). *The Demand for Hospital Nurses in England in the Late 1980's,* (ORS /3/80), DHSS, London.

DHSS/MAPLIN (1981). *Extracts from Wessex Strategic Planning User Manual,* Manpower Planning Department, Wessex RHA, (MAPLIN paper 81/13) DHSS, London.

DHSS/Operational Research Service (1982). *ORS National Demand Model for Nurses: Review of the Model,* (ORS/NURS D2), DHSS, London.

DHSS/Operational Research Service (1983). *Nurse Manpower Planning: approaches and techniques*, HMSO, London.

Dodd, A. (1987). *English National Board Cohort Study, 1986 Interim Report*, ENB, London.

Dolton, P.J. (1990). 'The Economics of Teacher Supply'. *Economic Journal*, 100, no.400, 91-105.

Downey, G. (1985). *National Health Service: control of nursing manpower*, Report by the Comptroller and Auditor General, London: HMSO, 36pp.

Dusansky, R., M. Ingber, A. Leiken and J. Walsh (1986). 'On Increasing the Supply of Nurses: an Interstate Analysis', *Atlantic Economic Journal*, 14, 34-44.

Eastaugh, S.R. (1985). 'The Impact of the Nurse Training Act on the Supply of Nurses 1974-85', *Inquiry*, 22, 4 (Winter), 404-17.

Eckstein, Z. and K. Wolpin (1989). 'Dynamic Labour Force Participation of Married Women and Endogenous Work Experience', *Review of Economic Studies*, 375-90.

Edmonstone, J. (1988a). 'Managing the Manpower Resource 1: the nature of the Problem', *Hospital and Health Service Review*, 84, 1 (Feb.), 13-5.

Edmonstone, J. (1988b). 'Managing the Manpower Resource 2: from analysis to action', *Hospital and Health Service Review*, 84, 2 (Apr.), 60-3.

Edwards, R. (1979). *Contested Terrain*, Heinemann, London (1974).

Edwards-Jones, I. (1991). School-leavers face jobs dearth, *Independent on Sunday*, 1 September, 8.

Elias, P.E. (1987). 'The Distribution of Persons with Nursing Qualifications in England and Wales', Institute for Employment Research, University of Warwick, Coventry.

Elias, P.E. and M. Rigg (eds.) (1990). *'The Demand for Graduates'*, Policy Studies Institute, London.

Elkan, R. and J. Robinson (1991). 'The Implementation of Project 2000 in a District Health Authority: The Effect on the Nursing Service', An Interim Report, Department of Nursing Studies, Univerrsity of Nottingham.

Employment Department (1989a). 'I Think I Could Resist Their Charms', *Employment Gazette*, March, 119, HMSO, London.

Employment Department (1989b). 'Women's Vital Role at Work', *Employment Gazette*, March, 118, HMSO, London.

Employment Department (1989c). 'Women at Work in Europe', *Employment Gazette*, June, 299-308, HMSO, London.

English National Board (1989-1990). *Annual Report*, ENB, London.

English National Board (1991a). *Applicant Handbook*, July Edition, ENB, London.

English National Board (1991b). *Annual Report 1990-1991*, ENB, London.

Equal Opportunities Commission (1991). *Equality Management: Women's Employment in the NHS*, EOC, Manchester.

Ermisch, J. and R. Wright (1989). 'Wage Offers and Full-time and Part-time Employment by Women', *NIESR Discussion Paper* no.164.

Feldstein, M.S. (1967). *Economic Analysis for Health Service Efficiency: Econometric Studies of the British National Health Service*, North Holland, Amsterdam.

Finniston, Sir M. (1980). *Engineering Our Future*, Report of the Committee of Enquiry into the Engineering Profession, Cmnd.7794, HMSO, London.

Firby, P.A. (1990). 'Nursing: a Career of Yesterday?' *Journal of Advanced Nursing*, 15, no.6, June, 723-37.

Firth, H. and P. Britton (1989). '"Burnout", absence and turnover amongst British nursing staff', *Journal of Occupational Psychology*, 62, no.1, 55-9.

Flood, S.D and D. Diers (1988). 'Nurse staffing, patient outcome and cost', *Nursing Management* 19, no.5 (May) 34-43.

Fogg, D. J. (1988). *A Study of Wastage in Nurse Education - No Way to Treat a Lady - or Man*, Unpublished M.Ed thesis, University of East Anglia.

Fordham, R. (1987). *Appraising Workload and the Scope for Change in Orthopaedics*, Centre for Health Economics, University of York, discussion paper no.25.

Francis, B.J., M.T. Peelo and K.L. Soothill (1988). *NHS Nurses Attitudes to Staff Turnover: An application of latent class analysis*, Centre for Applied Statistics/Department of Mathematics, Lancaster University, Statistics Group Research Report Series 88/02.

Gallagher, P. (1990). 'Project 2000 in Theory and in Practice'. *Nursing Standard*. 4, 50, 30-31.

Gallup (1984). Gallup Political Index. no.285. May.

Gallup (1985). Gallup Political Index. no.300. August.

Gallup (1987). Gallup Political Index. no.321. May. 35.

Gallup (1989). Personnel Directors Report, Social Surveys (Gallup Poll), London.

Gault, A.R. (1982). 'The Aberdeen Formula as an Illustration of the Difficulty of Determining Nursing Requirements', *International Journal of Nursing Studies*, 19, 2, 61-7.

Gibbs, I., D. McCaughan and M. Griffiths (1990). *Skill-mix in Nursing: A Selective Review of the Literature*, University of York, Centre for Health Economics, discussion paper no.69.

Gobbi, M. (1989). *Expectations, Experience and Responsibilities: A Study of Older Entrants in Two Schools of Nursing*', unpublished M.A. (ed.) dissertation, Faculty of Educational Studies, University of Southampton.

Gomulka, J. and N. Stern (1986). 'The Employment of Married Women in the UK', Discussion Paper no.98, Taxation, Incentives and Distribution of Income Programme, LSE.

Gomulka, J. and N. Stern (1990). 'The Employment of Married Women', *Economica*, 171-199.

Goode, R. (1988). Testing the Test, *Nursing Times*, 84, 36, 40.

Gray, A. and A. McGuire (1989). 'Factor Inputs in NHS Hospitals', *Applied Economics*, 21, 397-411.

Gray, A. and R. Smail (1982). *Why Has the Nursing Pay Bill Increased?*, Health Economics Research Unit, University of Aberdeen discussion paper 01/82.

Gray, A., C. Normand and E. Currie (1989). *Staff Turnover in the NHS: a preliminary economic analysis*, Discussion Paper no.46, Centre for Health Economics/Health Economics Consortium, University of York.

Greenhalgh, C. (1977). 'A Labour Supply Function for Married Women in Britain', *Economica*, 249-65.

Greenhalgh, C. (1979). 'Male Labour Force Participation in Great Britain', *Scottish Journal of Political Economy*, 275-86.

Greenhalgh, C. (1980). 'Participation and Hours of Work for Married Women in Britain', *Oxford Economic Papers*, 296-318.

Gregg, P. (1991). 'Is there a Future for Special Employment Measures in the 1990s?', *National Institute Economic Review*, November.

Grocott, T. (1989). A Hole in the Black Hole Theory, *Nursing Times*, 85, 41, 65-7.

Hall, J. (1976). 'Subjective Measures of Quality of Life in Britain: 1971 to 1975, Some Developments and Trends', *Social Trends,* 7. 47-60.

Hancock, C. (1989). Women, Power and Public Life, *Nursing Standard*, 4, 12, 18-9.

Hancock, R. (1988). Tailor-Made Training, *Nursing Times*, 84, 6, 40-1.

Hardy, L.K., H. Sinclair and J. Hughes (1984). 'Nursing Careers: findings of a follow up survey of graduates in nursing education and administration certificate courses of the Department of Nursing, University of Edinburgh, 1957-75', *Journal of Advanced Nursing*, 9, 611-618.

Harrison, S. and F. Brooks (1985). *Professional Manpower in the Yorkshire Region*, Nuffield Centre, University of Leeds.

Hart, E. (1989). *A Qualitative Study of Micro-level factors Affecting Retention and Turnover Amongst nursing Staff in Paediatrics and care*

288

of the Elderly, unpublished report for Trent RHA, Department of Nursing Studies, Queen's Medical Centre, Nottingham.

Hartley, K. and A. Shiell (1988a). Nurse Substitution and Training: Evidence from a Survey, *Health Care UK Policy Journal*, Policy Journals, Newbury, Berks, 84-9.

Hartley, K. and A. Shiell (1988b). 'Nurse Substitution and Training: Evidence from a Survey', *Health Care UK, 1988*, Policy Journals, Newbury, Berks, 84-9.

Hersley, J., W. Pierskalla and S. Wandel (1981). 'Nurse Staff Management', in Boldy D. (ed.) *Operational Research Applied to Health Services*, Croom Helm, Kent.

Heywood Jones, I. (1986). Late Starters, *Nursing Times*, 82, 52, 32-3.

Hirsh, W. (1986). Career Re-Entry: Driving the Talent Away, *Manpower Policy and Practice*, Spring, 12-4.

Hollister, R. (1967). *A Technical Evaluation of the First Stage of the Mediterranean Regional Project*, OECD, Paris.

Hooper, J. (1975). Training for Mature Entrants, *Nursing Times Occasional Paper*, 9 October.

Hoskins, M.D. (1982a). *The Supply of Nursing Staff to Non-Psychiatric Hospitals in England and Wales,* Discussion Paper no.23, Department of Economics, University of Leicester.

Hoskins, M.D. (1982b). *The Effect of Pay Changes on Cohort Survival: a study of the supply of midwifery staff to the NHS,* Discussion Paper no.26, Department of Economics, University of Leicester.

Hughes, G. (1991a). *Comprehensive Occupational Forecasts: A Review of Methods and Practice in Some OECD Countries*, Economic and Social Research Institute, Dublin, (mimeo.).

Hughes, G. (1991b). *Manpower Forecasting: A Review of Methods and Practice in Some OECD Countries*, Economic and Social Research Institute, Dublin.

Hughs, M.D. (1988). 'A Stochastic Frontier Cost Function for Residential Child Care Provision', *Journal of Applied Econometrics*, 3, 203-14.

Hunt, A. (1968). *A Survey of Women's Employment,* HMSO, London.

Hunt, P. (1980). *Gender and Class Consciousness,* Macmillan, London.

Hurd, R.W. (1973). Equilibrium Vacancies in a Labour Market Dominated by Non-Profit Firms: the 'shortage' of nurses', *Review of Economics and Statistics,* 55, 234-40.

Hutt, R. (1983). *Sick Children's Nurses: A Study for the DHSS of the career patterns of RSCNs.* IMS Report 78, Institute of Manpower Studies, University of Sussex, Brighton.

Hutt, R. (1988). Lasting the Course, *Senior Nurse,* 8, 12, 4-9.

Institute for Employment Research (1991). *Review of the Economy and Employment, 1991: Occupational Assessment,* University of Warwick, Coventry.

Institute for Manpower Studies (1989). *The Graduate Labour Market in the 1990s,* Report no.167, University of Sussex, Brighton.

Jack, W.H. (1990). *The Control of Hospital Based Medical and Nursing Manpower,* Report by the Comptroller and Auditor General for Northern Ireland, Department of Health and Social Services, HMSO, London.

Jones, K. (1989). *Towards a Regional Nurse Manpower Strategy 9: A study of DHA's nurse manpower plans for the general workforce in the Trent region for the period 1987/8-1993/4,* Trent RHA, Sheffield.

Joshi, H. (1984). 'Women's Participation in Paid Work', *Department of Employment Research Paper,* no.45., London: HMSO.

Joshi, H. (1985). 'Participation in Paid Work: Evidence from the Women and Employment Survey', in R. Blundell and I. Walker (eds.), *Unemployment, Job Search and Labour Supply,* Cambridge University Press, Cambridge.

Joshi, H., (1988). 'Female Participation in Paid Work' in R. Blundell and I. Walker (ed.), *Unemployment, Job Search and Labour Supply,* 217-42.

Joshi, H., S. Owen and R. Layard (1985). 'Why are more women working in Britain', *Journal of Labour Economics,* S147-86.

Jowell, R. and C. Airey (1985). 'British Social Attitudes', *Social Trends,* 15, 11-8.

Jowell, R., S. Witherspoon and L. Brook (eds.), British Social Attitudes: the 1987 Report, Social and Community Planning Research, Gower, Aldershot.

Jowett, P. and M. Rothwell (1988). *Performance Indicators in the Public Sector*, Macmillan, Basingstoke.

Jowett S., I. Walton and S. Payne (1991). *The NFER Project 2000 Research: An Introduction and Some Interim Issues*. Interim Paper no.2, National Foundation for Educational Research, Slough.

Kell, M. and J. Wright (1990). 'Benefits and the Labour Supply of Women Married to Unemployed Men', *Economic Journal*, 119-26.

Key, T. (1986). 'Nursing and the Need for Manpower Planning', in Harrison and Gretton, *Health Care UK, 1986*, Hermitage, Policy Journals, Berks.

Killingsworth, M.R. and J.J. Heckman (1986). 'Female Labour Supply: a survey', in O. Ashenfelter and R. Layard (eds.), *Handbook of Labour Economics*, 1, North Holland, Amsterdam.

Knapp, M. (1985). *The Turnover of Care Staff in Children's Homes*, Personal Social Services Research Unit University of Kent, Discussion Paper 382/2.

Knapp, M., K. Harissis and S. Missiakoulis (1981). *Labour Turnover and Wastage: the case of social work trainees and the usefulness of the polychotomous logit technique*, Discussion Paper 184/2, Personal Social Services Research Unit, University of Kent.

Knapp, M., K.Harissis and S. Missiakoulis (1982). 'Investigating Labour Turnover and Wastage Using the Logit Technique', *Journal of Occupational Psychology*, 55, 129-38.

Knapp, M. and S. Missiakoulis (1983). 'Predicting Turnover Rates Among the Staff of English and Welsh Old People's Homes', *Social Science and Medicine*, 17, 29-36.

Lavers, R. and D.K. Whynes (1978). 'A Production Function Analysis of English Maternity Hospitals', *Socioeconomic Planning Sciences*, 12, 85-93.

Layard, R. M. Barton and A. Zabalza (1980). 'Married Women's Participation and Hours', *Economica*, 47, 51-72.

Lee, K. and G. Hoare (1984). 'Towards a New Model of Health Manpower Planning', *Health Services Manpower Review*, 10, no.2, 4-8.

Lee, K., G. Hoare and A. Long (1984). 'Conceptual Orientation in the Planning of Health Manpower', *International Journal of Manpower*, 5, 3, 26-31.

Leenders, F. (1985). 'Stateside Staffing', *Nursing Times*, 81, no.38, 36-37.

LGC (1989). 'Nurseries Set to be the Perk of the 1990s', *Local Government Chronicle*, 7.

Lindley, R.M. (1987). *'New Forms and New Areas of Employment Growth: a Comparative Study'*, Programme for Research and Actions on the Development of the Labour Market, Commission of the European Communities.

Lindop, E. (1988). Giving Up, *Nursing Times*, 84, 5, 54-5.

Lindsay, C.M. (1980). *National Health Issues: The British Experience*, Roche Laboratories, Nutley.

Link, C.R. (1988). 'Returns to Nursing Education 1970-84', *Journal of Human Resources*, 23, 3, 372-87.

Link, C.R. and R.F. Settle (1979). 'Labour Supply Responses of Married Professional Nurses: new evidence', *Journal of Human Resources*, 14, 2, 256-66.

Link, C.R. and R.F. Settle (1981). 'Wage Incentives and Married Professional Nurses: a case of backward bending supply', *Economic Enquiry*, 19, 1, 144-56.

Littler, C. (1985). 'Taylorism, Fordism and Job Design', in D. Knights, H. Willmott and D. Collinson (eds.), *Job Redesign - Critical Perspectives on the Labour Process*, Gower, Aldershot.

Long, A.F. and G. Mercer (1987). *Health Manpower: Planning, Production and Management*, Croom Helm, Kent.

Long, A.F. and G. Mercer (eds.) (1981). *Manpower Planning in the NHS*, Gower Pub. Co. Ltd, Farnborough.

292

Long, A.F. and S. Harrison (1985). *Health Service Performance: Effectiveness and Efficiency*, Croom Helm, Kent.

Mackay, L. (1988). 'Career Women', *Nursing Times*, 84, (March 9th), 42-4.

Mackay L. (1989), *Nursing a Problem*, Open University Press, Milton Keynes.

Manpower Planning Advisory Group (1991). 'Operations Research Services: A Guide to Nurse Supply Modelling', Department of Health, London.

Market and Opinion Research International (1989). *'Students '89'*. Faxed information.

Marketing (1987). *'National Service'*. Marketing (UK). July 9, 20-1.

Martin, J. and C. Roberts (1984). *Women and Employment: a Lifetime Perspective*, Department of Employment, Office of Population Censuses and Surveys, HMSO, London.

Maxwell, R. (1988). *Reshaping the National Health Service*, Hermitage, Poicy Journals, Berks.

Maynard, A. (1987). 'What Nursing Shortage?', *The Health Service Journal*, Oct. 8th.

Mayston, D. (1990). 'NHS resourcing: a financial and economic analysis', in A.J. Culyer, A.K. Maynard and J.W. Posnett (eds.), *Competition in Health Care*, Macmillan, Houndsmill, Basingstoke.

McGuire and Westoby (1983). *A Production Function Analysis of Acute Hospitals*, Discussion Paper 04/83, Health Economics Research Unit, University of Aberdeen.

McNally, F. (1979). *Women for Hire: a Study of the Female Office Worker*, Macmillan, London.

McVey, S. (1991). Shift those Patterns, *Nursing Standard*, 5, 47, 53.

Meager, N., J. Buchan and C. Rees (1989). *Job Sharing in the National Health Service*, Institute of Manpower Studies, Research Report no.174, IMS, Brighton.

293

Menneymeyer, S.T. and G. Gaumer (1983). 'Nursing Wages and the Value of Educational Credentials', *Journal of Human Resources*, 18, 32-48.

Mercer, G. (1979). *The Employment of Nurses*, Croom Helm, Kent.

Mersey Regional Health Authority (1988). 'The Recruitment, Retention and Re-entry of Nurses, Midwives and Health Visitors: A Strategy for Action', Mersey RHA, Liverpool.

Miller, S.J. and W.D. Bryant (1965). *A Division of Nursing Labour*, Community Studies Inc., USA.

Missiakoulis, S., C. Hale, K. Harissis and M. Knapp (1980). *Hospital Employee Turnover: some methodological comments and a re-analysis*, Personal Social Service Research Unit, University of Kent, Discussion Paper 166.

Moore, J. (1988). A letter to Miss Audrey Emerton. Chairman, UKCC, 20 May, 1988, DHSS, London.

Moores, B. (1987). 'The Changing Composition of the British Nursing Workforce 1962-1984', *Journal of Advanced Nursing*, 12, no.4, 499-504.

Moores, B., B. Singh and A. Tun (1982). Attitudes of 2325 active and inactive nurses to aspects of their work, *J Advanced Nursing*, 7, 483-89.

Moores, B., A. Tun and B. Singh (1983). 'An Analysis of Factors which Impinge on a Nurse's Decision to Enter, Stay in, Leave or Re-enter the Nursing Profession', *Journal of Advanced Nursing*, 8, 227-35.

Mulligan, B. (1973). *Measurement of Patient Dependency and Workload Index*' (Kings Fund Project Paper), DHSS, London.

National Association of Health Authorities (1987). *Recruitment and Retention of Staff in the Professions Supplementary to Medicine: A summary of recent studies*, NAHA.

National Audit Office (1985a). *NHS: Control of Nursing Manpower*, Session 84/85, HC Paper 558.

National Audit Office (1985b). *NHS: Hospital Based Medical Manpower*, Session 84/5, HC paper 373.

National Audit Office (1987). *Control over Professional and Technical Manpower*, Session 86/87, HC Paper 95.

National Economic Development Office/Training Agency (1988). *Young People and the Labour Market*, NEDO/Training Agency, London.

National Union of Public Employees/Low Pay Unit (1989). *Nursing a Grievance: Low Pay in Nursing*, NUPE/LPU, London.

Nazarko, L. (1991). 'Outclassed and Uneducated', *Nursing Standard*, 6, 6, 54.

Nessling, R.C. and S. Boyle (1990a). *The Professional Nursing Labour Market: A District Perspective - North Hertfordshire*, Nursing Directorate, NW Thames RHA.

Nessling, R.C. and S. Boyle (1990b). 'A Welcome Return?', *Nursing Times*, 86, 44, 54-5.

Nursing Standard (1989a). Feature 'A Strategy for Nursing - Solving the Staffing Problem', *Nursing Standard*, 4, 4, 21.

Nursing Standard (1989b). Feature Job Focus, Angling for Success, *Nursing Standard*, 4, 10, 56.

Nursing Standard (1990). News - Staff Shortages - Reforms require 'National Strategy', *Nursing Standard*, 4, 35, 6.

Nursing Times (1989). News - ENB steps up pressure for conversion courses, *Nursing Times*, 85, 29, 11.

O'Donoghue, M. (1965). 'Manpower/educational activities of the Irish EIP Team', in OECD *Manpower Forecasting in Educational Planning*, Organisation for Economic Co-operation and Development, Paris.

Office of Population Censuses and Surveys (1973). General Household Survey, 1972 and Introductory Report, HMSO, London.

Office of Population Censuses and Surveys (1980). *Classification of Occupations 1980*, HMSO, London.

Office of Population Censuses and Surveys (1986). *Labour Force Survey*, 1983 and 1984, HMSO, London.

Office of Population Censuses and Surveys (1990). *Standard Occupational Classification*, HMSO, London.

Oxford Regional Hospital Board (1967). *Measurement of Nursing Care*, Operational Research Unit Report no.9, Oxford RHB, Oxford.

Parnes, H.S. (1962). *Forecasting Educational Needs for Economic and Social Development*, Paris: Organisation for Economic Co-operation and Development.

Pearce, C. (1988). 'The Nursing Workforce', *Senior Nurse*, 8, 3 (Mch.), 25-7.

Pearson, R. and G. Pike (1989). *The Graduate Labour Market in the 1990s*, Institute of Manpower Studies, Report no.167, IMS, Brighton.

Pembrey, S. and S. Punton (1990). 'Nursing Beds', *Nursing Times*, 86 no.14, 44-5.

Perry, S. (1990). 'Returning to Work after the Birth of the First Child', *Applied Economics*, 1137-48.

Pfeffer, J. and C.A. O'Reilly (1987). 'Hospital Demography and Turnover among Nurses', *Industrial Relations*, 26, no.2, 158-73.

Phillips, V. (1989a). 'Labour Supply Estimates for Nurses: A Review of the Literature' in *Human Resources in Child Care*.

Phillips, V. (1989b). 'The Labour Supply of Nurses in the UK; Evidence from the Women and Employment Survey', *Centre for Socio-Legal Studies*, Oxford.

Phillips, V.L. (1989c). 'A review of the existing literature on nurses' labour force participation and of the general literature on female labour supply', paper presented at the Health and Human Resources Conference, Antwerp (revised version).

Phillips, V.L. (1990). 'An analysis of the participation and hours of work decision with fixed costs for nurses in Great Britain', paper presented at the Health Economists' Study Group meeting, Dublin. (revised version).

Pollert, A. (1981). *Girls, Wives, Factory Lives*, Macmillan, London.

Poulton, K. (1987). 'Nursing Manpower in the European Region'. Geneva: CIOMS Conference, Acapulco, Mexico, CIOMS, Geneva.

Price Waterhouse (1987). *Report on the Costs, Benefits and Manpower Implications of Project 2000*, UKCC, London.

Price Waterhouse (1988). *Nurse Retention and Recruitment*, Price Waterhouse, London.

Rajan, A. and R. Pearson (eds.) (1986). *UK Occupation and Employment Trends to 1990: An employer-based study of the trends and their underlying causes*, Butterworths for the Institute of Manpower Studies, London.

Reid, N. (1985a). *Wards in Chancery? Nurse Training in the Clinical Field*, RCN, London.

Reid, N. (1985b). 'The Effective Training of Nurses: manpower implications', *International Journal of Nursing Studies*, 22, 2, 89-98.

Reid, N.G. (1986). 'Nursing Manpower: the problems ahead', *International Journal of Nursing Studies*, 23, 3, 187-97.

Reid, N.G and M. Melaugh (1987). 'Nurse Hours per Patient: a method for monitoring and explaining staffing levels', *International Journal of Nursing Studies*, 24, no.1, 1-14.

Resource Analysis Team, Wessex RHA (1987). 'Qualified Nurse Manpower: Report on Demand, Supply and Training', Wessex RHA, Southampton.

Review Body for Nursing Staff, Midwives, Health Visitors and Professions Allied to Medicine (1984a). *First Report on Nursing Staff, Midwives and Health Visitors*, Cm.9258 Session 83/4.

Review Body for Nursing Staff, Midwives, Health Visitors and Professions Allied to Medicine (1984b). *First Report on PAMs*, Cm.9257, Session 83/4.

Review Body for Nursing Staff, Midwives, Health Visitors and Professions Allied to Medicine (1985a). *Second Report on Nursing*, Cm.9529, Session 84/5.

Review Body for Nursing Staff, Midwives, Health Visitors and Professions Allied to Medicine (1985b). *Second Report on PAMs*, Cm.9528 Session 84/5.

Review Body for Nursing Staff, Midwives, Health Visitors and Professions Allied to Medicine (1986a). *Third Report on Nursing*, Cm.9782, Session 85/6.

Review Body for Nursing Staff, Midwives, Health Visitors and Professions Allied to Medicine (1986b). *Third Report on PAMs*, Cm.9783, Session 85/6.

Review Body for Nursing Staff, Midwives, Health Visitors and Professions Allied to Medicine (1987a). *Fourth Report on Nursing*, Cm.129, Session 86/7.

Review Body for Nursing Staff, Midwives, Health Visitors and Professions Allied to Medicine (1987b). *Fourth Report on PAMs*, Cm.130, Session 86/7.

Review Body for Nursing Staff, Midwives, Health Visitors and Professions Allied to Medicine (1988a). *Fifth Report on Nursing* Cm.360, Session 87/8.

Review Body for Nursing Staff, Midwives, Health Visitors and Professions Allied to Medicine (1988b). *Fifth Report on PAMs*, Cm.361, Session 87/8.

Review Body for Nursing Staff, Midwives, Health Visitors and Professions Allied to Medicine (1989a). *Sixth Report on Nursing*, Cm.577, Session 88/9.

Review Body for Nursing Staff, Midwives, Health Visitors and Professions Allied to Medicine (1989a). *Sixth Report on Nursing*, Cm.577, Session 88/9.

Review Body for Nursing Staff, Midwives, Health Visitors and Professions Allied to Medicine (1989b). *Sixth Report on PAMs*, Cm.578, Session 88/9.

Review Body for Nursing Staff, Midwives, Health Visitors and Professions Allied to Medicine (1990a). *Seventh Report on Nursing Staff, Midwives and Health Visitors*, Cm.934, Session 89/90.

Review Body for Nursing Staff, Midwives, Health Visitors and Professions Allied to Medicine (1990b). *Seventh Report on PAMS*, Cm.935, Session 89/90.

Review Body for Nursing Staff, Midwives, Health Visitors and Professions Allied to Medicine (1991a). *Eighth Report on Nursing Staff, Midwives and Health Visitors*, Cm.1410, Session 90/1.

Review Body for Nursing Staff, Midwives, Health Visitors and Professions Allied to Medicine (1991b). *Eighth Report on PAMS*, Cm.1410, Session 90/1.

Rigg, M., P. Elias, M. White and S. Johnson (1990). *An Overview of the Demand for Graduates*, Policy Studies Institute/Institute for Employment Research, HMSO, London.

Robertson, D. and J. Symons (1990). The Occupational Choice of British Children' *Economic Journal*, 828-42.

Robinson, J., J. Stilwell, C. Hawley and N. Hempstead (1989). 'The Role of the Support Worker in the Ward Health Care Team', Nursing Policy Studies no.6, Coventry: Nursing Policy Studies Centre and Health Services Research Unit, University of Warwick, Coventry.

Robinson, J.C. (1988). 'Market Structure, Employment and Skill Mix in the Hospital Industry', *Southern Economic Journal*, 55, 315-25.

Robinson, S. (1980). 'Midwifery Manpower', NERU Occasional Paper 4, Chelsea College, Nursing Education Research Unit.

Rogers, J. (1991). The Lifeblood of the NHS, *Personnel Management*, June, 44-8.

Rogers, R.T. (1988). 'Information Requirements of Manpower Planning and Pay Determination: report of the working group', Department of Health, London.

Royal College of Nursing (1985a). *The Education of Nurses: a new dispensation* (Report of the Commission on Nursing Education, chairman: D. Judge) RCN, London.

Royal College of Nursing (1985b). *Annex of Research Studies for the Commission on Nursing Education*, RCN, London.

Royal College of Nurses (1987). *Shortage of Nurses in London* (Report of a Working Group), RCN, London.

Salvage, J. (1990). 'The Theory & Practice of the New Nursing', *Nursing Times*, 86 no.4, 42-5.

Scottish Home and Health Department (1969). *Nursing Workload per Patient as a Basis for Staffing* (Scottish Health Services Studies no.9) SHHD, Edinburgh.

Senior, E. (1988). 'Manpower Planning Objectives and Information Systems', in *Nursing Administration*, Delia Hudson (ed.), Church Livingstone, Edinburgh.

Sheldon, R. (1986). 'Control of Nursing Manpower', Fourteenth report from the Committee of Public Accounts, session 1985/86, Department of Health and Social Security, Scottish Home and Health Department, Welsh Office, HMSO, London.

Sheppard, H.L. (1973). 'Youth Discontent and the Nature of Work', in Gottlieb, D. (ed.) *Youth in Contemporary Society,* California: Sage, 99-112.

Simnett, A. (1986). The pursuit of respectability: women and the nursing profession 1860-1900 in R. White (ed.), *Political Issues in Nursing, 2*, Wiley and Sons, Chichester, 1-23.

Sloan, F. and R. Richupan (1975). 'Short-run Supply Responses of Professional Nurses', *Journal of Human Resources*, 10, 2, 241-57.

Sloan, J. and F. Robertson (1988). 'A labour market profile of nurses in Australia', *Australian Bulletin of Labour* 14, 507-28.

Smith, A. and D. Bartholomew (1988). 'Manpower Planning in the United Kingdom: An Historical View', *Journal of the Operational Research Society*, 39, no.3.

Smith, P. (1987). 'Performance Indicators: are they worth it?', in Harrison and Gretton, *Health Care UK: 1987*, Hermitage, Policy Journals, Berks.

Smithers, A. and P. Robinson (1989). *Increasing Participation in Higher Education,* BP Educational Services, London.

Social Services Committee (1987). *Fifth Report - The Future of the NHS*, Session 87/8, HC paper 613.

Social Services Committee (1989). *Resourcing the NHS.*

Sprague, A. (1988). 'Post-War Fertility and Female Labour Force Participation Rates', *Economica*, 682-700.

Stabler, C. and D. Justham (1987). *Men in Nursing: report of a survey of male nurses in two Health Authorities*, Rotherham HA and Doncaster HA.

Stilwell, J. and R.A. Wilson (1990) (eds.). *The National Health Service and the Labour Market*, Project Report, Institute for Employment Research, University of Warwick, Coventry.

Sullivan, D. (1989). 'Monopsony Power in the Market for Nurses', *Journal of Law & Economics* 32, S 135-78.

Sunday Times (1989). 'Bright Young Things Demand Golden Hello', London: *Sunday Times*, A3.

Taket, A., J. Beardsworth and V. Rushworth (1984). 'Nurse Manpower Project for NHS Management Inquiry: a comparison of some methods of estimating the requirement for nursing staff', Department of Health and Social Security.

Taylor, F.W. (1947). *Scientific Management*, New York: Harper & Row, (first published 1911).

Thomas, K.J., J.P. Nicholl and B.T. Williams (1988). 'A Study of the Movement of Nurses and Nursing Skills between the NHS and the Private Sector in England and Wales', *International Journal of Nursing Studies*, 24, 1, 1-10.

Training Agency (1989). Training in Britain: a Study of Funding, Activity and Attitudes - the Main Report, HMSO, London.

Trent Regional Health Authority, Manpower Studies Section (1990a). *Trent Region Manpower Summary*, Report no.24, Trent RHA, Sheffield.

Trent Regional Health Authority, Manpower Studies Section (1990b). *Trent Region Manpower Summary*, Report no.25, Trent RHA, Sheffield.

Trent Regional Health Authority/Trent Regional Nursing Officer's Department (1978). *An Analysis of Nursing Staffing Levels in Hospitals in the Trent Region*, Trent RHA, Sheffield.

United Kingdom Central Council for Nursing, Midwifery and Health Visiting (1986). *Project 2000: a new preparation for practice*, UKCC, London.

United Kingdom Central Council for Nursing, Midwifery and Health Visiting (1987a). 'Widening the Entry Gate', Topic Paper no.5, UKCC, London.

United Kingdom Central Council for Nursing, Midwifery and Health Visiting (1987b). *Project 2000, The Final Proposals*, Project Paper 9, London, UKCC.

Vousden, M. (1988). Please Put Your Son in the Ward, Mrs Worthington, *Nursing Times*, 84, 15, 35-6.

Wacjman, J. (1983). *Women in Control*, Milton Keynes: Open University Press.

Wadhwani, S. and M. Wall (1988). 'Tests of the Efficiency Wage Model', Centre for Labour Economics Discussion Paper 313.

Wagstaff, A. (1989a). 'Econometric Studies in Health Economics: A Survey of the British Literature', *Journal of Health Economics*, 8, 1-51.

Wagstaff, A. (1989b). 'Estimating Efficiency in the Hospital Sector: a comparison of three statistical cost frontier models', *Applied Economics*, 21, 659-72.

Waite, R.K., J. Buchan and J. Thomas (1990). *Career Patterns of Scotland's Qualified Nurses. A Report for the Scottish Home and Health Department*, Institute of Manpower Studies, University of Sussex, Brighton.

Waite, R. and R. Hutt (1987). *Attitudes, Jobs and Mobility of Qualified Nurses: A report for the RCN*, Report no.130, Brighton Institute for Manpower Studies.

Waite, R., J. Buchan and J Thomas (1989). *Nurses In and Out of Work*, Institute of Manpower Studies Report no.170, IMS, Brighton.

Walker, R. and M. Wren (1990). *Nurse Manpower Early Warning System*, Report no.1: Apr-Sept 1989, Trent RHA, Sheffield.

Watts, M. (1972). 'Training in a Time of Change' *Nursing Times*, March 30th.

Watts, M. (1984). 'Training for the Mature Entrant', *Senior Nurse*, 1, 38, 26-7.

Welsh Health Common Services Authority, Health Intelligence Unit (1989). *Project 2000 Nurse Supply Model for Wales: (version 2): Programme documentation and user notes*, WHCSA.

Welsh Health Common Services Authority, Health Intelligence Unit (1990). *Project 2000 Nurse Supply Model for Wales: First All Wales Scenario*, WHCSA, Cardiff.

Welsh Health Common Services Authority, Manpower Planning Division (1990). *Welsh National Health Service, Manpower Resource Plans 1989; Commentary and Plans*, WHCSA, Cardiff.

Welsh Office (1985). All Wales Nurse Manpower Planning Committee, *First Report*, Welsh Office, Cardiff.

Welsh Office (1987). *Nurse Supply Modelling: second report*, Cardiff: Cathays Park, 31pp.

West Midlands Regional Health Authority (1980). *Use of the Trent Nursing Formula*, (MAPLIN Paper no.80/10), DHSS, London.

West Midlands Regional Health Authority, Manpower Planning Section (1989). *Staying Power - A study of the West Midlands regional labour market, including projections and employer response*, West Midlands RHA, Birmingham.

West Midlands Regional Health Authority, Manpower Planning Section (1990). *Staying Power Report no.2: A profile of nursing and midwifery staff in the West Midlands*, West Midlands RHA, Birmingham.

Weston, C. (1989). 'What the Survey Said', Guardian Impact. London: *Guardian*, 12-3.

Whitfield, K. and R.A. Wilson (1991a). 'Staying On in Full-Time Education: The Educational Participation Rate of 16 Year Olds'. *Economic*, 58, 391-404.

Whitfield, K. and R.A. Wilson (1991b). 'Forecasting the Educational Participation Rate of 16 Year Olds in England and Wales: A Socio-Economic Approach', *International Journal of Forecasting* 7, 65-76.

Whyte, L. (1988). *Mature Students in Nurse Education*, unpublished paper, Sheffield City Polytechnic School of Health and Community Studies, Sheffield.

Wilson, R.A. (1986). 'Changing Pay Relativities for the Highly Qualified' *Review of the Economy and Employment* 1985/6, 2, 30-47, Institute for Employment Research, University of Warwick, Coventry.

Wilson, R.A. (1991). 'Prospects for the Labour Market for the Highly Qualified' (revised estimates for 1990-2000). Institute for Employment Ressearch, University of Warwick, Coventry.

Wilson, R.A. and D.L. Bosworth (1987). *New Forms and New Areas of Employment Growth,* European Commission, Brussels.

Wilson, R.A., D.L. Bosworth and P.C. Taylor (1990). *Projecting the Labour Market for the Highly Qualified,* Institute for Employment Research, University of Warwick, Coventry.

Wiseman, M. (1980). *Nurse Manpower Planning in Plymouth,* Institute of Biometry and Community Medicine, University of Exeter.

Witherspoon, S. (1988/9). 'Interim Report: A Woman's Work', in *British Social Attitudes: the 5th Report,* edited by R. Jowell, S. Witherspoon and L. Brook, 1988/89 edition, Social and Community Planning Research, Gower, Aldershot.

Worthington, D. (1988). *Nurse Manpower Planning (Supply Models and Quantitative Aspects of Recruitment, Retention and Return)* Report to Operational Research Service, DoH, London.

Worthington, D. (1990). 'Recruitment, retention and return - some quantitative issues', *International Journal of Nursing Studies,* 27, 199-211.

Wren, M.C. (1990). 'The Supply of Nurses and Midwives in the Trent Region', Trent RHA, Sheffield.

Wright-Warren, P. (1986). *Mix and Match: a review of nursing skill mix,* DHSS, London.

Yett, D., L. Drabek, M.D. Intriligator and L.J. Kimbell (1972). 'Health Manpower Planning: An Econometric Approach', *Health Services Research,* 7, 134-47.

Youdi, R.V. and K. Hinchliffe (eds.) (1985). *Forecasting Skilled Manpower Needs: The Experience of Eleven Countries,* UNESCO International Institute for Educational Planning, Paris.

Young, A. *et al.* (1983). *Factors Affecting the Recruitment and Wastage of Nurses in Northern Ireland,* New University of Ulster, Coleraine.

Zabalza, A. (1983). 'The CES Utility Function, Non-linear Budget Constraints and Labour Supply Results on Female Participation and Hours', *Economic Journal*, 312-30.